REALITIES OF CONTEMPORARY NURSING

S0-ADF-529

ABOUT THE AUTHOR

Dr. Persis Mary Hamilton recently retired from Napa Valley College. She has been a nurse for over 40 years, with clinical practice in psychiatric, obstetric, pediatric, medical-surgical and community health nursing. She has been a staff nurse, a supervisor and an administrator. Hamilton has taught in LPN, ADN, and BSN programs. Her dissertation work was on "features of textbooks that enhance learning." She currently has a private practice as a psychotherapist.

REALITIES OF CONTEMPORARY NURSING

Persis Mary Hamilton, BS, MS, EdD

Addison-Wesley Nursing
A Division of
The Benjamin/Cummings Publishing Company, Inc.

Dedicated to

NANCY EVANS
Mentor, supporter, friend

Sponsoring Editor: Mark McCormick
Production Editor: Gail Carrigan
Interior Designer: Eleanor Mennick
Cover Designer: Yvo Riezebos
Editorial Assistant: Wendy Gross
Timeline concept and research: Wendy Gross
Timeline design: Yvo Riezebos
Compositor: G & S Typesetters, Inc.
Text printer: R.R. Donnelley

Copyright © 1992 by Addison-Wesley Nursing, a Division
of The Benjamin/Cummings Publishing Company, Inc.
All rights reserved. No part of this publication may be
reproduced, stored in a retrieval system, or transmitted, in
any form or by any means, electronic, mechanical,
photocopying, recording, or otherwise, without the prior
permission of the publisher. Printed in the United States of
America. Published simultaneously in Canada.

Library of Congress Cataloging-in-Publication Data
Hamilton, Persis Mary.
    Realities of contemporary nursing / Persis Mary Hamilton.
       p.   cm.
    Includes bibliographical references and index.
    ISBN 0-201-06675-0
    1. Nursing—Practice. I. Title.
    [DNLM: 1. Education, Nursing—methods—United States.   2. Nursing.
WY 16 H219r]
RT82.H35 1991
610.73—dc20
DNLM/DLC
for Library of Congress   91-22235
                                                                        CIP

ISBN 0-201-06675-0
5 6 7 8 9 10-DOC-97 96 95 94

Addison-Wesley Nursing
A Division of the Benjamin/Cummings Publishing Company, Inc.

Preface

WHEN MARLENE KRAMER wrote her now classic *Reality Shock: Why Nurses Leave Nursing,* she identified a problem that had long troubled the profession, namely, that large numbers of nurses leave nursing after working for only a brief period of time. Why? Kramer's research revealed that nurses leave nursing because they are disillusioned by what they find in the real workaday world. She found that more realistic expectations would result if instructors exposed students "early to the potential conflicts they would encounter as graduate nurses . . . by attacking some of the idealized beliefs students receive from nursing faculty." *

In response to Kramer's findings, many nursing schools created or revised existing transition courses and curricular strands to better prepare their graduates for the realities of contemporary nursing. Changing the curriculum was fairly uncomplicated. Teaching it was more complex, mainly because of the number and diversity of "realities." Reference materials were scattered throughout the literature. A balanced, comprehensive, up-to-date text was sorely needed.

To fill the need, Addison-Wesley conducted a nationwide survey, asking nursing instructors and clinicians to identify the content of an "ideal" text for a transition course or strand. *Realities of Contemporary Nursing* was written to their specifications. As each chapter was drafted it was reviewed by up to five experts from across the country to ensure its appropriateness and accuracy. We are proud of the results. We believe the text meets the needs of students, instructors, and practicing nurses.

Philosophical and Theoretical Framework

The text presents nursing as a true, though emerging profession, encompassing all the characteristics of an authentic profes-

* Kramer M: *Reality Shock, Why Nurses Leave Nursing.* Mosby, 1974.

sion. Nursing has its own history, credentials, organizations, ethical codes, and educational system. It is based on science and functions within theoretical frameworks and legal constraints. Its members lead and manage others, use personal and professional power, and, to an increasing extent, practice autonomously. The text encourages nurses to acknowledge and assume their professional identity.

Each chapter begins with a vignette that captures a real-life nursing situation. The text then presents applicable philosophies and theories, followed by practical examples and exercises. Every effort was made to avoid sexist pronouns and to present topics from an attitude of caring and respect for human dignity.

Contents

Realities of Contemporary Nursing is about *being* a professional nurse in contrast to *doing* clinical nursing. It begins with the framework of nursing, its history, education, credentialing, organizations, and place in the health-care system. The text then explores nursing ethics, legal issues, change, power, politics, stress, collective bargaining, management-leadership, and managing a career. It concludes with a brief discussion of current realities of contemporary nursing, especially the prejudice these realities uncover. The appendices include a list of state licensing boards and nursing and health-related organizations. A more detailed description of the chapters follows.

Chapter 1: The Coming of Age of Nursing gives an account of the influences on nursing of religion-culture, war-politics, and science-technology from ancient to present times. The chapter includes a four-color timeline to illustrate and illuminate these influences throughout history. It concludes with a discussion of professionalism, the criteria of a profession, and how nursing meets those measures and is a true, albeit emerging, profession.

Chapter 2: Education for Nursing discusses nursing education for practical and registered nurses. The chapter presents both sides of the entry into practice controversy. It then describes advanced degrees, continuing education, educational preparation for nursing roles, literature, preceptorships and internships, research, and theories of nursing.

Chapter 3: Credentialing: Licensure and Certification describes licensure, the National Council Licensure Examination (NCLEX), and nurse practice acts. The chapter also discusses the certification of individuals and organizations. An appendix at the end of the book lists state licensing boards.

Chapter 4: Nursing Organizations discusses the purposes and activities of various types of nursing organizations. The chapter describes alumni organizations, the American Nurses' Association, the National Student Nurses' Association, the National League for Nursing, the International Council for Nursing, special interest and health-related organizations, and government agencies. It refers readers to an appendix for a list of these organizations.

Chapter 5: Health-Care Systems describes various health-care systems found in the world today. The chapter was co-written by Dr. Roberta O'Grady of the School of Public Health, University of California, Berkeley. In understandable terms it describes the United States health-care system, including Medicare, Medicaid, health-care policy, personal health care, and health-care trends.

Chapter 6: Ethical Concerns discusses values and the values clarification process. It examines belief systems, ethics, ethical principles, and ethical codes and offers a process for resolving ethical dilemmas. Case studies focus on real life situations and include ethical dilemmas about death, scarce resources, behavior control, and professional relations.

Chapter 7: Legal Issues reviews the organization of government, sources of law, and types of law in the United States. The chapter was co-written by Nancy J. Brent, a nurse-attorney practicing in Chicago, Illinois. It describes the trial process for both civil and criminal trials, Good Samaritan laws, violations of nurse practice acts, and malpractice. Selected cases involving nurses help illuminate the content. The chapter gives information about professional liability insurance and suggests actions to consider if accused of malpractice.

Chapter 8: Change, Power, and Politics addresses the concept of change as well as various models of planned change. It describes the types, sources, and uses of power, political strategies, and political action. The chapter discusses traditional women's roles and the nursing profession. It suggests strategies nurses can use to become powerful and take charge of their personal and professional lives.

Chapter 9: Managing Stress Effectively presents stress as stimulus, response, and transaction between an individual and the environment. It discusses stress management, burnout, and surviving shift work. A highly practical chapter, it offers several exercises to help the working nurse manage stress effectively.

Chapter 10: Management-leadership discusses a number of concepts vital to effective management-leadership, including systems theory, management, leadership, decision making, problem solving, creativity, and computer technology. It describes the management functions of planning, organizing, directing, and controlling, and gives practical examples and exercises.

Chapter 11: Collective Bargaining presents essential features of contracts: various types, their termination, and elements of a sound employment contract. It also covers labor unions, the collective bargaining process, grievances, arbitration, and what employers can do to reduce discontent.

Chapter 12: Career Management presents career management from a career perspective rather than a job perspective. It emphasizes the need for nurses to make autonomous choices and recommends systematic problem solving to collect data, set goals, plan, implement, and evaluate a work-life plan. The chapter describes management strategies of marketing, interviewing, relationships, production, and control, and recommends that nurses take charge of their lives to achieve career goals.

Afterword: Current Realities focuses on three compelling contemporary problems: homelessness, substance abuse, and sexually transmitted diseases, particularly AIDS. It addresses the prejudice these realities uncover and the conflict that nurses experience between their professional ethics and personal attitudes.

Teaching-learning Effectiveness

The effectiveness of the book as a teaching-learning tool is enhanced by many features. Each chapter opens with a powerful photograph that emphasizes an important concept. Then, a vignette of a real-life situation points to the practical value of the content. A comfortable reading level makes the prose easily understood. Unique terms are defined in vocabulary lists or by italics within the text. Numerous tables and figures illustrate concepts. Exercises and examples, such as resumes and letters of application, personalize the content. To illustrate the progression of nursing through the ages, Chapter 1 includes a full color detachable timeline. The use of sexist terms has been avoided throughout the book. Each chapter includes learning objectives, a summary of the content, learning activities, annotated readings of supplementary material, and a reference list.

An instructor's manual is available to provide suggestions for optimal use. Chapters in this manual match those of the text and include a chapter summary, learning objectives, lecture outline, learning activities, audiovisual instructional aids, and a testbank of multiple choice questions, keyed to the learning objectives. The test key includes rationales for distractors.

Acknowledgments

I am grateful for the contributions and efforts of the following people who provided their support, energy, knowledge, and talent to the project:

Debra Hunter, executive editor, for her enthusiastic support for the project, ongoing advocacy, and management skill.

Mark McCormick, editor, for his encouragement, persistence, sensitivity, intelligence, and just plain hard work.

Nancy Evans, former senior editor, for conceiving the project, conducting the nationwide survey, and trusting me to produce a quality text worthy of the Addison-Wesley reputation.

Armando Parcés-Enríquez, former editor, for his encouragement and assistance.

Wendy Gross, assistant editor, for her cheerful can-do spirit, sense of humor, competence, immediacy, and ready helpfulness.

Gail Carrigan and members of the production team for their exceptional skill and positive contributions.

Tia Hamilton O'Rear, RN, knowledgeable consultant, photographer, model, daughter, and source of great pride, for her time and effort on behalf of her Mom's project.

Chuck O'Rear, photographer par excellence and friend.

Susan G. Sisson, sounding board, reviewer, confidant, and daughter, for her continuing encouragement and support.

David F. Singletary, my husband, for his patience, acceptance, respect, ongoing support, and computer wizardry.

Contributors, for their insights and expertise, and reviewers, for thoughtful suggestions that guided me regarding depth, balance, and shade.

Countless patients and students, colleagues, mentors, instructors, family members, and friends who have left their marks on my life. Those human experiences, melded with many years of learning and teaching, created the examples and conclusions of this text.

CONTRIBUTORS AND REVIEWERS

Joyce Adriance, RN MS, Napa Valley College, Napa, CA
Candace Bartron, RN MS, Dade Community College, FL
Leslie Bonjean, RN MSN, Purdue University, Calumet Campus, Hammond, IN
Nancy J. Brent, RN, Attorney at Law, Chicago, IL
Pattie Bufalino, RN MS, Riverside City College, Riverside, CA
Emma F. Clark, RN MSN, Nicholls State University, Thibodaux, LA
Denise E. Collings, RN BSN, Eureka, CA
Kristine T. de Queiroz, RN MSN, Pasadena City College, Pasadena, CA
Wendy Earl, San Francisco, CA
Ruth Faur, RN MS, Purdue University, West Lafayette, IN
Jeanette Flanagan, RN MSN, Shepherd College, Shepherdstown, WV
Mary E. Foley, RN BSN, California Nurses Association, Oakland, CA
Karen Lee Fontaine, RN MSN, Purdue University, Calumet Campus,
    Hammond, IN
Patricia Hora, RN MS, Riverside City College, Riverside, CA
Sandy S. Joseph, RN MA, Santa Monica College, Santa Monica, CA
Ellen Logan, RN MSN, University of Toledo, Toledo, OH
Brenda L. Lyon, RN DNS, Indiana University, Bloomington, IN
Barbara Marckx, RN MS, Broome Community College, Binghamton, NY
Mary Lou Mayers, RN MSN, Greater South East Community Hospital, VA
Diana J. Mason, RN MSN, New York, NY
Milene Megel, RN MA PhD, New York State Board of Nursing, Albany, NY
Carol Nelson, RN MSN, Mead, WV
Roberta S. O'Grady, RN MA MPH DrPH, University of California,
    Berkeley, CA
Patricia Pierce, RN MSN DNS, Neward, DE
Nancy Plasse, RN, Attorney at Law, San Francisco, CA
Mary Rode, RN MSN PNP, University of Evansville, Evansville, IN
Sharon P. Shipton, RN MSN, Youngstown State University, Youngstown, OH
Dana Stahl, RN MS, El Centro College, Dallas, TX
Susan W. Talbott, RN MA MBA, Baltimore, MD
Judith Cavanah Turner, RN MS, Casper College, Casper, WY
Elizabeth Wajdowitz, RN PhD, St. Petersburg Junior College, St. Petersburg, FL
Verle Waters, RN FAAN MA, Ohlone College, Fremont, CA

Contents

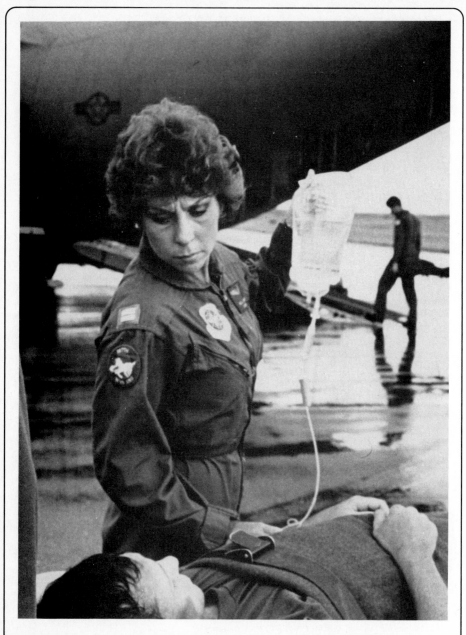

Using modern technology and medicine to reduce the casualties of war, a twentieth century flight nurse heads an aeromedical evacuation team. (Courtesy Air National Guard)

CHAPTER 1

Nursing Throughout History

LEARNING OBJECTIVES

1. Discuss how religion, culture, politics, war, technology, and medicine influence nursing throughout history.

2. Identify the predominant influences on nursing in prehistoric and ancient civilizations.

3. Explain the rationale for the development of feudalism, monasticism, and guilds in medieval Europe and how these institutions influenced nursing.

4. Describe how the Crusades affected nursing.

5. Discuss how the Renaissance and Reformation influenced the people and nursing care during and after that period.

6. Describe the "Dark Ages of Nursing" and explain its origin.

7. Identify some of the social reforms spurred by conditions of the Industrial Revolution.

8. Discuss the influence on nursing of Florence Nightingale, explaining her importance to modern nursing.

9. Describe the influences on nursing of the religion, culture, politics, war, technology, and medicine of Colonial America.

10. Discuss the effects on nursing of the Civil War and the great immigrations of people during the nineteenth century.

11. Describe some of the influences on nursing of World War I, II, and Vietnam.

12. Identify the influences on nursing that have resulted in it becoming a true profession.

" **Carol Baker,** " *the speaker announced. Carol walked stiffly to the podium wearing the official school cap and her new white uniform, her mind awhirl, her body on automatic. The long awaited moment had arrived. The dean attached the nursing school pin to her uniform, shook her hand, and paused for the obligatory photograph. Carol returned to her seat, so full of emotion she thought she would burst. When the last person had been pinned, the graduates rose together and recited a modern version of the Florence Nightingale Pledge. The lights were dimmed and, beginning with a candle held by a faculty member, a flame was passed along until each new nurse's candle was lit. The audience broke into applause and the new graduates filed out into the arms of proud family and friends. Compared to this moment of triumph, college commencement would be an anticlimax.*

Later, at the reception, Carol's mother said, "It was a beautiful ceremony, so much tradition, so much symbolism. Some day you must tell me what it all meant." Carol didn't answer.

The next day Carol reviewed the events of the night before. She thought of her enormous pride in being called "nurse," of the ceremony, the cap, the pin, the nursing oath, the candles. Somehow, the very existence of those symbols and her identification with them made Carol feel part of an elite company, part of history, part of a tradition thousands of years old. But what did all those symbols mean? Where did they originate?

The traditions of nursing are rooted in the distant past. Even the word *nursing* comes from the language of ancient Rome. In Latin *nutrire* means to nourish, nurture, or suckle a child. Because the need for nurturance and care is as old as humankind, nursing has been called the *oldest* of arts and the *youngest* of professions (Donahue 1985). Although its essential function—caring for those who cannot care for themselves—has not changed, the practice of nursing has changed, influenced by the prevailing religion and culture, politics and war, and technology and medicine of the times. Change continues to this day.

Influences on Nursing

Religion and Culture

Many people believe that the most important function of religion has been that of healing. From the earliest Neolithic evidence of *trephining* (skull drilling), to the techniques of contemporary religions, and from the *shaman's* (healer's) hut to the big city revival hall, healing and religion have been inextricably interrelated (Smith 1978). Since healing and care of those who need healing are bound together, nursing is significantly influenced by religion and culture.

Politics and War

When groups of people live together they devise systems of government. These systems are intended to provide order and to protect the rights of the citizens, the body politic. Because government has power over the lives and livelihood of its citizens, politics invariably influences nursing care. When differences arise between groups of people, conflict results. When conflict escalates to war nameless warriors are called upon to destroy each other on behalf of the government. The resultant injury, sickness, and death of war greatly influence nursing.

Technology and Medicine

Since the beginning of time, humans have been striving to meet basic needs for survival, security, acceptance, recognition, and self-actualization (Maslow 1967). Because survival is threatened by injury and illness, it is inevitably bound to health. Through trial and error, intuition, revelation, and experimentation humans have devised technology to meet their basic needs and medicine to treat their illnesses. Thus, both technology and medicine have influenced nursing care.

Times and Places

Prehistoric Civilizations

Although there are no written records of the earliest civilizations, it is speculated that the culture and religion of primitive tribes discovered in recent times reveal something of prehistoric civilizations. In these tribes, women assume major responsibility for nourishing, nurturing, and caring for children and incapacitated family members. Individuals who demonstrate special skill in caring for the 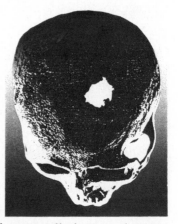 sick are called upon to help others and eventually become known as *shamans,* or healers. In the absence of scientific study, trial and error becomes the basis for practice. Treatment methods are imbued with a magical aura and passed along to apprentices. The belief that evil spirits cause illness influences nursing care. Thus, an important function of caregivers is to drive out, or *exorcise,* evil spirits by using various charms, incantations, massage, hypnosis, and herbal mixtures. Some ancient healers resorted to drilling holes in the skull, or *trephining,* to release the spirits. In time, historians believe that ritualistic ceremonies developed into religious rites, and eventually the role of healer was combined with that of priest. People constructed magical explanations for the cause of illness.

Ancient Civilizations

Egypt

The Egyptian civilization was developed by people who settled along the Nile River before 4000 BC. Its culture and religion greatly influenced health care. A record of these ancient people was found inscribed on five documents on papyrus paper, dating back to 1500 BC. They describe over 250 diseases, surgical and dental procedures, and more than 700 substances used as drugs. They tell of medical schools, at least one school of midwifery, and the first known physician, Imhotep, surgeon, priest, and architect. Advanced concepts of sanitation and hygiene prevailed and community planning helped maintain public health by protecting the water from pollution. Strict laws regulated food, drink, exercise, bodily cleanliness, and sexual relations. Dying persons were isolated in "houses of death," away from healthy people. Because of beliefs about life after death, embalming became a highly developed art, as did bandaging, seen in the intricate wrappings of mummies. Women of ancient Egypt enjoyed considerable freedom and dignity, managed the household, and cared for the sick and wounded.

Babylonia

Babylonia was located in what is now Iraq, an area called the Cradle of Civilization and the Fertile Crescent. The region is described in this way because its culture blossomed in the warm climate and fertile soil of the Tigris and Euphrates River Valleys. At first, separate city-states grew up, complete in themselves, with temples, workshops, granaries, and schools. By 2100 BC, the separate city-states had united into the Babylonian Empire. Babylonians were students of astronomy, mathematics, and numerology. Many of their religious beliefs came from observing the planets and stars. They assigned magical significance to numbers, such as 3 and 7, and developed horoscopes to predict the future. They believed that when people displeased the gods, evil spirits possessed them and made them ill. This belief influenced health care significantly. Evil spirits were banished with diet, rest, massage, purging, magical formulas made of vile-tasting plants, minerals, and excreta. Babylonian records describe child care, midwifery, and nursing care of plague, tuberculosis, fevers, jaundice, tumors, abscesses, and heart disorders.

Those who practiced medicine and surgery were held accountable for their actions. The laws were strict, especially the Code of Hammurabi, inscribed in stone in 1900 BC and now on display in the Louvre in Paris. Hammurabi, sixth king of Babylonia, created a criminal and civil code from older laws and customs. Among his edicts were laws regulating medical practice, including a sliding fee scale and penalties for malpractice, such as amputation of the hand of a surgeon who bungled an operation.

Israel and Judaism

As Semitic tribes moved into Babylonia, others settled in Palestine, a region near the Mediterranean Sea. These Hebrews, "people from beyond," descended from Abraham (also called Israel), a shepherd from Ur of Chaldea near the Persian Gulf. By the time of King Hammurabi, about 1950 BC, the Hebrews were well established in the Jordan River Valley. They built towns, collected water in cisterns, raised sheep, and cultivated olives and grapes. The country flourished and Jerusalem became a religious and political center of commerce. In the eighteenth century BC, famine drove the people of Jerusalem (Jews) to Egypt. There they prospered for a while, but eventually were taken captive, remaining as slaves for 400 years (Donahue 1985). Under the leadership of Moses, the adopted son of the Pharoah's daughter, the Hebrews escaped from Egypt and returned to Palestine to reestablish the nation of Israel.

Moses had been educated in the learning of Egypt. He was taught the history of the Hebrew people by his natural mother, who was also the wet nurse hired to care for him after he was discovered among the reeds of the river. His mother had hidden Moses there to escape the edict to kill all male Hebrew infants. He instituted a theocentric (god-centered) form of government and the Mosaic Code, which contained many Egyptian hygienic rules. Eventually the Hebrew kingdom fell to invading powers and the people were taken into slavery. In 1948, descendants of that ancient culture reestablished the nation of Israel in Palestine.

The Hebrews wrote historical narratives and detailed codes of conduct, as found in the Old Testament and the two Talmuds. These codes regulated every aspect of personal, family, and national life, significantly influencing health care. The sacred writings affirmed one all-powerful god who blessed obedience with long life and prosperity and punished disobedience with sickness and death. Blood had symbolic cleansing power; animal sacrifice was a regular priestly duty. Specific rules governed women during menstruation, pregnancy, and childbirth. Male infants were circumcised at eight days of age and persons with communicable diseases were isolated until they recovered. Relief for widows, orphans, and the poor was encouraged. Houses for strangers were built and expanded to include the sick. Dietary laws strictly forbade eating blood or creatures that were scavengers, had been torn by wild beasts or had died of disease, or had cloven hoofs but did not chew the cud. One day a week was set aside for rest and worship. Orthodox Jews follow these same laws to this day.

India, Hinduism, and Buddhism

The Himalayan mountains isolated India from the rest of the world until about 3000 BC, when Aryan people migrated there from the West. They found a warm climate, rich vegetation, and a race of dark-skinned people. By 2500 BC, an advanced culture emerged in which the people developed geometry, trigonometry, the decimal system, and a written script.

From about 1600 to 500 BC, the Vedic language and Brahman (Hindu) religion dominated. Hinduism divided the people into four *castes*, or social levels. It affirmed *pantheism* (everything is a part of god), *nihilism* (nothingness is desirable), and *transmigration* and *reincarnation* (rebirth of the soul into human or animal forms). Believers worshiped ancestors, revered animals such as cows and monkeys, and forbade the eating or killing of these animals. Priests directed the worship of numerous deities, interpreting and enforcing a Code of Conduct. The code was written in four *Vedas,* sacred books which served as historical documents. They greatly influenced health care, promoting hygienic practice and offering magical cures for injury, disease, and infertility. With time, supplemental Vedas were written which reveal a high level of surgical and medical knowledge. Following strict rules of cleanliness, surgeons excised tumors, repaired hernias and harelips, and performed Cesarean births and tonsillectomies, anesthetizing patients with hypnotic drugs and hypnosis. They used vaccination to produce immunity and treated tuberculosis, leprosy, neurologic disorders, diabetes mellitus, and hepatitis. In a team approach to health care, the document affirmed the interdependence of physician, drugs, nurse, and patient.

About 530 BC, Siddhartha Gautama, a Hindu priest, announced himself Buddha, the Enlightened. He taught that perfection consists of attaining nothingness by means of severe penance. His philosophy ignored the caste system and made inner peace available to everyone. Buddhism gradually gained acceptance and became the dominant religion, greatly influencing health care. Social programs were instituted and public hospitals built. Rules for ritual and daily life were dictated by the Laws of Manu, compiled between 200 BC and 200 AD. These laws, like the Mosaic Law and Code of Hammurabi, regulated dietary practice and family hygiene. They punished physicians for malpractice and expected them to maintain high standards of practice and morality. Physicians earned permission to practice from the king by a kind of licensing system. Nurses, too, were expected to maintain high standards and to be skillful and trustworthy. Usually they were men or older women, though midwives and some pharmacists were women.

China, Taoism, and Confucianism

About 3000 BC, Mongolian people from central Asia migrated to China, settling first in the lush Yellow River Valley, then south in the Yangtse River Valley and beyond. Over time three religious systems appeared in ancient China: Taoism, Confucianism, and Buddhism. Each one significantly influenced health care.

Taoism, the oldest religion, was based on Tao, the Way, a balance present in everything. The Tao was represented by the yin and yang, an intermingling of heaven and earth. Emperor Fi Hse is credited with creating the *pakua,* the symbol for yin and yang. Disease demons were combated in many ways, including frightening them with noisy firecrackers and banishing them by administering tea made of the ashes of paper on which magic symbols had been written.

Ancient Chinese health care was profoundly influenced by the Taoist concept of balance between health and illness. Huang Ti, the Yellow Emperor, is credited with writing the great medical compendium, *Nei Ching* (Veith 1966). It tells how to promote health and how to prevent, assess, and treat disease. Assessment consists of looking, listening, asking, and feeling, particularly feeling the pulse, which is a primary diagnostic gauge. Recommended treatment is to cure the spirit, nourish the body, give medicine, treat the whole person, and use acupuncture and moxibustion. *Acupuncture* is the insertion and twisting of needles in areas along 12 meridians of the body. *Moxibustion* uses the same meridians but involves placing mounds of powdered plant on the skin and burning them until a blister forms. Medicinal herbs were widely used and smallpox vaccination was described. Surgery was limited to repairing wounds and castrating males for work in the palace. Halls of healing were praying areas near temples, but little is recorded of hospitals, probably because families were expected to care for their own. Women managed the home, but their value was measured by their ability to produce sons.

About 500 BC, Confucius became prominent as a political reformer, basing his reforms on moral principles. He taught a negative version of the Golden Rule: "What you do not wish done to you do not do to others." He stressed the value of knowledge and etiquette, family cohesion, ancestor worship, and he viewed women as inferior to men. His teachings were generally approved, but they failed to stimulate change and personal ambition.

By 200 BC, Buddhism from India had gained widespread acceptance. It had many of the same influences on health care in China that were described for India.

The Americas

The American continents probably were settled before 10,000 BC by people from Central Asia who crossed the Bering Strait into what is now Alaska. They migrated toward food, water, and favorable climates, leaving traces of their cultures on the

Atlantic and Pacific coasts of North and South America. Aztec, Mayan, Incan, and Toltec civilizations flourished in the Americas, influencing health care. The people believed sickness resulted from displeasing the gods. Health was achieved by maintaining a balance between the body, nature, and the supernatural by wearing protective charms and purifying the body with sweats and mineral baths. Shamans and priests chanted prayers and performed healing rituals, including human sacrifice and the symbolic transfer of disease to animals. Aztec medicine, surgery, and midwifery were highly developed. The Aztecs built hospices for the sick and treated illness and injury with minerals and herbs, massage, trephining, bloodletting, suturing, amputation, and tooth extraction. In the southwestern part of North America, sand painting became a unique form of therapy. The shaman created intricate designs of colored sand to effect specific cures (Smith 1978). Within their designated role, women were respected, held authority over their homes, assisted with childbirth, and cared for the sick and elderly.

Greece and Greek Polytheism

Ancient Greece was built by people of the Aegean peninsula on the ruins of a civilization that began before 4000 BC. In about 1400 BC, Aryan tribes from the north, called Helenes, invaded the land, conquering the city-states they found along the Mediterranean coastline and mountainous interior. There the Greeks built a new civilization that was to influence human affairs for centuries to come, especially health care. The society was linked by a common language, religion, literature, and Olympic Games, held every four years dating from 776 BC.

The Greeks recounted many mythical tales of gods who acted more like glorified humans than powerful deities. Apollo was the god of health and medicine. Asklepios, son of Apollo and a human mother, was the chief healer. He was pictured holding the wand of Mercury, a wayfarer's staff entwined by sacred serpents of wisdom. The modern symbol of medicine, or caduceus, came from this portrayal. In places of great beauty, splendid temples served as shrines to Asklepios. Managed by priests and nursing attendants, these health resorts became social and cultural centers. Care for the sick and injured was provided in *iatrion* (clinics for ambulatory patients) and *xenodochia* (shelters for strangers), which were precursors to hospitals.

In time, one branch of priests became itinerant physicians. Their findings were combined into the first general medical text, long viewed as the standard for practice. This comprehensive text was credited to a priest named *Hippocrates* (about 450–377 BC), called the "Father of Medicine." It taught that disease is not the work of spirits, demons, or deities, but the result of breaking natural laws. The true art of a physician is to assist nature to effect a cure. Hygiene is a way of life, involving diet, exercise, and avoidance of excess. The body has four humors: blood, phlegm, yellow bile, and black bile. Balance between the humors produces health; excess or deficiency causes illness. Case histories described subjective symptoms, objective signs, and the environment. The Hippocratic Method came to mean intellectual honesty, careful observation, study of the patient rather than the disease, assisting nature to effect a cure, and ethical practice as defined by the *Hippocratic Oath*. Greek literature refers to caregiving and describes various nursing procedures, including directions for poultice application, bathing, diets for heart and kidney cases, and comfort measures such as smoothing bed linens. Since women were not admitted to the "mysteries" of any art, men probably provided such nursing care as was given outside the home.

The unique culture and religion of the Greeks lead to the "birth of reason," characterized by Socrates, Plato, and Aristotle. These philosophers sought truth through observation and reason rather than through intuition and revelation.

Italy and Roman Polytheism

Ancient Italy was settled by peoples of Asia Minor, Aryans of northern Europe, and seafarers of other lands. The city of Rome was built in about 753 BC, on the banks of the Tiber River on ruins of an ancient Etruscan city. In time, the Roman army became a dominant force, conquering and absorbing other city-states. By 290 BC, Rome was the chief city of central Italy. By 31 BC, under a succession of aggressive leaders, it had become an empire, including most of the lands around the Mediterranean Sea. But by 476 AD, the Empire had crumbled and waves of Huns, Goths, and Vandals occupied the land.

During the height of its power, the culture and religion of the Roman Empire greatly influenced care of the sick and injured. Its brutal culture approved of slavery, crucifixion, gladiator contests, and human sacrifice. The difference between citizen and non-citizen, bond and free was immense. Caesars ruled the empire and Roman governors and armies occupied conquered lands. The gods of Roman polytheism included Jupiter, Juno, Janus, and Mars. Later, the Romans added the Greek gods Hygeia and Asklepios. There was a god or goddess for almost every physiological function or disease, such as Scabies who cured scabies and Febris who reduced fevers. Pleasing the gods brought prosperity; displeasing them brought destruction.

The Romans borrowed the cultural achievements of the peoples they conquered. From Greece they acquired money, textiles, sailing ships, art, and religion, and they adapted the Greek alphabet to the Latin tongue. After conquering Greece in 146 BC, the Romans sent enslaved Greek physicians throughout the Empire to provide medical care to the soldiers. Pedanius wrote *De Materia Medica*, a compendium of over 600 preparations of medicinal herbs used to treat Nero's armies. Using the Hippocratic method of observation Aretaeus described diphtheria, pneumonia, emphysema, epilepsy, tetanus, and diabetes. Physicians performed Cesarean births for prolonged labors, tracheostomies for respiratory distress, and physical therapy for muscle and joint disorders. Celsus, a physician of the first century AD, wrote a medical text in which he described the four cardinal signs of infection: heat, pain, redness, and swelling. Pliny reported various occupational diseases such as mercury poisoning and asbestosis. Galen, a Greek assigned to care for gladiators and athletes, described numerous surgical procedures and his understanding of physiology. His medicinal prescriptions were used for centuries. Midwives assisted at births and women nursed sick family members in the home. Less restricted than in other cultures, they dined with men, engaged in activities outside the home, and owned property.

Roman culture was renowned for its laws, monetary system, and military strategy, but its greatest achievements were in engineering, many of which affected public health. Marshes were drained, and aqueducts, good roads, baths, central heating systems, and cemeteries were built. Roman interest in military might led to improved medical care for soldiers, first aid on the battle field, ambulance service to carry wounded men to field hospitals, *nosocomi* (trained orderlies) to provide nursing care, and *valetudinaria* (military hospitals) equipped to house the sick and wounded.

Christianity

At the height of Roman imperial power, in about 3 BC, Jesus of Nazareth was born in the conquered province of Palestine. The religion he began would profoundly influence nursing care for centuries to come. When Jesus was about 30 years of age he gathered 12 disciples and began to preach. He proclaimed the fatherhood of a loving God and a kingdom of heaven available to all by a life of inner purity and service to others. He taught in parables and gave a positive version of the Golden Rule: "Whatsoever ye would that men do to you, do ye even so to them" (Matthew 7:12). Jesus healed the sick and berated Jewish pharisees for hypocrisy. When the crowds hailed him "the Messiah," both Jewish and Roman officials decided this Christ had become dangerous. As a result, Jesus was arrested, tried, and crucified. His disciples buried his body, reported his resurrection and ascension into heaven, and began to spread his teaching throughout the Roman Empire.

People from every walk of life became converts: physicians like Luke, leaders like Paul, and notable women like Phoebe. In 312 AD, Emperor Constantine espoused Christianity and established himself as absolute ruler. "By 400 AD, it was probably as dangerous *not to be* a Christian as it had been *to be* one in 100 AD" (Donahue 1985, p. 93).

At first, Christianity was a simple faith, but with time its doctrine, rituals, and organization grew more complex. As the Roman Empire declined, the power of the church increased, and a rigid male hierarchy took control. The bishop of Rome, the Pope, became the supreme ruler of the "Holy Roman Empire." In 330, Emperor Constantine split from Rome, moved to Istanbul and established the Eastern branch of the church.

As Christianity gained acceptance many women of wealth and influence devoted themselves to its teachings to care for the poor and sick. Marcella made her home into a monastery for women. In 385, Paula, a learned woman, assisted Jerome with a Latin translation of early church writings known as the Vulgate. In 390, Fabiola founded the first free Christian hospital of Rome in her palace.

Islam

In 570 AD, the founder of Islam was born in Mecca, the commercial and religious center of Arabia. Muhammad, an ambitious but uneducated shepherd, became a servant of a rich widow, married her, and gained for himself community status. At that time Mecca was the site of the black stone of Kaaba and the chief god of Arabia to which Arabs made annual pilgrimages. Muhammad rejected Kaaba and became convinced that there was but one true god, Allah. He preached physical and spiritual death awaited unbelievers, and one brotherhood of men with direct access to god without priests. Women had identity only as adjuncts of men. Dietary restrictions of Islam included refraining from alcohol and pork. These and other doctrines of the faith are found in the sacred book of Muslims, the *Koran*. The culture and religion of Islam influenced nursing, the status of women, and world history for centuries.

After Muhammad's death in 632, a power struggle between his heirs resulted in the Shiite and Sunite schism which continues to this day. Regardless of this division, the faithful set out to spread the new religion by force. Armed with the sword of Islam they conquered Turkey, Persia, Arabia, Egypt, Palestine, North Africa, and Spain, instituting the Byzantine Empire (Wells 1956).

Nestorians and Arabian Medicine

Nestorians were an early group of Christians who founded hospitals and medical schools in Greece. By a twist of fate they greatly affected health care for many centuries. When the Roman Pope declared them heretics in 450, the Nestorians went to Persia, taking along Greek and Roman literature. There they built medical schools in which the learning of ancient Greece, India, China, and Arabia was valued and where Arabs, Christians, and Jews studied together. Although the study of anatomy was suppressed because of Islamic teachings, the Arabs excelled in clinical medicine, chemistry, and drug therapy. Lepers and the mentally ill were treated kindly. Patients were separated according to diagnosis and attended by male nurses because women were not permitted outside the home. Rhazes, 860–932, the "Father of Pediatrics," studied childhood communicable diseases. Avincenna, 980–1037, authored the *Canon of Medicine,* a text used in medical schools for 600 years. For 1000 years eastern schools maintained leadership over the decaying western branch of medicine. Traditional Greek medicine was thus preserved, to return to Europe many centuries later.

Medieval Europe

The years between the fall of Rome in 476 and the fall of Constantinople in 1453 divide ancient and modern times. The interval between is known as the Middle Ages or medieval period. The first 500 years is called the Dark Ages because world conditions were so chaotic. There was war, lawlessness, exorbitant taxation, abysmal poverty and huge wealth, ignorance, superstition, sickness, and misery.

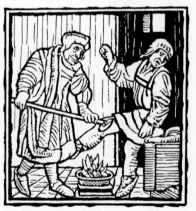

The bubonic plague, called the Black Death, swept across Europe at intervals for 300 years. In the pandemic of 1348, about one-third to one-half of the population died. To forestall spread of the disease, maritime cities of the Mediterranean adopted a *quaranta,* a 40-day detention period for vessels entering their ports. Thus, isolation for a set period of time became known as *quarantine.* Communicable diseases such as smallpox, syphilis, leprosy, and diphtheria ravaged the population.

During the Middle Ages there was no personal security or safety. As a consequence, three social systems grew up by which people exchanged autonomy for safety. They were: feudalism, monasticism, and guilds.

Feudalism

Feudalism was based on a lord-vassal relationship. The lord owned the land but was expected to protect his vassals from outside harm. The lady bore and reared his children, ran the manor, and cared for the sick, serving as nurse and physician. Vassals (serfs) worked the land, paid fees and services to their lord, and fought in his militia. Female serfs were valued for work and childbearing. Both lords and serfs honored the Catholic church and those who gave their lives to its service.

Monasticism

Monasticism reflected a widespread belief that salvation required self-denial and withdrawal from the world. Monastic orders for both men and women grew up around strong leaders. Each had its own rules of conduct and dress. *Novitiates,* new members, entered as probationers and, after a period of testing, took vows of the order. To symbolize humility and obedience, women shaved their heads and wore a cloth veil as a covering. Each order developed a unique *habit* (uniform) and representation of the crucifix which hung from the *rosary* (prayer beads). The cap, uniform, and pin of modern nursing schools are modifications of the veil, habit, and crucifix of Medieval nursing orders.

The church recognized four types of monastic orders named for their founders: Basil, Augustine, Francis, and Benedict. Benedictine rules were less severe than those of the other orders and allowed for a more balanced life of work, rest, and prayer. As a result, these monasteries become centers of learning and culture. In time, care of the sick became an important function of every type of religious community. However, care was not based on scientific principles. Caregivers used untested treatments, including cautery, enemas, bloodletting, leeching, diet, and baths.

Nursing orders such as the Parabolani brothers of Rome cared for bubonic plague victims; Augustinian sisters established Hotel Dieu in Lyons in 542, Hotel Dieu in Paris about 650, and Santo Spirito Hospital in Rome in 717. In 848, a medical school was established at Salerno which was affiliated with the Benedictine Abbey at Monte Cassino. One of its highly respected physicians was a German abbess named Hildegarde (1099–1179). There were also secular orders such as the Alexian brothers and Bequines of Belgium. These orders operated much like religious orders except that members had more freedom to offer care to the sick because they were not bound by monastic vows.

Guilds

Guilds were unique social organizations that came into being about 750 in England and 1050 on the continent. At first they were voluntary associations formed for mutual protection and assistance of the members and their families. Master craftsmen operated an apprenticeship system in which youths contracted to work in exchange for bed and board and an opportunity to learn a trade. Craft guilds held a near-monopoly on all trades from 1350 to the rise of the factory system about 1700. They served as models for the health care societies of modern Germany. Their apprenticeship method of learning provided the model for nursing education well into the twentieth century.

The Crusades

From 700 to 1000 both the Holy Roman and Byzantine Empires coexisted. In both, bloody conflict between various dominions continued. In 1094, when the Turks mounted a particularly threatening force against Greece, Emperor Alexius Comnenus of Constantinople appealed to Pope Urban II for help. The Pope seized the opportunity to draw together Christians for a Holy War against Islam. The object was to recapture the site of the holy sepulchre in Jerusalem from "infidel Seljuk Turks." In 1097, he organized the first crusade. Knights looted and captured city after city until they reach Jerusalem, taking it in 1099. The second crusade was organized to consolidate initial gains. It provoked the Muslims to mount a counter crusade, a *Jehad* (holy war), against the Christians which ended in 1187 when the Muslims recaptured Jerusalem. The loss provoked a third crusade. A fourth and fifth followed. The sixth and final crusade ended in 1244, with Jerusalem, the battered prize, in Muslim hands. There it remained until 1918, when British and French forces recaptured the city, only to give it back to Muslim Jordan.

Christian churches and enclaves were built along the route of the crusades. Military nursing orders evolved to care for the sick and wounded. The Knights Hospitallers of St. John was one such order. Over their armor, the knights wore a habit adorned with a Maltese cross, a symbol the Nightingale School of Nursing adopted many years later. This order of knights continued for centuries, becoming so expert in disaster relief that when the International Red Cross was formed in 1864, the order's representatives were consulted.

Renaissance and Reformation

During the years between 1350 and 1600, two great social movements occurred, the Renaissance (reawakening) and Reformation (correction). The forces that produced the Renaissance brought discontent with the Roman Catholic church and led to the Reformation. As a result, enormous change took place in the political, economic, intellectual, and religious arenas of life. The Western world be-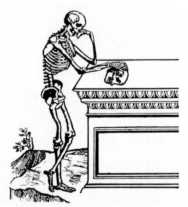 came aware of the larger world of Marco Polo and Columbus, experimental evidence replaced intuition in the intellectual community, and printing allowed the widespread distribution of information. Existing social institutions changed and new ones emerged, especially those involving care of the sick.

The intellectual revolution began in Italy about 1350 and spread to Western Europe. Copernicus, Descartes, Galileo, and Newton made revolutionary discoveries. The telescope, microscope, barometer, thermometer, and pendulum clock were invented. Leeuwenhoek, using the microscope, described protozoa, bacteria, and human spermatozoa. Falopio discovered the fallopian tubes. Vesalius, a Flemish anatomist, published the first authoritative text of human anatomy. Pare, a French surgeon, used ligatures to tie off bleeding vessels. Harvey demonstrated the circulation of blood with animals, initiating experimental physiology. Art expanded from religious subjects to living people. Leonardo da Vinci, Michelangelo, and Raphael depicted anatomically correct figures, as did the Dutch master Rembrandt, whose "Lesson in Anatomy" became a classic.

The religious revolution, called the Reformation, began as a result of theological debate and in response to abuses of the Roman church. The spread of ideas quickened as the result of two inventions: manufacture of paper from China via Arabia, and printing with movable type introduced in the Western world by Gutenberg. By the time the church initiated reform, a mendicant monk named Martin Luther (1483–1546) had led a rebellion against church rule. His followers, called Lutherans, and other "Protestants," declared independence from the Pope and the right of nations to choose religious affiliation. The Western world divided into Catholic and non-Catholic nation-states. Within a few years Northern Europe was Lutheran. Many other groups arose: Calvinists, Presbyterians, Anabaptists, Mennonites, Anglicans, Quakers, and Puritans. Though all groups called themselves Christians, each interpreted scripture differently and believed it possessed the truth. Bitter hatred arose, leading to the Thirty Years' War (1618–1648) and to immigration of many groups to the New World to practice their faith without interference.

The Dark Ages of Nursing

The Reformation had no direct effect on hospitals in Catholic countries, but in Protestant nations most hospitals operated by Catholic orders were closed or taken over by the government. In England in 1525, Henry VIII confiscated the property of some 600 charitable endowments. Monks and nuns of nursing orders were expelled. No one was prepared to take their place. Women of the lowest social strata in society were recruited to fill nursing positions. The work was strenuous, the hours long, the pay poor, and corruption rampant. Thus, the period from 1550 to 1860, 310 years, is called the Dark Ages of Nursing. It was associated with the rise of the factory system, which replaced cottage industry throughout Europe and England. In 1844, in the novel *Martin Chuzzlewit,* Charles Dickens describes the sorry state of nursing through the characters of Sairey Gamp, a home nurse, and Betsy Prig, a hospital nurse:

She was a fat old woman, this Mrs. Gamp, with a husky voice and a moist eye. . . . She wore a very rusty black gown, rather the worst for snuff, and a shawl and bonnet to correspond. . . . The face of Mrs. Gamp—the nose in particular—was somewhat red and swollen, and it was difficult to enjoy her society without becoming conscious of a smell of spirits. . . . Mrs. Prig was of the Gamp build, but not so fat; and her voice was deeper and more like a man's. She had also a beard. (Dickens 1936)

Industrial Revolution and Social Reform

During the period called the Industrial Revolution, Europe was devastated by famine, plague, and poverty. Life was cheap and ignorance widespread. Factories gave starvation wages for long hours of dangerous work. Child labor, disease, alcoholism, and squalor abounded. Social reform was desperately needed. Several groups formed to minister to the sick and poor, including the Order of the Sisters of Charity of St. Vincent de Paul and the Brothers of St. John of God. The Sisters developed an educational program for women which included a two-month probation followed by a five-year training period. In 1640, the Sisters established the Hospital for Foundlings in Paris for abandoned children.

Many individuals were stirred by the desperate social conditions and began to work for change. One of the best known was John Howard (1727–1789), an Englishman who spent his life and fortune investigating prisons, pesthouses, asylums, and hospitals. His vivid portrayals shocked public consciousness and helped bring about change. Although slow, interest in reform grew. Elizabeth Guerney Fry, a deeply religious Quaker, was especially concerned for women prisoners and their children. She helped form the Society of Protestant Sisters of Charity.

Kaiserswerth

Inspired by prison reforms in England and Holland, Pastor Theodor Fliedner and his wife Frederike established the Deaconess Institute at Kaiserswerth, Germany in 1836. Originally a refuge for released prisoners, it expanded to become a hospital and training school for deaconesses. The three-year program included pharmacology, teaching, and home and hospital nursing. Graduate deaconesses took no vows nor earned wages, but were taken care of for life in an arrangement known as the *motherhouse system*. Kaiserswerth's influence spread to all corners of the globe. Branches were established in many nations and emissaries from abroad came to Germany to learn from the program. In 1849, a motherhouse was founded in Pittsburgh, Pennsylvania.

Florence Nightingale

A reformer of health care and the founder of modern nursing, Florence Nightingale, was born May 12, 1820, the second daughter of prominent English parents. She was reared in wealth and social position and probably better educated than most men of her day (Donahue 1985). At an early age Florence expressed interest in becoming a nurse, but her parents disapproved, expecting her to marry, bear children, and take her place in society. Instead, Florence began a systematic study of public health, hospitals, and nursing orders of the Roman Catholic church. She traveled widely. In Rome, she met Sir and Mrs. Sidney Herbert, prominent Britishers who were interested in hospital reform. In 1847, Florence took a condensed three-month course of study at Kaiserwerth, later calling it her "spiritual home." In 1853, she took additional training with the Sisters of Charity in Paris. On returning to London, Florence began working with the committee that supervised the Establishment for Gentlewomen During Illness, a hospital for women. In 1853, she became its superintendent and within one year transformed it into a model institution for that day.

Reports from the Crimean War of appalling conditions for soldiers in field hospitals brought public outrage and demand for change. In 1854, Sir Sidney Herbert, then Secretary of War, commissioned Nightingale to go to Crimea and institute reform. With energetic commitment and 37 select nurses from various nursing orders, Nightingale accepted the challenge. Within six months, the death rate in one hospital of 3500 patients dropped from 42.7% to 2.2%. Obstacles of every kind created enormous demands of time and energy. Florence contracted Crimean fever, nearly died, and remained a semi-invalid the rest of her life. In 1856, she returned to London, a national heroine. The Nightingale Fund was established in her honor and she was immortalized by Longfellow's poem, "The Lady with a Lamp."

Florence was appointed to many commissions and wrote extensively on health, statistics, sanitation, hospitals, and nursing education. The two best known of her books are *Notes on Hospitals* (1858) and *Notes on Nursing: What it Is and What it Is Not* (1860). She affirmed that nurses should spend their time caring for patients, not doing menial jobs, that they should be educated, use their knowledge to improve patient care, have social standing, and continue to learn throughout life. Nightingale declared that nursing schools should be run by nurses, independent of hospitals and physicians. She opposed state licensure for nurses, arguing that individual merit would be "leveled down." She insisted on cleanliness and order but never accepted the germ theory, believing to her death in the spontaneity of disease (Dock and Stewart 1938).

In 1860, The Nightingale Training School for Nurses opened as an entirely independent educational institution financed by the Nightingale Fund. It was strongly opposed by physicians who wrote, "nurses are in much the same position as housemaids and require little teaching beyond that of poultice-making." In spite of opposition, the school prospered, serving as a model for nursing education, with graduates in demand around the world. Until her death in 1910, Nightingale worked to improve health care. With all her imperfections, Florence Nightingale was a remarkable woman. Because of her life the status of nursing rose from degradation to honor.

International Red Cross

The International Red Cross was established in 1864, through the efforts of J. Henri Durant, a Swiss banker. He credited Nightingale's work in Crimea as the inspiration for his idea of a humanitarian agency to provide care for war casualties. Twelve nations signed the original Treaty of Geneva, agreeing to honor Red Cross nurses as noncombatants, respect their hospitals, and permit humanitarian services for either side in a war. The treaty recognized a common flag, a red cross on a white background, the reverse of Switzerland's flag. (Muslim countries use a red crescent.) The treaty was ratified in England in 1870. At the urging of Clara Barton, the United States signed it in 1882.

Colonial America

Exploration and colonization of the New World came in the wake of the Renaissance and Reformation. Nations sought power, trade, and wealth in the New World. Colonists sought religious freedom and economic opportunity. Beginning in 1519, Spain founded colonies from Mexico to Peru, establishing the first hospital on the continent in Mexico City in 1524 and the first medical school 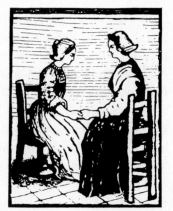 in 1578. France established colonies in Nova Scotia, Canada, and New Orleans. In 1617, Maria Hubou, the first woman to nurse in North America, arrived in Canada with her husband, a surgeon. In 1639, Augustinian sisters arrived in Quebec to staff the Hotel Dieu. Soon thereafter, Ursuline sisters came to open the first training school for nurses in North America. In 1642, Jeanne Mance, one of the most romantic figures in the history of Canadian nursing, founded Hotel Dieu of Montreal (Donahue 1985). A century later, the Order of Grey Nuns became Canada's first district nurses. In 1725, Jean Louis, a Frenchman, endowed L'Hospital des Pauxres de la Charite in New Orleans.

Beginning in 1607, England laid claim to Atlantic coastal lands, exchanging colony charters for taxes. Slaves began arriving from Africa in 1619, and in 1620, Pilgrims and Puritans settled the Massachusetts Bay Colony. Soon the Dutch East India Company established New Amsterdam on Manhattan Island, English Catholics took refuge in Maryland, dissident members of the Massachusetts Colony founded Connecticut and Rhode Island, and William Penn founded Pennsylvania, a Quaker colony. Although English colonists came to America for similar reasons and endured common hardships, for 150 years they remained isolated and antagonistic toward one another. Indian massacres, starvation, nutritional disorders, infectious diseases, and complications of pregnancy took a high toll. Nursing and medical care consisted of prayer and folk remedies. Quacks abounded. Any educated man was considered prepared to be a physician. In the years before the American revolution, there were only five "hospitals." In fact, these were almshouses with infirmaries for the homeless poor where other inmates nursed the sick. One of the first, Bellevue Hospital on Manhattan Island, was founded in 1658 by the Dutch East India Company to care for sick sailors and African slaves arriving on company ships. Donahue (1985) describes Bellevue as a "house of horrors" with a death rate of more than 50%. Not until the city hired Alice Fisher, a Nightingale nurse from England in 1884, did the quality of nursing care improve.

The first hospital in the United States solely dedicated to treatment of the sick was Pennsylvania Hospital, founded in 1751 at the urging of Benjamin Franklin. There, patients were segregated according to diagnosis; insanity was considered an illness rather than a moral defect. In that day the typical treatment of insane people was to house them in filthy dungeonlike rooms in shackles. For a fee the public could visit, stare, and laugh. In his famous work, *Medical Inquiries and Observations upon the Disease of the Mind* (1812), the highly respected Dr. Benjamin Rush proposed humane treatment for the mentally ill. In 1786, Quakers founded the Philadelphia Dispensary to provide outpatient care for the poor, offering free obstetrical, medical, and surgical services. In 1791, New York Hospital opened, gaining attention because its attendants received lectures on anatomy, physiology, maternity nursing, and child care. During the 1800s many religious nursing orders began work in America, including the Dominicans, Irish Sisters of Mercy, Episcopal Sisterhood of the Holy Communion, Lutheran deaconesses from Kaiserswerth, and the Sisters of Charity, begun by Mother Seton in Emmitsburg, Maryland.

Revolutionary War

In 1776, the colonies declared independence from England. Their hastily mobilized army had no medical or nurse corps and volunteers nursed the wounded in private homes and public buildings. Smallpox, dysentery, and scarlet fever ravaged the camps. Food was scarce, clothing meager, ether unknown, and amputation the most common surgery. In spite of all these obstacles, the beleaguered army prevailed and the United States became a separate nation.

Medical Practice and Education

In colonial America medicine was much as it had been in medieval Europe. As discoveries of Pasteur, Lister, Koch, and others became known, treatment and hygienic practice began to change. Tincture of opium, coca, ipecac, and digitalis were introduced. In 1796, Jenner demonstrated that cowpox was a safe and effective smallpox vaccine. Although some physicians were trained in Europe, most were self-taught or learned from established physicians as apprentices. By 1800, there were only four medical schools in United States. Then, for-profit schools began to appear, many granting degrees in but one year of lecture-only study. Soon more than 400 such schools emerged. Formation of the American Medical Association (AMA) in 1847 led to reform. The Flexner Report of 1910 gave a damning indictment of medical education, grading each school. As a result, better schools attracted foundation grants and poor ones closed. During this period, men took control of medicine, excluding even midwives from practice. A Boston physician gloated, "one of the first and happiest fruits of improved medical education in America [is] that females are excluded from practice" (Robinson 1946). A notable exception was Elizabeth Blackwell (1821–1910), the first woman physician in the United States. After being denied admission to 29 medical schools, she was accepted "as a lark" by Geneva College in New York. Although ridiculed, she graduated first in her class, only to find that no hospital would admit her patients. In 1857, she founded New York Infirmary, a 40-bed hospital staffed solely by women, and in 1868 it became the first medical school for women (Sigerist 1934).

War Between the North and South

As the United States grew, adding territories that became states, a profound difference developed between the South, with a landed gentry supported by slave labor and the North, with a citizenry of free individuals. When the South seized federal forts in 1861 and seceded from the Union, the Civil War began. Neither side had field hospitals, a medical corps, nurse corps, or ambulance service. Although ether and chloroform were first used as general anesthetics in the 1840s, they were often unavailable in the battlefield. The need for nurses was critical. Sisters from various religious orders offered their services, as did hundreds of volunteers, managing as best they could, dressing wounds, serving food, and giving medicine. *Red Rover,* the first hospital ship, was staffed by Catholic Sisters of Mercy who thus became the first navy nurses. Dorothea Dix, a school teacher and reformer, was appointed superintendant of the first army nurse corps, and Clara Barton founded the American Red Cross. Walt Whitman and Louisa May Alcott wrote of their experiences nursing the sick and wounded. Mother Mary Ann Bickerdyke challenged corrupt medical officers, and Jan Stuart Woolsey and her sisters worked for standards of selection and training of army nurses. Harriet Tubman and Susie Taylor, Afro-American nurses, served with the Union army. They and many others supported antislavery activities. In the end, more than 618,000 men died from battle injuries or disease. The Union was preserved and slavery abolished, but the South was ravaged and legal segregation of the races continued for another century.

Nineteenth Century

Between 1800 and 1900, 30 million immigrants arrived in America
from all parts of the world. The population of coastal cities exploded and
the economy industrialized. A network of railroads was built from coast
to coast. Thousands of people migrated to the West in search of gold
and land. A series of inventions significantly changed life, including processes for steel making, refrigeration,
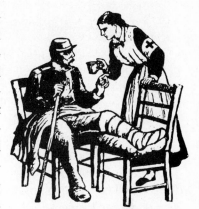
the linotype, electric light, typewriter, telephone, phonograph, and
automobile. Discovery of the alkaloid of morphine in 1815 led to
research on vegetable drugs, including quinine, strychnine, atro-
pine, and codeine.

Graduate nurses were in demand to work in hospitals, homes,
factories, and out of charitable centers called "settlement houses"
located in the ghettos of Eastern cities. Nurses worked 12- to 15-
hour days, often lived in dormitories controlled by hospitals, and
had no job security or retirement plan other than their own savings
(Table 1-1). In 1893, Lillian Wald began the famous Henry Street
Settlement in New York. She was the first president of the National
Organization for Public Health Nursing (NOPHN) and is known
as the founder of school and community health nursing. In 1888
and 1895 the first occupational health nurses, Betty Moulder
and Ada Stewart, were hired to care for industrial employees and
their families. In 1898, while serving in Cuba during the Spanish-
American War, Clara Maas became a yellow fever research subject. Her death ten days after the bite of an infected mosquito led
to the conquest of that disease.

Twentieth Century

At the dawning of the new century the optimism of advancing
technology was soon clouded by World War I and an influenza epidemic. In the United States these events greatly affected nursing

Job Description of Hospital Staff Nurses in 1887 *

In addition to caring for your 50 patients, each nurse will follow these regulations:

1. Daily sweep and mop the floors of your ward. Dust the patient's furniture and window sills.
2. Maintain an even temperature in your ward by bringing in a scuttle of coal for the day's business.
3. Light is important to observe the patient's condition. Therefore, each day fill kerosene lamps, clean chimneys, and trim wicks. Wash windows once a week.
4. The nurses' notes are important in aiding the physician's work. You may whittle nibs [pencil points] to your individual taste. Keep pencil handy.
5. Each nurse on duty will report every day at 7 am and leave at 8 pm except on the Sabbath, on which day you will be off from 12 noon to 2 pm.
6. Graduate nurses in good standing with the director of nurses will be given an evening off each week for courting purposes, or two evenings a week if you go to church regularly.
7. Each nurse should lay aside from each payday a goodly sum of her earnings for her benefit during her declining years so she will not become a burden. For example, if you earn $30 a month, you should set aside $15.
8. Any nurse who smokes, uses liquor in any form, gets her hair done at a beauty shop, or frequents dance halls will give the director good reason to suspect her worth, intentions, and integrity.
9. The nurse who performs her labors and serves her patients and doctors faithfully and without fault for a period of five years will be given an increase of five cents a day by the hospital and administrator, provided there are no outstanding hospital debts.

*Source: An advertisement in a Western newspaper, 1887.

Reproduced from Collins J: *California Nurses' Association Bulletin*, Sept–Oct 1962.

and the role of women. The League of Nations was instituted to "end all wars." Many women worked against great odds to give women more political and personal power. In 1916 Margaret Sanger was imprisoned for opening the first birth control information clinic in America. In 1920 the nineteenth Amendment to the Constitution was ratified, giving women the right to vote. In 1925, Mary Breckinridge founded the Frontier Nursing Service, providing the first organized midwifery service in the Appalachian Mountains of Kentucky.

The depression and drought of the 1930s wrought social and economic havoc in the United States. Thousands of families migrated to western states. Although nursing services were needed, jobs were scarce, and wages low; yet nurses were unwilling to join the strident labor movement of the day. The government, under the "New Deal," instituted many social programs, notably the Social Security system to which Medicare was added in 1965.

World War II and Its Aftermath

During the 1930s, dark clouds of antisemitism, greed, and nationalism in Germany, Italy, and Japan intensified. They led to World War II, a conflict destined to change every area of life, including nursing. In 1941 the United States entered the war, and in 1945 dropped the first atomic bombs. As in other wars, qualified nurses were acutely needed. The US Cadet Nurse Corps was created to increase the number of nurses. It consisted of a 30-month basic program paid for by the government and offered by existing schools of nursing. Participating schools had to meet National League of Nursing Education (NLNE) criteria and admit all qualified students, regardless of race or religion. Graduates, when registered, were commissioned as military officers. They served in medical units throughout the world. Newly introduced sulfonamide antibiotics, penicillin, prepackaged intravenous plasma and blood, anesthetics, physical therapy, and group psychotherapy significantly improved the prognosis of the sick and wounded.

At war's end in 1945, the United Nations and the World Health Organization were formed. But peace did not come. Communist nations, led by the Union of Soviet Socialist Republics, and non-communist ones, led by the United States, began a "cold war" that lasted until 1990. During that time both sides squandered human and environmental resources on huge weapons arsenals. In 1949 Congress created the US Air Force Nurse Corps, and between 1950 and 1953 the US Army Nurses served in the Korean War in Mobile Army Surgical Hospitals (MASH).

A soaring birth rate following World War II created the "baby boom" that ended with the advent of the oral contraceptive "pill" in the late 1950s. A poliomyelitis epidemic paralyzed and killed thousands before vaccines developed by Salk in 1955 and Sabin in 1961 halted its spread. Because the disease paralyses breathing muscles, the first respirators, "iron lungs," were invented. Sister Kenny, an Australian nurse, antagonized physicians by introducing a system of hot wet packs to relieve the painful muscle spasms. The treatment eventually was endorsed by members of the medical establishment. However, nursing leaders of that time did not approve of such autonomous nursing action and Sister Kenny remained a maverick to her death.

In 1956, Russia launched "sputnik" and the world entered the space age. The United States initiated an ambitious space exploration program, landing men on the moon in 1969. The technology that was developed greatly affected nursing care. It included information retrieval and storage, robotics, electronic communication, computers, food preservation, monitoring devices, and lightweight materials.

Vietnam and Civil Rights

During the 1960s the United States was embroiled in a civil war in Vietnam and a civil rights movement at home. People demonstrated en masse against the war and for civil rights. President John F. Kennedy, civil rights leader Martin Luther King, and presidential candidate Robert Kennedy were assassinated. Uncounted numbers of young people dropped out of work or school and "tuned in" to street drugs. In 1973, the troops came home from the war, but thousands suffered post-traumatic stress syndrome, drug addiction, and damage from substance abuse.

The war demonstrated the value of specialized physician-nurse teams working together in intensive care units and recovery rooms. Hospitals throughout the land installed such units. Disposable supplies replaced reusable ones, sophisticated diagnostic and therapeutic machines were purchased, and health care costs soared. Research brought advances in genetics, pharmacology, organ transplantation, immunology, and every medical specialty. Life-prolonging technology and patient rights issues created ethical dilemmas never before encountered.

After nurses demonstrated their ability to care for acutely ill patients in intensive care units, other "expanded roles" opened for nurses. In 1973, the American Nurses' Association initiated the certification program in specialty practice. Masters programs in clinical specialties opened in major university centers as did doctoral degrees in nursing. By 1982, certified clinical nurse specialists worked in every health care setting and by 1990, nurses worked individually and in joint practice with physicians across the nation.

Contemporary United States

As the twentieth century draws to a close, religion and culture, politics and war, and technology and medicine continue to influence nursing care. In the United States, religious groups opposed to abortion attempt to restrict a woman's access to abortion. Organized medicine opposes "socialized medicine." The epidemic of acquired immune deficiency syndrome (AIDS) spreads unchecked around the globe. Continuing war in the Middle East and violence around the world leave people hungry, homeless, injured, and sick. At the same time technology and medical research make constant advances in the diagnosis and treatment of disease and injury.

Professionalism

As a result of the influences of religion, war, and technology on nursing care, the image nursing holds of itself is changing. Uprichard (1973) suggests that throughout history nursing has had succeeding images of itself. During primitive times it had a folk image of itself. During medieval times nursing had a servant image of itself. In recent years nursing has developed a new image of itself, a professional image.

Professionalism, by definition, is a set of attributes that are valued by a profession, such as commitment to one's work and orientation to service rather than personal profit. Nurses who consider themselves "professional" have a different self-image than those who do not. Margretta Styles suggests that "professionalism is something that comes from within the individual, a self-image which nurses have of themselves, a way of life, a commitment to the ideals of the profession" (1982).

Professionalization, by definition, is the process by which an occupation develops the characteristics of a profession. Ever since Abraham Flexner compared social work to law, medicine, and the religious ministry, people have been debating the professional status of various occupations. A profession, said he, is (1) basically intellectual, carrying with it great responsibility; (2) learned in nature, because it is based on a body of knowledge; (3) practical, rather than theoretical; (4) well-organized internally; (5) motivated by altruism; and (6) can be taught through educational discipline (1915).

Since Flexner's time, many people have proposed lists of criteria they believe characterize professions. Moloney (1986) compared the lists of 14 distinguished persons and found 12 criteria all 14 had included. She concluded that "nurses might advance nursing's move toward professionalism if they thoroughly understood the definition and meaning of *profession* and the individual responsibilities required . . . to achieve professional status." Using Moloney's 12 criteria, let us evaluate nursing to see if it can be called a profession.

(1) *Knowledge-based.* Scientific research is the most reliable means of gaining knowledge. Nursing has developed a whole body of knowledge through scientific research. In addition, nursing practice uses knowledge from the chemical, mathematic, biologic, behavioral, physical, and social sciences. Indeed, nursing is knowledge-based.

(2) *Theory-based.* The development of nursing theory requires broad scholarship in the sciences, recognition of a phenomena, creation of new connections or concepts, and the careful design

and control of research studies. For many years nurse theorists have been developing a body of theory on which nursing practice is based. Yes, nursing is theory-based.

(3) *Altruistic.* Throughout history, unselfish caring has been the hallmark of nursing. In fact, if altruism were the sole criteria, nursing would have been a profession from its inception. But altruism is not enough. Modern nursing uses both "heart" and "head." It employs knowledge and theory together with unselfish caring to assist patients and their families to adapt effectively and attain maximum wellness. Indeed, nursing is altruistic.

(4) *Codes of ethics.* The American Nurses' Association, Canadian Nurses' Association, and the International Council of Nurses all have codes of ethics which nurses endorse. (See Chapter 6.) While the words may differ, the standards and principles these codes affirm are the same. Yes, nursing has a code of ethics.

(5) *Autonomy.* Autonomy is the freedom to make prudent and binding decisions consistent with the scope of practice and freedom to implement those decisions (Batey and Lewis 1982). Autonomy requires that nurses be responsible and accountable for their clinical decisions and the outcomes of those decisions (Moloney 1986). Even though licensure confers accountability, of all the criteria of a profession, autonomy has been most difficult to achieve. As Sister Kenny found, even nurses have not always supported it. This was true in part because they did not conceptualize their role as different from physicians. In part, it was because most nurses were women and employees, therefore dependent and subservient. Change has come slowly. The women's movement has taught nurses independence and assertiveness. Today, to ensure autonomy, nurses work under contract or practice independently. Indeed, nursing is becoming autonomous.

(6) *Service.* The essence of nursing is service, caring for people who cannot care for themselves. Service does not mean martyrdom. It means assisting others to adapt more effectively, helping them attain maximum wellness, and meeting needs they cannot meet themselves. Yes, nursing is service.

(7) *Competence.* Nurses value clinical competence. It is essential for safe practice. Competence is achieved through education and experience. To maintain high standards of competence,

nurses and their professional organizations support mandatory licensure, accreditation of nursing programs, and continuing education. Indeed, nursing values competence.

(8) *Commitment.* Commitment connotes dedication to a calling in contrast to working at a job. Nursing requires dedication. It is too demanding and complex to be anything less. Yes, nursing means commitment.

(9) *Professional association.* For more than a century nurses in America have supported their own professional organizations. (See Chapter 4.) These organizations provide structure and leadership for nursing. Indeed, nursing has its own professional organizations.

(10) *Prestige.* In the days when nurses were members of religious orders, nursing had a degree of prestige and a mystical aura. In modern times, the public image of nurses is not always positive. The public has not known what responsibilities nurses carry and what rewards they receive. As nurses define their roles and functions, gain more autonomy, and demand greater remuneration, they will achieve the acknowledgment they deserve. Yes, nursing is a prestigious calling.

(11) *Authority.* Nurse practice acts give nurses authority to practice nursing. Physicians are not licensed to practice nursing, social workers are not licensed to practice nursing, physician's assistants are not licensed to practice nursing. Only nurses are licensed and have the authority to practice nursing. Since nurse practice acts differ from state to state, it behooves nurses to know exactly what their license authorizes them to do. "Physicians are authorized to practice medicine, which is to diagnose, treat, prescribe, and operate on disease, not people. Everything else is nursing" (Diers 1989). Indeed, nursing has authority.

(12) *Trustworthiness.* Trustworthiness means being accountable for one's acts. Nurses are legally and ethically responsible for their practice. As licensed professionals, nurses must meet standards of practice; failure to do so may lead to charges of malpractice. As ethically responsible citizens, nurses faithfully fulfill their commitments to employers and patients. Yes, nurses are trustworthy.

Indeed, nursing meets all 12 criteria of a profession. As Thelma M. Schorr, editor of the *American Journal of Nursing,* said in her succinct editorial of May 1981, "Yes, Virginia, nursing is a profession."

Summary

Nursing is the art and science of caring for those who cannot care for themselves. Throughout history nursing has been influenced by the religion and culture, politics and war, and technology and medicine of each age. These influences have left their mark in the traditions that remain, reminding us that while nursing is the oldest of arts it is the youngest of professions.

Learning Activities

1. Select ten events of history that you believe had the greatest influence on nursing. Were they from religion, culture, politics, war, medicine, or technology?

2. In a group discussion, compare the life and teachings of Jesus, Muhammad, and Gautama relative to care of the sick.

3. Visit a Roman Catholic monastery or interview someone who has experienced monastic life.

4. Read *Martin Chuzzlewit*, by Charles Dickens.

5. In a discussion group, consider the question, "If Florence Nightingale could visit a nursing school today, what would surprise, please, and displease her most?"

6. Debate the proposition: "Nursing has achieved the status of a profession."

7. Role play explaining the meaning of the symbolic traditions of Carol Baker's pinning ceremony as described in the vignette at the beginning of this chapter.

Annotated Reading List

Donahue MP: *Nursing: The Oldest Art, An Illustrated History*. Mosby, 1985.

This beautifully illustrated text traces the history of nursing from ancient civilizations to the present. The author, an authority on nursing history, writes well, using appropriate quotes from original sources. About 400 illustrations, 200 in full color, show some of the world's most famous paintings, objects of art, and photographs.

Kalisch PA, Kalisch BJ: *The Changing Image of the Nurse*. Addison-Wesley, 1988.

This book looks at portrayals by the media of nursing and the public image that results. It describes concepts and theories concerning the image of the nurse, how mass communications depict nursing, and the socialization process of nurses. The authors describe five images of the nurse in the mass media since the mid-nineteenth century. They identify a new and ideal image for the future, a "nurse careerist," and suggest ways to cultivate this new image.

Moloney MM: *Professionalization of Nursing: Current Issues and Trends*. Lippincott, 1986.

In this readable text the author addresses the degree to which nursing has become a profession. She presents this still-debated issue in five parts: an introduction to professionalization of nursing, perspectives on professionalization of nursing, control of nursing education, control of nursing practice, and strategies to advance the professionalization process.

References

Batey MV, Lewis FM: Clarifying Autonomy and Accountability in Nursing Service: Part I. *J Nurs Admin* 1982; 9:15.

Dickens C: *Martin Chuzzlewit*. In: *The Works of Charles Dickens*, Vol II, p 318. Books, 1936.

Dier D: *1989 Calendar*. Addison-Wesley, 1989.

Dock LL, Stewart IM: *A Short History of Nursing*, 4th ed. Putnam's Sons, 1938.

Donahue HP: *Nursing: the Oldest Art, an Illustrated History*. Mosby, 1985.

Flexner A: Is Social Work a Profession? *School Society* 1915; 1:26.

Maslow A: A Theory of Metamotivation: The Biological Roots of the Value of Life. *J Human Psych* 1967; 7:93–127.

Moloney MM: *Professionalization of Nursing; Current Issues and Trends.* Lippincott, 1986.

Nightingale F: *Notes on Hospitals.* Appleton & Co., 1858.

Nightingale F: *Notes on Nursing.* Appleton & Co., 1860.

Robinson V: *White Caps: The Story of Nursing.* Lippincott, 1946.

Rush B: *Medical Inquiries and Observations Upon the Diseases of the Mind.* Philadelphia PA, Kimber and Richardson, 1812.

Schorr TM: *Yes, Virginia, Nursing is a Profession.* (editorial). *Am J Nurs* May 1981; 959.

Sigerist HE: *American Medicine.* Norton, 1934.

Smith JZ: Healing cults. In: *The Encyclopaedia Brittanica,* Vol 8. WE Preece, Editor, pp 685–687, 1978.

Styles M: *On Nursing: Towards a New Endowment.* Mosby, 1982.

Uprichard M: Ferment in nursing. In: *The Challenge of Nursing,* Auld E, Birum LH. Mosby, 1973.

Veith I: *Huang Ti Nei ching Su Weň, The Yellow Emperor's Classic of Internal Medicine.* New Edition, Univ. of Calif. Press, Berkeley, 1966.

Wells HG: *The Outline of History,* 5th ed. Vol 1 and 2. Doubleday, 1956.

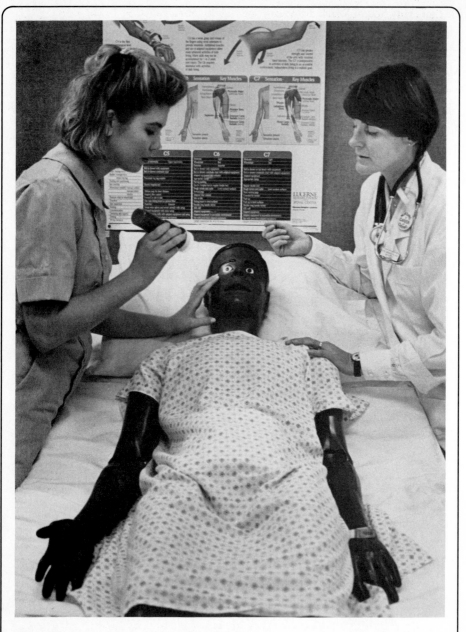

A student demonstrates neurological assessment on a mannequin under the watchful eye of her instructor. By doing so, students are able to apply knowledge to practice in a skills laboratory before caring for patients. (Photograph by Tia O'Rear)

CHAPTER 2

Education of Nurses

LEARNING OBJECTIVES

1. Compare the educational preparation and scope of practice of licensed practical nurses with that of certified nurse's aides.

2. Compare diploma, associate degree, and bachelor's degree nursing programs relative to their history, administration, length, and licensure.

3. Discuss educational articulation between practical nurse, associate degree, and bachelor's degree programs.

4. Discuss factors that motivate ADN and diploma graduates to enroll in bachelor's degree programs.

5. Discuss the concepts of role and expanded role as they relate to nursing.

6. Differentiate between clinical nurse generalist, clinical nurse specialist, and nurse practitioner.

7. Compare preceptorship and internship programs, discussing their value to new nurses and hospitals.

8. Discuss entry into practice relative to grandfathering, interstate endorsement, scope of practice, titling, and competency expectations.

9. Discuss mandatory versus voluntary continuing education requirements for licensure.

10. Describe types of nursing literature and ways to select it.

11. Discuss the process, written report, ethical considerations, and evaluation of nursing research.

12. Compare the central theme, definition, and nursing process of three conceptual models of nursing practice.

Alicia's large family had gathered for the annual spring dinner at Gramma's home. Three generations were there, soon to be four. They had stuffed themselves on shared delicacies and sat back to visit. Aunt Joan turned to Alicia and said, "Won't you be graduating from nursing school pretty soon?"

Alicia replied proudly, "I certainly will be, in six weeks, two days, and about two hours! You'll all get invitations." Alicia's cousin, Tom, leaned forward and said, "I know a girl who went to nursing school for only one year; how come you've been going for so long?" Before Alicia could reply, someone else said, "I thought nursing schools were in hospitals; how come you go to a community college?" Alicia's pregnant cousin brightened, "I see a nurse practitioner at the prenatal clinic almost every visit. Is that what you're going to be when you graduate?" Alicia tried to explain that she was going to be a registered nurse. One-year nursing programs usually are for licensed practical nurses. I do go to hospitals for clinical experience, but my classes are at the college. No, I won't be a nurse practitioner. That takes much more education."

As Alicia attempted to enlighten her family she realized how little she knew about nursing education. She was relieved when the conversation shifted to other topics. However, the questions people asked left her wondering. Why are there so many levels of nursing? What are the differences between them? Just what is a nurse practitioner?

Unlike medicine, which focuses on disease and injury, nursing focuses on human responses to health problems. As a result, nursing provides a broad range of health care services, from the most basic to the most complex. To deliver these services, a wide spectrum of caregivers have evolved, from the least to the most highly skilled and educated. These caregivers include nurse's aides, orderlies, nursing assistants, practical-vocational nurses, registered nurses, clinical nurse specialists, and nurse-practitioners. Historically, caregivers divided into two groups: *practical nurses* and *trained (registered) nurses*. At first, practical nurses learned their skills by "practical experience" with little or no formal education, while registered nurses learned their skills in three or more years of training within formal educational programs. The two divisions of nursing remain to this day, but they have changed significantly.

Practical Nursing

Nursing Assistants

The first practical nurses in the United States worked in the homes of people in the community, bathing, cooking, keeping house, and giving nursing care to new mothers, babies, and sick family members. They were self-taught or learned from other caregivers. In time, hospitals hired these workers in low-paying jobs as nurse's aides, orderlies, and nursing assistants. To this day, this branch of practical nursing continues, unlicensed and relatively invisible. While some of these workers take brief courses in basic skills, most have no formal nursing education.

In recent years some states have begun regulating the practice of these workers. In California, the Department of Health Services (DHS) accredits programs for Home Health Aides (HHA) and Certified Nursing Assitants (CNA). These programs are offered by long-term care facilities and adult education units. The HHA pro-

41

gram is 120 hours in length. The CNA program is 150 hours and includes basic nursing skills such as bathing, personal hygiene, and food preparation. On completion, graduates receive a certificate of completion from the DHS. They work under the direct supervision of licensed nurses and physicians (California Department of Health Services 1985).

Licensed Practical Nurses

The first formal preparation for practical nurses in the US began in 1890 at the YWCA in Brooklyn, New York. It was known as the Ballard School, after Miss Lucinda Ballard who provided the operating funds. The course of study was about three months long. Students learned to care for invalids, the aged, and children in home settings. Other early practical nursing programs included the School of Practical Nursing in Brooklyn, New York, founded in 1893; the Thompson School for Practical Nurses in Brattleboro, Vermont, begun in 1907; and the Household Nursing Association in Boston, now called Shepard-Gill School of Practical Nursing (Johnston 1966). In 1908, the American Red Cross began teaching classes in home nursing. In 1918, the Surgeon General of the US Army asked the Red Cross to begin training nurse's aides for military hospitals. The number and reputation of practical nursing schools grew, and before long civilian hospitals were hiring graduates.

In the mid-1930s the American Nurses' Association (ANA) became aware of increasing numbers of "subsidiary" workers. As a result, representatives of the ANA, National League of Nursing Education (NLNE), and National Organization for Public Health Nursing (NOPHN) formed a Joint Committee to Outline Principles and Policies for the Control of Subsidiary Workers in the Care of the Sick. The committee recommended that "workers of this type should be subject to control under compulsory licensure to provide satisfactory control of their use." In 1938, New York enacted the first practical nurse practice act. By 1949, 28 states, Hawaii, and Puerto Rico had passed licensing laws. By 1959, all 50 states and Canada had Licensed Practical Nurses (LPN) or Licensed Vocational Nurses (LVN), as they are called in Texas and California (Johnston 1966).

Currently, the scope of practice of practical nurses consists of meeting the health needs of patients in stable conditions in hospitals, homes, and long-term care facilities, under the supervision of registered nurses and physicians. Graduates of state accredited programs take a National Council Examination for Practical Nurses (NCLEX-PN) and work under provisions of their state nurse practice act.

In 1941, the Association of Practical Nurse Schools was founded. A year later membership was opened to individuals and the name was changed to the National Association of Practical Nurse Education (NAPNE). NAPNE developed the first nationally endorsed curriculum for practical nurses. In 1949 the National Federation of Licensed Practical Nurses (NFLPN) was organized. The National League for Nursing (NLN) established a Council on Practical Nursing (CPN), and in 1966 the Chicago Public School Program became the first NLN accredited practical nurse program in the US.

In the US today, practical nurse education varies from state to state and school to school. Programs are offered by high schools, hospitals, adult education departments, trade-technical schools, community colleges, and universities. Usually curricula are one year long and counted in clock hours rather than credit hours. Clinical experience occurs in structured settings such as hospitals and extended care facilities.

Various career ladders have been devised to assist LPN-LVNs to become RNs. These plans seek to avoid duplication by giving credit for past education. In some colleges, *articulation* (joining together) of practical-vocational and registered nurse education is built into the curriculum plan, with all nursing students taking a one-year core nursing course. At the end of the year they can stop and seek licensure as a LPN-LVN or continue for an additional year, completing RN licensing requirements. In other schools, LPN-LVNs are credited with the first year of a degree nursing program. When they have completed prerequisite courses LPN-LVNs may enroll as second-year students. In California, this option is mandated by regulation of the RN licensing board, permitting LVNs to take the NCLEX-RN when they have completed 30 semester units of additional nursing course work (Board of Registered Nursing 1989).

Registered Nurse Education

Early Schools of Nursing

The first European nursing schools began in hospitals of religious and secular orders. When student novices completed their study they took vows and became full members of the order. When the Florence Nightingale school was established in London in 1860, students who completed the prescribed course of study were awarded a diploma. When nursing education entered colleges and universities, students who completed the nursing curriculum were granted academic degrees. Thus, hospital-based nursing education became known as *diploma programs* and college-based education became known as a *degree programs*.

The United States was nearly 100 years old when the Civil War (1861–1865) demonstrated a desperate need for prepared nurses. In 1869, a committee of the American Medical Association said "it is just as necessary to have well-instructed nurses as to have intelligent and skillful physicians" (Dolan 1978). They recommended that county medical societies supervise nurse education. Nightingale would have agreed that nurses need quality instruction, but she would have insisted that nursing schools operate independently of both hospitals and physicians.

Finally, in 1872, the New England Hospital for Women and Children (NEHWC) established the first nursing school. When Linda Richards graduated from the 12-month program, she became the first "trained" nurse in America. In 1873, programs designed after the Nightingale school (except that they were not autonomous) were founded at Bellevue, Massachusetts General, and New Haven Hospitals. In 1874, Canada founded its first "Nightingale" school at General and Marine Hospital in the city of St. Catherine's. Other schools began at Toronto General, Children's Hospital at Toronto, and Winnipeg General. In 1879, Mary Eliza Mahoney became the first "trained" Afro-American nurse when she completed the NEHWC program. In 1888, Mills School, a nursing school for men, was organized at Bellevue Hospital.

The success of these early programs and the fact that students provided nursing service at minimal cost to hospitals, led to a massive proliferation of schools. By 1909, there were 1105 hospital-based, two- and three-year diploma schools in the US and 70 in Canada. The Nightingale principle that student experience was for learning, not service, was forgotten. There was no standard curriculum or accreditation of schools. Each program was developed to meet the service needs of hospitals rather than the educational needs of students. Thus, curricula differed widely from school to school. The school superintendent often served as the hospital director of nurses. Instructors were graduates of the very same school. Few were educated beyond basic nursing, yet they taught most of the courses, including the biologic sciences. Sometimes the hospital dietitian taught nutrition and medical staff members gave lectures about diseases. Typically, the curriculum was laid out in blocks of study paralleling medical specialties, with rotations through the diet kitchen and operating room. Courses in anatomy, physiology, pharmacology, nutrition, history of nursing, and professional adjustment rounded out the curriculum. If the host hospital could not provide a specialty experience, such as psychiatry, students might not get it or were sent to other hospitals on affiliation.

Students worked split shifts on hospital units during the early and late hours of the day with classes in between. Most days were 12 to 15 hours long with one day off per week. Many students contracted communicable diseases. There was no sick leave and all lost time had to be made up before they could graduate. Juniors and seniors worked evening and night shifts but were expected to attend classes that met during the day. In these early schools almost all students were single young women who entered soon after high school graduation. They lived in dormitories near hospitals and their social lives were controlled by strict rules. Marriage was grounds for dismissal.

By 1912, most programs were three calendar years in length. Students were probationers (probies) for four to six months, during which instructors evaluated their aptitude and ability. If they survived this period, they were "capped" at a symbolic ceremony resembling the taking of religious vows, after which they were called freshmen, then juniors, and finally seniors. Status was designated by uniform changes, such as adding ribbons to the cap or wearing white instead of black stockings. Completion was marked by the awarding of a diploma and a school pin. Since hospitals were not degree-granting institutions, a diploma was not an academic degree and no college credit was given. Except for a few segregated schools, most programs barred all men and Afro-American women. In spite of these hardships, women continued to enter nursing. Few other occupations were open to them.

Studies Bring Change

As the nation matured and medical science and technology developed, nursing education needed to change. World War I dramatized the need for more and better educated nurses. In 1917, the NLNE, led by Isabel M. Stewart, published the first of three studies entitled *Standard Curriculum for Schools of Nursing* (Stewart 1943). It contained a systematic plan of instruction, outlining courses in detail. In 1927, the second study, entitled *Curriculum for Schools of Nursing* used job analysis to define the qualifications and functions of nurses. The third study of 1937, entitled *A Curriculum Guide for Schools of Nursing*, involved nurse educators throughout the nation in the curriculum development process.

In 1923, the Winslow-Goldmark Survey (Winslow-Goldmark Report, 1923) entitled *Nursing and Nursing Education in the United States*, concluded that public health nurses, supervisors, and instructors needed additional study beyond basic nursing. It recommended endowment for university schools of nursing (Committee for the Study of Nursing Education, 1923). Soon thereafter, Yale University School of Nursing was founded under the leadership of Annie W. Goodrich, followed by Western Reserve University under Frances Payne Bolton, Vanderbilt University, University of Toronto, and others. By 1932, the Association of Collegiate Schools of Nursing was established to promote nursing education at the college level and to encourage research.

In 1925, the Committee on the Grading of Nursing Schools began an eight-year study of nursing education. In 1928, in its first report, the committee concluded that the "need of a hospital for cheap labor should not be considered a legitimate argument for maintaining a . . . school. The decision . . . to conduct [a school of nursing] should be based solely upon the kinds and amounts of educational experience . . . [a] hospital is prepared to offer" (Committee on the Grading of Nursing Schools, 1928). In 1934, in its final report, the committee recommended that a collegiate level of education be instituted "dominated neither by hospital, nor treasury, nor nursing traditions" (Stewart, 1943).

In 1932 in Canada, a joint committee of the Canadian Nurses' Association and Canadian Medical Association led by Dr. George Weir studied nursing education (Gibbon and Mathewson, 1947). It recommended higher standards for graduation and better qualified instructors.

In 1948, Esther L. Brown studied society's need for nursing and published her findings in a book entitled *Nursing for the Future*. She recommended that basic schools of nursing be placed in colleges and universities, not hospitals, and that men and members of minority groups be recruited into nursing. In that same year, the Ginzberg Report studied problems of nursing shortages, publishing their conclusions in a book entitled *A Program for the Nursing Profession* (Kelly, 1985). The study recommended that nursing teams consist of four-year professional nurses, two-year registered nurses, and one-year practical nurses. Looking back, these recommendations seem remarkably prophetic.

In 1963, the Consultant Group of Nursing presented their two-year study commissioned by the US Public Health Service to advise the surgeon general of national nursing needs and identify the role of the federal government in meeting these needs. The report, entitled *Toward Quality in Nursing* (Kelly, 1985), recommended a study of nursing education that would yield criteria for quality care. In response, in 1967 the ANA and NLN set up the National Commission for the Study of Nursing and Nursing Education. It probed the supply and demand of nurses, their roles, functions, and education, and nursing as a career. The final report, entitled *An Abstract for Action* (National Commission, 1970), called for greater government funding for nursing research and for states to set up master planning committees for nursing education.

In 1983, the National Commission on Nursing published a three-year study that identified major issues in nursing. These issues were the status and image of nursing, relationships between health care personnel, the interface of nursing education and practice, effective management of nursing resources, and nursing as a self-determining profession.

In 1985, the National Commission of Nursing Implementation Project began its efforts to seek consensus about suitable education and credentialing for basic nursing practice, effective models for care, and ways to develop and test nursing knowledge.

Space does not permit a description of many other studies, but this sampling shows something of their nature and importance.

Diploma Programs

Diploma programs of today differ greatly from the service-oriented ones of yesteryear. They meet NLN accreditation criteria and are associated with colleges and universities. Since each school has unique historic roots, it is difficult to generalize. However, diploma programs typically: (1) are administered, controlled, and housed near to or in a sponsoring hospital; (2) charge tuition; (3) take three academic or three calendar years to complete; (4) meet accreditation standards of the state licensing boards; (5) employ faculty with bachelor's and master's degrees in nursing, some of whom have dual assignments in the school and the hospital; (6) use community agencies and the sponsoring hospital for clinical experience; (7) use nationally published professional nursing textbooks; (8) have a clearly stated philosophy, conceptual framework, learning objectives, and evaluation criteria; (9) prepare students to take the National Council Licensure Examination for Registered Nurses (NCLEX-RN); and (10) award a diploma on completion.

As educational standards have risen, so have costs. In the past 20 years diploma school education has become expensive and the number of schools has declined. Still, diploma education provides a unique learning experience. Because of the hours spent in direct patient care, students become skilled in basic nursing functions. They learn how to work within the bureaucratic structure of a hospital and how to function in the role of a staff nurse, a process called *professional socialization*. As a result, graduates of diploma schools make the transition from student to professional nurse with relative ease, rapidly becoming productive members of the health care team. Competencies of graduates of diploma programs have been identified by the National League for Nursing (NLN) Council of Diploma Programs. A list of these may be purchased from the NLN, 350 Hudson Street, New York, NY 10014.

Associate Degree in Nursing Programs

The Associate Degree Nursing (ADN) program is a relative newcomer to nursing education and is the first educational program established on the basis of research. It was suggested in 1951 by Mildred L. Montag in her doctoral dissertation as a solution to the shortage of nurses after World War II. In her proposal, ADN programs were to be theory-based, offered in community colleges, two years in length, and were to prepare graduates to take the licensing examination for registered nurses. Employing hospitals were to provide supervision of new graduates while they refined their clinical skills. Such supervision was to be given by experienced nurses, similar to supervision found in diploma school.

In 1952, a pilot project called the Cooperative Research Project in Junior and Community College Education for Nursing was begun by Teachers College, Columbia University. The five-year project included seven colleges and one hospital school located in six regions of the US. The results of the project showed that, indeed, programs could be established in community colleges, use clinical facilities in the community, attract quality students, and be cost effective. Graduates met learning objectives and passed the registered nurse licensing examination.

ADN programs were so successful that by 1988 there were 776 programs in the US, and ADN graduates made up the majority of RNs in the US (Anastas 1988). Jody K. Williams found that students are attracted to this type of education because of its short duration, quality, relatively low cost, and location near their homes (1989). While most ADN programs are in community colleges, some are in four-year institutions that also offer a bachelor of science in nursing (BSN) degree. The University of the State of New York offers an ADN through the Regents External Degree Program described later in this chapter.

ADN students differ from the traditional young, single white women who once characterized nursing students. Currently, the average age of ADN students throughout the US is 30 years; most work part or full time; half have children; many are single parents and have other interests, abilities, and degrees; and there are more men and racial minorities than in other programs (Williams 1989). Many ADN programs grant credit to LPN-LVNs for the first-year nursing courses, permitting them to enter as second-year students if they have met science and general education prerequisites.

Typically, ADN curricula build on a high school diploma that includes chemistry, mathematics, and English. Programs (1) are departments within community colleges, controlled, financed, and housed on college campuses; (2) charge minimal tuition in public colleges, more tuition in private institutions; (3) include four semesters or six quarters of nursing, communication, mathematics, humanities, and physical, social, and biological sciences; (4) meet standards of state licensing boards and regional higher education accrediting agencies; (5) use nationally published professional nursing textbooks; (6) have masters- and doctorate-prepared faculty who meet both college and licensing board qualifications; (7) use community hospitals and agencies for clinical experience; (8) are based on a philosophy and conceptual framework with clearly stated learning objectives and evaluation criteria; (9) accord students the same rights and responsibilities as other college students; (10) prepare students to care for individuals in structured settings, using the nursing process, decision-making, and management skills; (11) prepare graduates to take the NCLEX-RN; and (12) meet associate degree requirements of the college. Competencies of graduates of ADN programs have been identified by the NLN Council of Associate Degree Programs. A list of these may be purchased from the National League for Nursing, 350 Hudson Street, New York, NY 10014.

Bachelor of Science Degree in Nursing Programs

Near the end of the nineteenth century, the increasing complexity of nursing led to preparatory courses of theoretical instruction. One of the earliest was taught at St. Mungo's College in

Glasgow, Scotland in 1883. In 1887 the University of Texas assumed responsibility for the John Sealy Hospital in Galveston and its nursing school. Although the superintendent occupied a place on the university committee, students were not enrolled in the university. In 1901, a true prenursing course was developed by M. Adelaide Nutting at Johns Hopkins School of Nursing at Baltimore, Maryland. This six-month course offered basic sciences and nursing principles with related clinical practice. Within ten years similar preparatory courses were required in 86 schools of nursing in the United States and Canada.

Between 1907 and 1910, many hospital nursing schools were taken over or established by university hospitals. Some were placed under the auspices of medical schools. Nursing students were admitted and registered as regular students, but the school was not an independent unit within the university and some did not offer college degrees. By 1917, several universities granted graduates of nursing programs other-than-nursing degrees. By 1919, eight universities offered bachelor of science in nursing (BSN) degrees. These consisted of two academic years of liberal studies followed by a typical three-year diploma program. In 1923, Yale University School of Nursing became the first independent school of nursing within a university.

Considering that women did not have the right to vote until 1920, these early baccalaureate programs were exceptional. Many people of the day believed that higher education was wasted on women. Still others viewed nursing as an unacceptable vocation for women of social standing and moral character. In spite of these attitudes the number of BSN programs grew. By 1986, there were 459 BSN programs in the United States (Anastas 1988).

Generic (Standard) Baccalaureate
Programs

Following World War II, curricula of BSN programs began to resemble majors of other four-year professional degrees. Today these programs typically (1) build on lower-division humanities, mathematics, language, and physical, social, biological, and behavioral science courses; (2) are concentrated in the upper-division and emphasize research findings and collaboration with other disciplines; (3) are departments or schools within colleges and universities and are controlled, financed, and housed on college campuses; (4) charge tuition in accord with policies of the parent institution; (5) meet accreditation standards of state licensing boards, regional higher education accrediting agencies, and the NLN; (6) use nationally published professional nursing textbooks; (7) have master's and doctorate prepared faculty who meet both college and licensing board regulations and enjoy the same rights and responsibilities as other faculty members; (8) use community agencies for clinical experience; (9) are based on a philosophy and conceptual framework with clearly stated learning objectives and evaluation criteria; (10) prepare graduates to provide nursing care for individuals, families, groups, and communities using the nursing process; and provide critical decision-making, and leadership skills to address complex nursing problems; (11) accord students the same rights and obligations as other college students; (12) prepare students to take the NCLEX-RN; and (13) meet college requirements for a baccalaureate degree.

Alternative Baccalaureate Programs

In recent years several alternative baccalaureate nursing programs have appeared. Some build on a diploma or associate degree in nursing and some build on a bachelor's degree in another subject. Some programs are called *external,* because classes meet outside the walls of the sponsoring institution.

Programs that offer a BSN to diploma and ADN registered nurses have various names, such as Capstone, Two Plus Two, and Second Step. These programs provide baccalaureate education for ADN and diploma nurses. Several factors motivate nurses to enroll in these programs, namely (1) the 1965 ANA position paper stating that a BSN should become the minimum entry level for professional nursing practice; (2) upward mobility of hospital staff nurses to administration, education, community health, and clinical specialty areas; (3) societal approval of lifelong learning; (4) mandated continuing education for licensure; and (5) self-actualization.

Baccalaureate programs for registered nurses vary greatly. In some institutions RN students enter as lower division students and take all but basic nursing courses. In other programs, they receive credit for all academic and nursing courses. Still other BSN programs admit only ADNs and the major is entirely in upper division. Courses include pathophysiology, nursing theory, advanced nursing practice, statistics, research, leadership-management, and community health.

Many universities have developed innovative programs to meet the needs of working nurses seeking advanced education. In the California Statewide Nursing Program, courses are taught year round at sites throughout the state. They are designed for adult learners in one-unit modules with in-class learning activities and out-of-class assignments. Curricula and course content are standardized and required courses are offered on a rotating basis. Faculty members come from local universities and colleges. California State University awards a BSN degree to graduates (Degree and certificate programs for RNs 1989).

New York Regents External Degree program offers both an ADN and BSN degree. The program is designed to enable students to earn a college degree by using college courses, proficiency examinations, and/or special assessments. Fees are charged for enrollment, examinations, and record maintenance. The ADN curriculum is equivalent to a generic two-year nursing program and the BSN is equivalent to a generic four-year nursing program. Both programs are accredited by the NLN. There are no prerequisites, although nursing experience is an advantage. Clear learning objectives for each unit of study are measured by written tests and performance examinations at testing centers throughout the US (New York Regents External Degree 1988).

Master's Degree Programs

Master's degree programs prepare nurses for careers in education, administration, consultation, and advanced clinical practice. Curricula include specialization in such areas of nursing practice as maternal-child health, community health, psychiatric-mental health, adult health, and anesthesia. Many programs include study of both a clinical realm and a functional area, such as administration. Some programs emphasize clinical practice, preparing clinical specialists and nurse practitioners in such areas as midwifery, anesthesia, and gerontology.

Typically, master's degree programs require 24 to 48 semester units (30 to 60 quarter units) of graduate study. Entrance requirements include a bachelor's degree in nursing from an NLN-accredited program with a 3.0 grade point average, RN licensure, at least a year of work experience, completion of a prerequisite course in statistics, and a Graduate Record Examination or Miller Analogy test score. The goals of the applicant must match the goals and resources of the school. To accommodate students who work while pursuing advanced education, graduate schools have begun offering classes at off-campus sites, in the evening, on weekends, and by means of telecommunication systems.

Generic master's degree programs teach basic nursing theory and practice at the master's degree level. Prerequisites vary and include a bachelor's degree in a field other than nursing. After the two- to three-year program, graduates earn a master's degree in nursing and are eligible to take the NCLEX-RN. Several universities have begun offering these programs.

Doctoral Degree Programs

Doctoral degrees in nursing are relative newcomers to graduate education. Prior to their appearance, nurses who wished to pursue doctoral study earned degrees in related fields such as sociology, education, psychology, and physiology. Many nurses continue to do so. Thus a variety of degrees can be found among nursing leaders, including doctor of education (EdD), doctor of philosophy (PhD), doctor of public health (DPH), doctor of nursing science (DNSc), doctor of science in nursing (DSN), and doctor of nursing (ND). Regardless of the name, the essence of doctoral study is in-depth inquiry and scientific research into a particular area of learning in order to extend knowledge. Doctoral dissertations report research findings in a formalized pattern.

Generic doctoral programs in nursing admit students with bachelor's and master's degrees in fields other than nursing. The curriculum includes basic nursing theory and practice and completion of a research project in nursing. Graduates earn a doctoral degree and are eligible to take NCLEX-RN for licensure as registered nurses.

Entry into Practice

For many years nursing leaders have been debating minimum educational preparation for entry into practice. Although the NCLEX-RN test plan sets the content, and everyone supports quality, not everyone agrees on the quantity of education necessary for "professional" nursing.

In 1923, the Winslow-Goldmark Survey concluded that schools of nursing need to be "recognized and supported as separate educational components with, not just training in nursing, but also a liberal education" (Committee for the Study of Nursing Education 1923). In 1948, Esther L. Brown recommended that the term "professional" apply to nursing education that takes place in schools "able to furnish professional education as that term has come to be understood by educators." In 1951, Mildred Montag identified a *technical nurse* as one whose scope of practice is narrower than that of a *professional nurse* and broader than that of a *practical nurse*. Her study launched associate degree nursing programs across the land (1959).

In 1965, the ANA House of Delegates adopted the position that "minimum preparation for beginning professional nursing practice . . . should be baccalaureate degree education in nursing and minimum preparation for beginning technical nursing practice should be associate degree education in nursing" (ANA 1965). In 1978, the ANA House of Delegates adopted a resolution that "by 1985, the minimum preparation for entry into professional nursing practice would be the baccalaureate in nursing and . . . ANA would work with state nurses' associations to identify and define two categories of nursing practice by 1980" (ANA Commission on Nursing Education 1979). In 1984, the ANA established a timeline for implementing their goal to establish the baccalaureate for professional nursing practice in 5 percent of the states by 1986, 15 percent by 1988, 50 percent by 1992, and 100 percent by 1995 (ANA Cabinet on Nursing Education 1983).

In 1985, the ANA House of Delegates agreed that the term *registered nurse* be reserved for a professional nurse prepared with a baccalaureate degree and the term *associate nurse* be reserved for a technical nurse prepared with an associate degree (ANA Delegates 1985). That same year the National Organization for the Advancement of Associate Degree Nurses was organized to support the continued status of ADNs as professional nurses. In 1986, while many nursing organizations voted to support the ANA positions, the National Council of State Boards of Nursing, the organization responsible for writing NCLEX-RN, voted to take a position of neutrality regarding educational requirements for entry into practice (Hartung 1986). In 1987, the NLN membership voted to postpone indefinitely resolutions concerning the issue of entry into practice.

In 1987, North Dakota became the first state to change its nursing education rules to require that after January 1987, nurses would have to have a BSN degree to apply for RN licensure and an ADN to apply for LPN licensure (North Dakota 1986). In 1989, the rule was modified. The Board began issuing temporary RN licenses to graduates of ADN programs, giving them four years to obtain a BSN. They also began issuing temporary LPN licenses to graduates of practical nursing programs, giving them two years to obtain an ADN (Sage 1990).

By 1989, the nationwide shortage of nurses slowed the drive, but the effort of nursing leaders to require a BSN for RN licensure continues.

Controversial Issues

Whenever nursing leaders consider changing educational preparation for entry into practice, several controversial issues appear, namely, titling, grandfathering, endorsement, scope of practice, and competency expectations.

Titling is perhaps the most controversial issue. Even though the ANA position statement calls for two levels of nursing, professional and technical, agreement has not been reached as to the titles each should use. Some suggested titles are: professional/technical, registered/associate, registered/licensed practical, and nurse/

nurse associate (Edge 1986). The problem, of course, is that the term "registered nurse" is the traditional title, the one that commands the highest respect. No one wants to be downgraded from RN to anything else, least of all diploma and AD nurses who have passed the same licensing examination and work as peers and supervisors of BS nurses.

Grandfathering means allowing persons to continue to practice their profession or occupation when new qualifications, which they do not meet, become law. Legally, licensing of professional and occupational groups falls within the police power of the states. The power to license health professionals is used to safeguard the health and welfare of citizens. When a new state law is enacted, or if a law changes, a "grandfather clause" must be included because the Fourteenth Amendment to the US Constitution guarantees that a state cannot deprive a person of life, liberty, or property without due process. The Supreme Court has ruled that a license to practice is a property right as long as the licensee practices within the law. When applied to entry into practice, a grandfather clause guarantees that RNs with a diploma or an ADN have the right to continue to be licensed and practice under the law (Waddle 1986). However, a grandfather clause protects only the license. It does not guarantee job advancement or intangibles such as respect.

Endorsement for licensure between states becomes complicated if the states change their requirements one by one over time. Currently, nursing is one of the few occupations to have developed a process by which national examinations with standardized scores (NCLEX-RN and NCLEX-PN) are administered and accepted by each state or jurisdiction. Both registered nurses and practical nurses are able to move from state to state without having to retake and pass another examination. When one state requires a BSN for RN licensure and an AD for a PN licensure, AD and diploma RNs who move would not have reciprocity as RNs, but they might not meet requirements for a PN license either. Whether the Fourteenth Amendment would guarantee the right to a license in the new state has not been tested.

Scope of practice refers to the legally sanctioned functions of licensed persons. As nurses consider the implications of two new categories of nurses, scope of practice is a matter of great concern.

It was of such importance to the ANA that in 1985 its House of Delegates charged a special task force to delineate the scope of practice for future professional and technical nurses. The group concluded that "nursing has but one scope of practice made up of four components: a core (diagnosed human responses to acute or potential health problems), a boundary (dynamic perimeters), intersections (interaction within nursing and between nursing and other health care professionals), and dimensions (characteristics: knowledge base of nurse, role of nurse, nature of clients, and practice environment)." They also concluded that "differences between professional and technical nursing practice are found in all four dimensions" (ANA Task Force 1986). They did not, however, delineate the differences.

Competency expectations for the two categories of nursing are related to the scope of practice and are critical to the issue of entry into practice. At present there are two recognized, clearly identified sets of competencies, one for registered nurses and one for practical nurses. There are two licensing examinations that measure those competencies: NCLEX-RN and NCLEX-PN. However, even though many studies have been done, no difference in quality has been found between AD, diploma, and BS registered nurses. Despite efforts to identify a relationship between competencies and educational preparation, none has been found, except as relates to involvement with research (A Study 1986).

The Two Positions

Those who are committed to the ANA position believe a change in basic educational requirements is necessary if nursing is to achieve the status of a profession (Moloney 1986). In fact, some believe that nursing will not become a true profession until a doctorate is the entry level degree. The first step, they maintain, is to raise the entry level to a bachelor's degree.

Those who oppose the ANA position believe a change in basic education requirements for registered nurses is unnecessary and disruptive. They cite a lack of objective evidence that bachelor's-prepared nurses score higher on NCLEX-RN or perform better in clinical settings than associate degree or diploma graduates. They note that ADN programs are community-based, cost-effective, accessible, maintain high standards, and attract disadvantaged populations. They see a critical need for more registered nurses, not less. They propose that the present educational system continue and additional learning be recognized by continuing education and certification.

Continuing Education

One of the characteristics of a profession, as described in Chapter 1, is *competence*. Nurses must continually update their knowledge, skills, and attitudes to be competent in their ever-changing field. To do this some nurses enter formal academic degree programs, some take short-term courses and workshops, and some undertake independent study. "Continuing education in nursing," stated the ANA, "consists of planned, organized learning experiences designed to augment the knowledge, skill, and attitudes of registered nurses for the enhancement of nursing practice, education, administration, and research, to the end of improving health care to the public" (1978).

Continuing education (CE) is not a new idea. In about 1882 Nightingale wrote, "Nursing is, above all, a progressive calling. Year by year nurses have to learn new and improved methods as medicine, surgery, and hygiene improve" (1954). In 1899, Columbia University offered the first "postgraduate" nursing course of record in the United States. In the 1920s, nursing organizations began offering conferences and institutes.

In 1967, the ANA published its first clear statement on CE. In 1973, the ANA established the Council on Continuing Education. By 1974, most states had devised ways to recognize CE, and the ANA Council published *Standards for Continuing Education in Nursing*. It developed a system of accreditation, approval of CE courses, and a standard unit of measurement. *A continuing education unit (CEU)* equals ten hours of participation in an organized learning experience offered by a responsible sponsor, capable director, and qualified instructor (Facts about Nursing 1985).

In 1987, ANA established a new system whereby organizations can seek accreditation as either providers or approvers or both.

A *provider* is any organization that is responsible for offering a course of instruction. An *approver* is an organization that is responsible for recognizing courses, such as state nurses' associations and specialty organizations.

Some states have made CE mandatory for renewal of both registered nurse licenses and practical nurse licenses. Some have not. Many states are moving toward mandatory CE for all licensed professionals, including physicians, lawyers, and nurses. The licensing board of each state sets the number of required CEUs, designs a process for enforcing the regulations, and sets standards for approval of acceptable courses. It is the responsibility of registered nurses to meet requirements of the state in which they seek license renewal.

Nursing Literature

Nursing literature fills an important role in the education of nurses and the transmission of knowledge and culture. In 1885, Clara Weeks Shaw wrote the first US nursing text entitled, *A Textbook of Nursing for the Use of Training Schools, Families, and Private Students*. In 1890, Lavinia Dock wrote *Materia Medica for Nurses*. Later she wrote a four-volume *History of Nursing* with M. Adelaide Nutting. Other early nursing authors were Isabel Hampton and Diana Kimber. By 1930, over 700 texts had been written for nurses and published in the United States (Donahue 1985). By 1980, there were over 20,000 nursing texts and the number grows each year.

With so many texts, how do nurses choose what to read? Here are some suggestions: (1) Read book reviews and publisher advertisements in nursing magazines. (2) Read the list of "Books of the Year" selected by experts for the *American Journal of Nursing*. (3) Browse through bookstore and library stacks of colleges where there are nursing schools. (4) Ask nurse faculty members for suggestions; they receive copies of many new texts. (5) Consult *Books in Print*, a mammoth reference work that lists books by title and author; it is available in most libraries and bookstores.

Textbooks are but one way to gain nursing knowledge. Periodicals are an important way for nurses to stay abreast of the ever-changing health care field. Perhaps the oldest nursing periodical in the United States is the *American Journal of Nursing,* first published on October 1, 1900. Today there are more than 80 periodicals published for and about nursing. Many of these publications are official organs of a professional organization. For example, *Occupational Health Nursing* is the official journal of the American Association of Occupational Health Nurses.

Because of the great number of periodicals, nurses must choose those that meet their needs. Libraries of colleges and universities with nursing schools subscribe to the most widely read periodicals and usually can obtain others by interlibrary loan. Often libraries subscribe to the *Cumulative Index to Nursing and Allied Health Literature* and *Index Medicus,* where articles are listed by author and topic.

Although not classified as "literature" in the traditional sense, audiovisual and computerized data are a valuable source of information for nurses. Audiocassettes, videocassettes, and computer software are produced by multimedia and textbook publishers. They are indexed in the *Cumulative Index to Nursing and Allied Health Literature* and are available for purchase or loan from libraries. These materials are especially useful because they are convenient and use sound, sight, and interaction in addition to the written word.

Educational Preparation for Nursing Roles

Because nursing is knowledge-based and theory-based, education is essential to the preparation of its practitioners. As the profession grows and expands, various roles and levels within those roles emerge, each with its own educational requirements. In the vignette Alicia realized how little she knew of nursing roles and the preparation needed to fill them.

A *role* is a set of behaviors expected of people who hold a position; often it has a title, such as *mother.* A *work role* is a set of behaviors individuals are paid to perform, such as *staff nurse.* An *expanded role* is a set of more complex work behaviors requiring additional education and experience, such as *nurse practitioner.* A *functional role* is a set of behaviors that fulfills certain purposes. Key functional roles in nursing are: clinical (patient care), administrative (management), educational (teaching), and research. Basic nursing education prepares students for clinical roles. Clinical roles are divided into various levels, including staff nurses, clinical nurse generalists, clinical nurse specialists, and expert clinicians (nurse practitioners and clinical nurse specialists). Table 2-1 shows these roles relative to educational practice and focus of clinical care. Chapter 3 describes the certification of nurses in various roles.

Staff nurses in acute care setttings at the entry level give care to patients with acute or chronic illness, make nursing judgments based on scientific knowledge, and rely on standardized nursing care plans and procedures. As they gain experience, staff nurses rely less on standardized plans and procedures and more on individualized plans. Many hospitals use clinical steps to recognize and promote these nurses, such as Staff Nurse I, II, and III. Usually, the highest work role a nurse can attain without a master's degree is clinical nurse generalist.

Clinical nurse specialists (CNS) have advanced expertise in a nursing specialty and understand a broad range of theories that apply to clinical practice. While their practice encompasses preventative care, CNSs focus their practice on acute and rehabilitative care. They have master's or doctorate degrees in a clinical specialty plus additional experience. At the highest step CNSs are called *clinicians,* able to "observe, conceptualize, diagnose, and analyze complex clinical or nonclinical problems related to health . . . consider a wide range of theory relevant to understanding those problems, and . . . select and justify application of theory deemed to be most useful in understanding problems and in determining the range of possible treatment options" (ANA 1980).

Nurse practitioners (NP), as providers of primary (first-line) care, emerged in the 1960s to meet the health care needs of underserved people in rural areas. Though the term was new, the role was not. Nurses had served as primary caregivers in the United States since Mary Breckinridge began the Frontier Nursing Service in 1925. The first official program began in Colorado in 1965 in

Educational Preparation, Work Roles, and Clinical Practice

Roles and Focus of Clinical Nursing Practice

Education	Health Promotion & Primary Care	Acute Care	Long-term Care & Rehabilitation
Doctoral degree in nursing or related field	Expert clinician, clinical nurse specialist, nurse practitioner	Expert clinician, clinical nurse specialist, nurse practitioner	Expert clinician, clinical nurse specialist, nurse practitioner
Master's degree in nursing	Nurse midwife, nurse anesthetist, nurse practitioner: pediatric, family, gerontological, adult, school nurse	Clinical nurse specialist: mental health/psychiatric, medical-surgical, gerontological	Clinical nurse specialist: mental health/psychiatric, medical-surgical, gerontological
Bachelor's degree in nursing	Clinical nurse generalist: mental health/psychiatric, medical-surgical, gerontological, pediatric, school, perinatal	Clinical nurse generalist: mental health/psychiatric, medical-surgical, gerontological, pediatric, school, perinatal	Clinical nurse generalist: mental health/psychiatric, medical-surgical, gerontological, pediatric, school, perinatal
Diploma & Associate degree in nursing		Staff nurse: mental health/psychiatric, medical-surgical, gerontological, pediatric/perinatal	Staff nurse: mental health/psychiatric, medical-surgical, gerontological, pediatric/perinatal

Adapted from Henderson FC, McGettigan BO: *Managing Your Career in Nursing*, p 143, Addison-Wesley, 1986.

pediatrics. Physicians taught nurses to conduct physical examinations, interpret laboratory tests and x-rays, make judgments about health status, teach health, provide care, and collaborate with other providers. Other programs followed, with a duration of study lasting 6 to 18 months, where graduates received certificates from sponsoring medical and nursing schools and public health agencies. (McGettigan 1986). By 1991, many state licensing boards defined practice, assumed responsibility for accrediting programs, and issued certificates to graduates. By 1981, about 5600 NPs worked in hospitals, 4500 in public or community health agencies, and 4000 in health maintenance organizations and physicians offices (Institute of Medicine 1983).

Preceptorships and Internships

Nursing education began as apprenticeship training, with task-based learning measured by months and years. When nursing education moved to universities and colleges, learning became concept-based, measured by achievement of behavioral objectives. Clinical hours shrank. Graduates of associate degree and baccalaureate programs entered the work world with a fraction of the clinical time of diploma school graduates. They could analyze, synthesize, and evaluate, but had little experience in doing. Even though Montag's original proposal for ADN education hinged on a period of clinical supervision for new graduates, that part of her plan had not been implemented. By 1970, the need to ease the transition from student to staff nurse became apparent. Many institutes began offering preceptorships and internships.

Preceptorships are training periods for students nearing the end of a professional education program. Often preceptorships for nursing students are cooperative arrangements between colleges and hospitals. The college provides instructors to organize and monitor learning experiences and hospitals provide *preceptors* to model and teach the role of a staff nurse. Some programs build preceptorships into the basic curriculum.

Internships are training periods provided by employers for neophyte professionial employees (Nurse intern programs 1986). Internships vary in length from a few days to several months. They are called "new graduate," "orientation," and "permittee" (new graduates who have taken NCLEX-RN and have a permit to practice until they are licensed) programs. In some programs a patron-protégé system provides advisory support for new graduates in a range of involvement, from *mentor* to *sponsor* to *guide* to *peer pal* (Kelly 1987).

Preceptor and intern programs benefit hospitals, staff members, and new graduates. Staff morale increases as preceptors and mentors gain recognition, new graduates adjust to their role with greater ease, retention rates improve, policy and procedure manuals are updated, standards of care rise, and performance evaluations become more objective. The value of these programs is so well documented that they have become standard in nursing education.

Research in Nursing

Research in nursing focuses on building a body of knowledge about human responses to actual or potential health problems and to the effects nursing actions have on those responses (ANA 1980). Research is basic to nursing practice, education, and administration. Thus, in 1985, the US Congress established the National Center for Nursing Research under the National Institutes of Health. However, if knowledge gained by research is to be used, nurses must understand something of the process of conducting research, the written report, ethical considerations, and the means to evaluate findings.

The *process of conducting research* involves moving back and forth between ideas, hunches, existing knowledge, and observation (Wilson 1985). That process involves (1) stating the research question, (2) describing the purpose of the study, (3) reviewing relevant literature, (4) formulating hypotheses and defining variables, (5) deciding on a research design, (6) selecting a population, sample, and setting, (7) conducting a pilot study, (8) collecting data, (9) analyzing data, and (10) communicating conclusions and implications in a standardized report.

Ethical considerations are of special concern to nurses, mainly as they affect the rights of clients to (1) physical, emotional, financial, and social safety; (2) full disclosure regarding the nature, duration, purpose, methods of data collection, use to which data will be put, benefits that could be derived, inconveniences, side effects or results, alternatives to participation, identities of investigators, and how to contact investigators; (3) self-determination and freedom from coercion; (4) confidentiality and privacy; and (5) explanation of how these rights will be insured.

Evaluation of nursing research requires effort and practice, but its benefits are manifold. As nurses learn to read research reports they find that the mystique dissipates and their ability to evaluate findings grows. This is critical, because if nursing is to build a scientific body of knowledge, and if nursing practice is to be shaped by research findings rather than tradition, intuition, or habit, then the investigative skills of all nurses, regardless of their educational level, must be as integral to their repertoire as communication skills and sterile technique (Wilson 1985).

Theories of Nursing

True professions, we learned in Chapter 1, are knowledge-based and theory-based. Before a profession selects a theory as the basis for practice, however, it must define its purpose. Medicine defines its purpose as diagnosing and treating disease. The theory that "all disease is caused" leads the profession to adopt, although unconsciously, the "medical model" for practice.

What is the purpose or function of nursing? How is it defined? In 1860, Nightingale defined nursing as the "act of using the environment of the patient to assist him in his recovery" (Nightingale 1954). She believed a clean, well-ventilated, quiet environment was essential to healing. More recently, Virginia Henderson said, "The unique function of the nurse is to assist the individual, sick or well, in the performance of those activities contributing to health or its recovery (or to a peaceful death) that he would perform unaided if he had the necessary strength, will, or knowledge, and to do this in such a way as to help him gain independence as rapidly as possible" (1966). The ANA defined nursing as the diagnosis and treatment of human responses to actual or potential health problems (1980).

Many scholars see nursing as more complex than the ANA definition. Their models and theories address human responses to health problems from several viewpoints. Before comparing some of these models, let us agree on terminology.

- *Concepts*   Constructs or ideas such as person, goal, and health

- *Conceptual framework*   A set of concepts that fit together into a meaningful form, organizing information into a unique perspective or set

- *Model*   A representation of an object or an idea that shows only those features a model builder considers relevant

- *Conceptual model*   A configuration that gives clear and explicit directions for nursing practice, education, and research with assumptions, a value system, and major units representing important features of the model

- *Metaparadigm of nursing*   A global perspective on the discipline of nursing, including the person receiving care, goal of care, environment of person, health at the time of the interaction with a nurse, and nursing actions (Kozier and Erb 1987)

- *Nurse theorists*   Nurses who systematically define the basis and principles of nursing practice by grouping together related concepts to describe nursing functions, components, and dimensions, and to predict the effect of nursing actions

- *Theory*   An abstract explanation for an observable fact that is more specific than a model or framework, but because it is abstract—not directly applicable to practice—it is made up of concepts, propositions, and hypotheses

Many conceptual models for nursing practice have been and are being developed. Unlike medicine, nursing has not decided on a single model. In fact, because of its very nature, an exclusive model for nursing practice might not be ideal. Some well-known models are compared in Table 2-2.

Comparison of Selected Conceptual Models for Nursing Practice

Author	Central Theme	Definition-function of Nursing	Nursing Process
Imogene King (1981)	Goal attainment	A process of human interaction between nurse and client whereby each perceives the other and the situation, and through communication they set goals, explore and agree on means to achieve goals	Human interpersonal process of action, reaction, interaction, and transaction between individuals and groups in social systems, as illustrated by interlocking circles
Betty M Neuman (1980)	Systems	Concerned with all the variables affecting an individual's response to stressors; nursing function is to attain and maintain a system of stability by identifying stressors and assisting individuals to respond to stressors	Assessment: • Biologic data • Stressors as perceived by client • Stressors as perceived by caregivers • Identifying intra-, inter-, and extrapersonal factors Statement of problem Summary of goals Intervention plan Evaluation
Dorothy Orem (1980)	Self-care: universal and health deviation	A creative effort of one human being to help another; goal is to provide and manage self-care action on a continuous basis in order to help others sustain life and health, recover from disease or injury, and cope with their effects; to move the person toward responsible action in	Interpersonal process; a cycle of assisting, checking, adjusting, and readjusting Step 1: Nursing diagnosis Step 2: Planning a system of nursing Step 3: Actions of nurse

Table 2-2 (continued)

Comparison of Selected Conceptual Models for Nursing Practice

Author	Central Theme	Definition-function of Nursing	Nursing Process
		matters of self-care and family members toward increasing competence in making decisions relative to the continuing daily care of the person	
Martha Rogers (1980)	Unitary man and life processes	A science and art; nursing seeks to promote symphonic interaction between man and the environment, to strengthen the coherence and integrity of the human field, and to direct and redirect patterning of the human and environmental fields for realization of maximum health potential	Setting: life process and human field; nursing diagnosis; intervention; evaluation
Callista Roy (1984)	Adaptation	A scientific discipline that is practice-oriented and concerned with man as a total being at some point along the health-illness continuum; goal is to bring about an adaptive state in all four modes, thus to contribute to the person's health, quality of life, and dignified dying	Six steps: 1. Assessment in four modes of behaviors (physiologic, self-concept, role function, and interdependence) 2. Assessment in four modes of stimuli (possible causes) 3. Nursing diagnosis 4. Goal setting 5. Interventions 6. Evaluation

Summary

Because nursing focuses on caring for people with health problems rather than disease, its educational programs prepare a wide range of caregivers. Traditionally, caregivers were divided into practical and registered nurses. AD education for RNs blurred the division. Beginning in 1965, the ANA supported the BSN as the minimum education for entry into professional nursing practice. But not everyone agreed. The controversy continues, but the impetus for career-long learning brought about innovative advanced degree programs, mandatory continuing education, and expanded clinical practice roles. Nursing literature and multimedia provide valuable tools. Schools and hospitals offer preceptorships and internships to ease the transition from student to practitioner. Research provides the knowledge and theory base for nursing and has produced several conceptual models for nursing practice.

Learning Activities

1. Interview five registered nurses, asking each one at which level they began practicing nursing (aide, LPN, ADN, BSN), how their work role has changed, and if they plan to earn further degrees in nursing.

2. Survey education opportunities for nurses at all levels in your community, obtaining specific program descriptions; compare entrance requirements, length, cost, accreditation, options for part-time study, diploma, or degree, and licensing on completion.

3. From your community hospital and clinics obtain job descriptions and qualifications for staff nurses, clinical nurse specialists, and nurse practitioners.

4. In a group discussion, compare the concept of technical and professional nursing practice with job descriptions and qualifications of staff nurses in your community hospital.

5. Discuss entry into practice issues as they would impact nurses in your community, including grandfathering, interstate endorsement, scope of practice, competency expectations, and titling.

6. What are the continuing education requirements of your state? How do licensees prove they have met them? Who accredits courses?

7. Make a literature search of a topic such as asthma, using the *Cumulative Index to Nursing and Allied Health Literature* to identify articles written during the past three years.

8. Read a nursing research report in a nursing journal. What parts of the report were easily understood? What parts were not? What precautions were taken to insure that the rights of human subjects were observed? Did you understand the findings?

Annotated Reading List

Anastas L: *Your Career in Nursing,* 2nd ed. Publ. No. 41–2216. Natl. League for Nursing, 1988.

This readable source of information gives a general picture of nursing as a profession. It is especially helpful for recruiters, counselors, and nurses as they advance in their careers. Chapter titles suggest its content: What's it like to be a nurse? What is a Nurse? Who should be a Nurse? Education, the real world of nursing. Hospital specialties. Nonhospital careers. Specialists. New trends in nursing.

Buckwalter KC: Is nursing research used in practice? Chapter 9 in: *Current Issues in Nursing,* 2nd ed. Blackwell Scientific, 1985.

This chapter examines issues about the application of new knowledge to practice. It addresses the question, "Are research findings influencing the quality of patient care?" The format of the chapter is a debate. Arguments both for and against the question are stated. The author concludes that "resolution of the issue is perhaps premature and inappropriate."

She decries a lack of institutional support for research and suggests planned change strategies to better implement research-generated knowledge to nursing practice.

Lenburg CB: The New York Regents external degree assessment model: Basis for creating alternative nursing programs for adult learners. Chapter 18 in: *Current Issues in Nursing,* 2nd ed. Blackwell Scientific, 1985.

In this chapter Carrie Lenburg tells about the external degree program she played such a large part in developing. She suggests that the "assessment model can be adopted and adapted in a variety of ways" to solve educational needs of many kinds. She describes regional performance assessment centers and how they are used in the program. She concludes that by combining the best of adult education, competency-based education, and objective assessment philosophies, an external degree program "allows maximum flexibility and individualized learning while ensuring academic quality and integrity."

Waters V, Limon S: *Competencies of the Associate Degree Nurse: Valid Definers of Entry Level Nursing Practice.* Pub No. 23-2172. Natl. League for Nursing, 1987.

This concise pamphlet describes a study that was designed to see if 1978 NLN competency statements accurately describe current entry-level performance of ADNs. It took place at six sites: five colleges and the state nursing board. The study found that the NLN competency statements do accurately describe current entry-level ADN performance in California. The project leaders recommend that across the nation similar studies take place for both ADN and BSN entry level functions.

References

American Nurses' Association: *Educational Preparation for Nurses.* ANA, 1965.

American Nurses' Association: *Self-directed Continuing Education in Nursing.* ANA, 1978.

American Nurses' Association: *Nursing: A Social Policy Statement.* ANA, 1980.

American Nurses' Association Cabinet on Nursing Education: *Education for Nursing Practice in the Context of the 1980s.* Publ. No. NE-11 5M4183. ANA, 1983.

American Nurses' Association Cabinet on Nursing Education Task Force: *The National Plan to Implement ANA's Educational Goal.* ANA, 1985.

American Nurses' Association Commission on Nursing Education: *A Case for Baccalaureate Preparation in Nursing.* Publ. No. NE-6 ANS, pp 5–7. ANA, 1979.

American Nurses' Association Task Force on Scope of Practice: *The Scope of Nursing Practice, Draft II.* ANA, 1986.

ANA delegates vote to limit RN title to BSN grad; "associate nurse" wins vote for technical level. *Am J Nurs* 1985; 85:1016–1017.

Anastas LL: *Your Career in Nursing.* Publ. No. 14–2216. Natl. League for Nursing, 1988.

Board of Registered Nursing: *Laws Relating to Nursing Education, Licensure-Practice with Rules and Regulations,* p 104. Sacramento, CA: Department of Consumer Affairs, 1989.

Brown EL: *Nursing for the Future.* Russell Sage, 1948.

California Department of Health Services: *Manual for Nurse Assistant Training Programs in Long Term Health Care Facilities.* Sacramento: State of California, 1985.

Committee for the Study of Nursing Education: *Nursing and Nursing Education in the US.* The Committee, 1923.

Committee on the Grading of Nursing Schools: *Nurses, Patients, and Pocketbooks,* p 447. The Committee, 1928.

Degree and certificate programs for registered nurses. Long Beach, CA: Statewide Nursing Program, 1989.

Division of Research: *Education for Nursing: the Diploma Way.* Publ. No. 16–1314. Natl. League for Nursing, 1989.

Dolan JA: *Nursing in Society,* 14th ed., p 175. Saunders, 1978.

Donahue MP: *Nursing: the Oldest Art, an Illustrated History.* Mosby, 1985.

Edge S: State positions on titling and licensure. In: *Looking Beyond the Entry Issue: Implications for Education and Service.* Publ. No. 41–2173, p 129. Natl. League for Nursing, 1986.

Facts About Nursing '84–'85. ANA, 1985, p 109.

Gibbon JM, Mathewson MS: *Three Centuries of Canadian Nursing.* Macmillan of Canada, 1947.

Hartung D: Organizational positions on titling and entry into practice: A chronology. In: *Looking Beyond the Entry Issue: Implications for Education and Service.* Publ. No. 41–2173. Natl. League for Nursing, 1986.

Henderson V: *The Nature of Nursing.* Macmillan, 1966.

Institute of Medicine: *Nursing and Nursing Education: Public Policy and Private Actions,* p 27. Washington, DC: National Academy Press, 1983.

Johnston DF: *History and Trends of Practical Nursing.* Mosby, 1966.

Kelly LY: *Dimensions of Professional Nursing,* 5th ed. Macmillan, 1985.

Kelly LY: *The Nursing Experience: Trends, Challenges, and Transitions.* Macmillan, 1987.

Kozier B, Erb G: *Fundamentals of Nursing: Concepts and Procedures,* 3rd ed. Addison-Wesley, 1987.

McGettigan BO: Assessing the options. Chapter 6 in: *Managing Your Career in Nursing,* Henderson FC, McGettigan BO. Addison-Wesley, 1986.

Moloney MM: *Professionalization of Nursing and Nursing Education: Summary Report and Recommendations.* Lippincott, 1986.

Montag MM: *The Education of Nursing Technicians,* p 70. Putnam, 1951.

National Commission for the Study of Nursing and Nursing Education: Summary, Report, and Recommendations Feb 1970; *Am J. Nursing,* 70:270–289.

New York Regents external degree, bachelor of science (nursing) degree description. U of NY Regents External Degree, 1988.

Nightingale F: Nursing the sick. In: *Selected Writings of Florence Nightingale,* Seymer LR, p 349. Macmillan, 1954.

North Dakota rule changes require associate, baccalaureate education. *Issues* 1986; 7(2): 1–3.

Nurse intern programs. *Nurs Health Care* May 1986; 7(5): 270–271.

Sage I: Telephone communication regarding status of N. Dakota licensure for LPNs and ADNs. Oct 1990.

Stewart IM: *The Education of Nurses,* p 214. Macmillan, 1943.

A Study of Nursing Practice and Role Delineation and Job Analysis of Entry Level Performance of Registered Nurses. National Council of State Boards of Nursing, 1986.

Waddle FI: The grandfather concept: A simple process. *Oklahoma Nurse* Sept 1986.

Williams JK: Nursing education: Why students choose ADN programs. *Am J Nurs* March 1989; 89:396.

Wilson HS: *Research in Nursing.* Addison-Wesley, 1985.

Winslow-Goldmark Report: *The Study of Nursing and Nursing Education in the United States.* Macmillan, 1923.

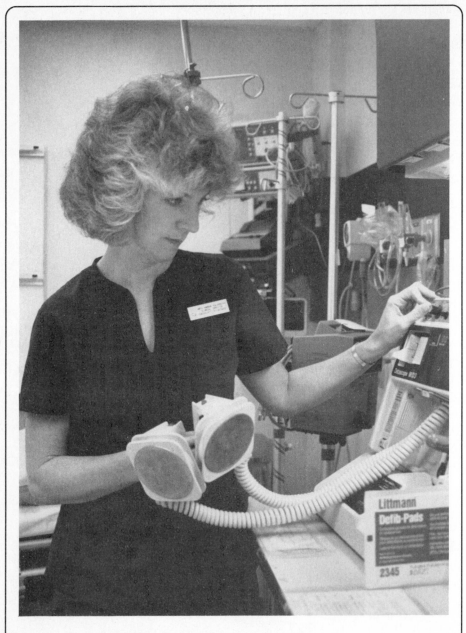

A registered nurse (RN) checks the equipment in the hospital emergency unit at the beginning of her shift. She is a Certified Emergency Nurse (CEN), a Certified Critical Care Nurse (CCRN), and Advanced Cardiac Life Support (ACLS) certified. (Photograph by Tia O'Rear)

CHAPTER 3

Credentialing: Licensure and Certification

LEARNING OBJECTIVES

1. Explain the difference between certificates and licenses, giving examples of each.

2. Describe the origin and current use of registration.

3. Trace the history of licensure, comparing permissive and mandatory licensure.

4. Describe the current NCLEX-RN examination, its content, who may take it, when it is given, and how the results are reported.

5. State the purpose of nurse practice acts, rules, and regulations and explain exemptions from licensure.

6. Describe requirements for licensure, the application process, and the purpose of interim permits.

7. Discuss the causes and consequences of disciplinary actions and rehabilitation programs for impaired nurses.

8. Discuss the reasons nursing organizations oppose regulation by licensing boards of expanded roles for nurses.

9. Describe the purpose and process of certification, giving examples of certificates offered by professional organizations and government bodies.

10. Discuss issues involved in creating a uniform credentialing system.

11. Describe the accreditation process, giving examples of both governmental and nongovernmental accreditation.

77

Dana *poured over the want-ad section of the newspaper. "Wow, look at all these jobs for nurses!" She fell silent for a minute, then asked, "What do you suppose all these initials mean: FNP, CEN, CNM, PHN, ACLSC?"*

Dana's roommate, Sarah, looked up from the NCLEX-RN review book she was studying and said, "They're special credentials you've got to have to get those jobs."

"I know that, but what do they mean?"

"I don't know, but if you don't get busy and study for the state board examination, you won't need to know!"

"True, but I'd still like to know what they mean. My aunt used to tell me that if I got my "RN degree" I'd be set for life. But since I've been a student nurse nobody ever mentions such a degree. They talk about associate degrees and bachelor's degrees, but not RN degrees. Maybe there is a degree I haven't heard about. . . . I wonder if that's what these initials stand for. Are they degrees, licenses, certificates? What are they?"

"They're just credentials, all kinds of credentials," Sarah replied impatiently. "Now please, if you're not going to study, you can at least be quiet and let me!"

Dana went back to searching the want ads. She didn't want to bother Sarah, but she felt even more perplexed. What were credentials? What was the difference between degrees, licenses, and certificates? Who awarded them? What did they mean?

Credentials

Before learning the meaning of specific titles, nurses like Dana and Sarah need to know the definition of some general terms, including credential, certificate, license, and registration.

Credentials are proof of qualifications, usually in writing, stating that individuals or organizations have met specific standards. There are two types of credentials: certificates and licenses.

Certificates are credentials verifying that individuals or organizations have met certain standards. They are issued by governmental (public) and nongovernmental (private) agencies. While both types of certificates give professional status, those issued or endorsed by governmental agencies also have legal status. Examples of certificates include nursing school diplomas, college degrees, nurse practitioner certificates, nurse-midwife certificates, and hospital accreditation certificates.

Licenses are credentials issued by governmental agencies. They are enforced by the police power of the state to protect public health and safety. Licenses verify that individuals and organizations have met minimal standards, and give licensees permission to carry out prescribed functions. For example, a registered nurse (RN) license signifies that a person has met minimum entry-level requirements and may practice within the scope described by the nurse practice act (NPA) of the state. A long-term care facility license verifies that a hospital has complied with certain minimum requirements and may operate according to the prescribed conditions of the law governing long-term care facilities.

Institutional licensure is an alternative to individual licensure for professionals. Typically, licenses of health-care institutions give them permission to operate, making them responsible for such things as sanitation, fire safety, staffing, and equipment. Institutional licensure gives these facilities the added responsibility and right to decide *who* is qualified to perform *what* tasks, awarding licenses as they see fit. Proponents of institutional licensure argue that it is only reasonable to give these facilities such a right since they are accountable for employee performance. Opponents argue that agreement between institutions about standard criteria would be difficult, if not impossible. Employee mobility between agencies would be complicated and professional autonomy would be lost. Nursing organizations consider institutional licensure to be an ongoing threat, especially with the growth of for-profit health-care corporations (Kelly 1979).

Registration is the creation of an official register or roster of names of persons, places, or things meeting certain criteria. When requested, the registering agency verifies that particular registrants have met the criteria necessary for inclusion on the roster. Where there are large numbers of registrants the process is cumbersome. Before licensure laws, graduates of nursing schools were registered in official rosters, hence the term "registered nurse." Modern state licensing and certification procedures have replaced nurse registration except for professional employment registries.

Licensure

Historical Background

Credentials for nurses have not always existed as we know them today. In medieval times members of nursing orders were known by their reputation and identified by the insignia of the order displayed on their habit. When the Nightingale school was established, its reputation for high standards spread throughout the world. Its graduates were in great demand, but they did not wear religious habits and there was no licensing system. Instead, the school wrote personal letters of recommendation for each graduate, verifying their abilities. As other schools were established they began awarding certificates of completion, or diplomas, to graduates.

With the proliferation of schools in the United States during the late 1800s and early 1900s, standards for nursing schools and nursing practice varied greatly. Programs differed in length from 6 to 36 months; service rather than education dominated many schools. In

1894, the Society for Superintendents of Training Schools in the United States and Canada was founded, and in 1896, the Nurses' Association Alumnae of the United States and Canada was established to gain control over the profession and stem the growth of substandard nursing schools. Both groups saw licensure for nurses as the way to accomplish these goals. Hospitals opposed any form of regulation. After a struggle, organized nursing prevailed. The first nurse practice act was passed in the United States in North Carolina in 1903 and in Canada in 1914. By 1923, all 48 states, the District of Columbia, and territory of Hawaii had licensure laws (Bullough 1980).

Permissive Licensure

The first licensure laws could more accurately be called nurse registration acts than nurse practice acts. The term *registered nurse* was defined as a person who had graduated from an acceptable nursing program and passed an examination, rather than a person who engaged in a specific type of practice. These first laws provided for *permissive licensure.* They offered a voluntary process by which nurses who met predetermined standards could obtain a license and have their names registered with the states. Those who did not meet the standards or did not want to bother with registration could still practice nursing and call themselves "nurse."

Mandatory Licensure

In 1938, New York became the first state to pass a *mandatory licensure* law requiring a license of all persons working as nurses. This law established two levels of nurses, registered and practical, restricting specific nursing functions to these two groups. The significance of this law was that for the first time a *scope of practice* was written into law. The process of defining nursing and passing mandatory nurse practice acts was facilitated in 1955, when the Board of Directors of the American Nurses' Association adopted a model nurse practice act for professional and practical nursing. In 1976, they revised the model to reflect expanded roles in professional nursing, and in 1980 and 1990, they revised it again (*The

Nursing Practice Act 1990). In 1982, the National Council of State Boards of Nursing published an alternate model nurse practice act (*The Model Nurse Practice Act* 1982).

Licensure Examinations

By 1923, even though every state provided for licensure for nurses by examination, the states differed greatly. In 1945, the American Nurses' Association Council of State Boards of Nursing was organized. It assumed responsibility for developing a uniform state board test pool examination. By 1950, all states used the same test, which was prepared by the National League for Nursing (NLN) Testing Division. The examination was divided into the subject areas of medical, surgical, obstetric, pediatric, and psychiatric nursing.

In 1978, the National Council of State Boards of Nursing (NCSBN) was formed, with representatives from 53 jurisdictions of the United States. A new test plan was developed to follow the steps of the nursing process and NLN prepared the first test. Beginning with the examination of February 1983, the test was prepared by CTB Testing Service, a subsidiary of McGraw-Hill Publishing Company. Besides preparing and scoring the test, the company provides a statistical analysis of test results to the NCSBN, the states, and individual schools. In 1987, the test was revised to reflect the findings of a study that analyzed the tasks of entry-level RNs (*Test Plan of the NCLEX-RN* 1987). The current test is a paper and pencil test. However, NCSBN is studying clinical simulation testing (CST) and computer-adaptive testing (CAT), a technique for administering multiple-choice questions via computer. Nationwide implementation of computerized testing is not yet scheduled (New computer formats forseen for NCLEX 1988).

National Council Licensure Examination for Registered Nurses

The name of the current test is the National Council Licensure Examination for Registered Nurses (NCLEX-RN). Written to follow a test plan designed by the NCSBN, the test includes two components: phases of the nursing process (assessment, analysis, planning, implementation, and evaluation) and client needs (environment, physiologic integrity, and psychosocial integrity). It is administered on two days in February and July each year in locations throughout the United States and consists of a four-part test of about 370 questions from which a single composite score is calculated (State board failure rate 1988). The score is derived from a complex process of weighting test questions. It measures knowledge, skills, and abilities as follows:

42–47% — meeting needs for physiologic integrity
25–31% — meeting needs for a safe effective care environment
12–18% — health promotion and maintenance
 9–15% — meeting needs for psychosocial integrity

Although each state retains the right to set its own passing score, to date all states have used the suggested 1600 of a possible 3200. Beginning with the February 1989 test, candidates and schools received only a pass or fail result. This was done to prevent the inappropriate use of test scores for such things as employee screening.

To help students prepare for the examination, the NCSBN offers a booklet entitled *Specific Nursing Behaviors to be Measured in NCLEX-RN (Detailed Test Plan)*. It can be obtained from the National Council of State Boards of Nursing, 625 N. Michigan Avenue, Suite 1544, Chicago, IL 60611.

Nurse Practice Acts and Rules and Regulations

A *Nurse Practice Act* (NPA) is a law made by the state legislature to regulate nursing practice, protect the public, and make nurses accountable for their actions. Each NPA authorizes an administrative body, often called a board of nursing, to implement provisions of the act. The board writes a set of *rules and regulations* (R&R) that become administrative law (see Chapter 7). Both NPAs and R&Rs are enforced by the police power of the state. Periodically, nurses should read a current copy of these documents. They can be obtained from their state licensing board. (See Appendix A for state board addresses.)

Both the American Nurses' Association and National Council of State Boards of Nursing published model nurse practice acts, but no two state acts are the same. Some states have one act for both registered nurses and practical nurses; others have two separate acts. Some acts are broad in scope, leaving details to the rules and regulations. Others are quite specific, requiring legislative action for minor changes. Regardless of their differences, nurse practice acts and rules and regulations address similar issues, discussed below:

Definition of Nursing

To avoid misinterpretation, legislative acts begin with a definition of terms. Perhaps the most important definition of all is the *definition of nursing*. In 1990, the ANA revised their model nurse practice act and definition of nursing practice to reflect their position, differentiating professional from technical nursing practice. The definition does not address practical nursing practice (Table 3-1).

Scope of Practice

The *scope of practice* is a statement delineating the range of responsibility of nursing. Although the wording differs from state to state, most state acts refer to the specialized knowledge of nurses, use of the nursing process, and performance of service for compensation. Several states include some reference to treating human responses to actual and potential health problems. About half of state nurse practice acts describe expanded roles for nurses.

Titling

Nurse practice acts make it illegal for persons to represent themselves by the title registered nurse (RN) if they do not meet stipulated requirements. Other titles may also be protected by nurse practice acts, such as nurse-midwife, nurse anesthetist, and nurse practitioner.

Administrative Board

The administrative board (board of nursing or licensing board) is the body legally empowered to carry out the intent of a nurse

Definition of Nursing from the American Nurses' Association

Model Nurse Practice Act of 1990

(c) the "practice of nursing" means the performance of services for compensation in the provision of diagnosis and treatment of human responses to health or illness;

(d) "professional nursing practice" encompasses the full scope of nursing practice and includes all its specialities and consists of application of nursing theory to the development, implementation, and evaluation of plans of nursing care for individuals, families, and communities. Professional nursing practice requires substantial knowledge of nursing theory and related scientific, behavioral, and humanistic disciplines. Professional nursing practice includes, but is not limited to:

(1) assessment, diagnosis, planning, intervention, and evaluation of human responses to health or illness;

(2) the provision of direct nursing care to individuals to restore optimum function or to achieve a dignified death;

(3) the procurement, coordination, and management of essential client resources;

(4) the provision of health counseling and education;

(5) the establishment of standards of practice for nursing care in all settings, including the development of nursing policies, procedures, and protocols for a specific setting;

(6) the direction of nursing practice, including delegation to those practicing technical nursing;

(7) the supervision of those who assist in the practice of nursing

(8) collaboration with other independently licensed health care professionals in case finding and the clinical management and execution of intervention as identified to be appropriate in a plan of care; and

(9) the administration of medication and treatments as prescribed by those professionals qualified to prescribe under the provision of (*cite state statute[s]*);

(e) "technical nursing practice" includes the skilled application of nursing principles in the delivery of direct care to individuals and families within organized nursing services. Technical nursing practice requires the study of nursing within the context of the applied sciences. Technical nursing practice includes, but is not limited to:

(1) participation in the development, evaluation, and modification of a plan of care;

(2) the provision of direct care to individuals to restore optimum function or to achieve a dignified death;

(3) patient teaching;

(4) the supervision of those who assist in the practice of nursing;

(5) the administration of medications and treatments as prescribed by those professionals qualified to prescribe under the provisions of (*cite state statute[s]*).

This portion excerpted from *Suggested State Legislation: Nursing Practice Act, Nursing Disciplinary Diversion Act, Prescriptive Authority Act,* © 1990 by American Nurses' Association, Kansas City, MO, pp 8–9. Reprinted with permission.

practice act. The makeup of boards varies from state to state. They range in size from 7 to 17 members. Often their membership is stipulated by the NPA according to occupations, such as a staff nurse, nurse educator, hospital administrator, physician, and public member. Board members are appointed by the state governor, except in North Carolina, where registered nurses elect the RN members of the board. In all but six states there is a combined board for registered nurses and licensed practical nurses. In those six states there are two separate boards. While all boards function within the framework of their own state government, they all are represented on the NCSBN and cooperate with the NLN and ANA. As mentioned above, the board writes the rules and regulations that become administrative law, enforced by the police power of the state.

State boards of nursing hire an executive director who is responsible for administering the work of the board and seeing that the nurse practice act and rules and regulations are followed. The American Nurses' Association recommends that boards of nursing: (1) govern their own operation and administration; (2) approve or deny approval to schools of nursing; (3) examine and license applicants; (4) review licenses, grant temporary licenses, and provide for inactive status for those already licensed; (5) regulate specialty practice; and (6) discipline those who violate provisions of the licensure law through court hearings, issue subpoenas to witnesses, revoke, suspend, or refuse to renew a license, and set limitations or conditions on practice.

Requirements for Licensure

Since the granting of licenses is a function of the state, not the federal government, nurses must meet the requirements of the state where they wish to practice. However, the states may not make age, residence, or citizenship a licensure requirement since such restrictions have been judged unconstitutional. Typical licensure requirements include the following:

1. *Education.* An applicant must have completed an educational program in a state-approved school of nursing and re-

ceived a diploma or degree from that program. Transcripts must be submitted directly to the board of nursing. Some exceptions exist. California allows persons who have completed certain required nursing courses in BSN programs to apply for licensure even though they have not yet earned the degree. North Dakota requires a bachelor's degree for an RN license and associate degree for a PN license, but issues temporary licenses, giving RNs four years and PNs two years to earn required degrees. Some states also require evidence of high school education.

2. *Examination.*   The applicant must pass the NCLEX-RN or NCLEX-PN.

3. *Health.*   Some states require evidence of physical and mental health.

4. *Moral character.*   Many states require a statement that the applicant is of good moral character as determined by the licensing board. In practice, this means that persons convicted of a felony must provide a description of the offense, the penalty, and evidence of rehabilitation with their application for licensure.

5. *Payment of fees.*   Applicants pay fees for processing their application, for the NCLEX-RN or NCLEX-PN, and for interim work permits.

Application Procedure

State licensing boards develop their own application forms, which they send to accredited nursing programs several months before the end of the school year. If graduates wish to begin practice in another state they should write to that state for forms. This is necessary because applicants must take the examination in the state where they first seek licensure. (See Appendix A for addresses.) Application forms include specific instructions about the examination such as dates, location, fees, and identification process; requests for information regarding conviction of a felony, transcripts to verify completion of a nursing program; procedures for applying for a temporary permit; and deadlines for application. Currently, test results are mailed four to six weeks after the test.

Exemptions from Licensure

In what is termed an *exception clause,* NPAs and R&Rs include provisions to allow certain people who are not licensed in the state to perform nursing functions. Since every exemption from licensure weakens mandatory aspects of the law and reduces the protection of the public it must be justified on the basis of overriding factors. Exemptions usually include (1) students enrolled in nursing programs, (2) unpaid people caring for friends or family members, (3) caregivers conducting religious rites who do not claim to be RNs, (4) RNs licensed in other states who are employed by patients temporarily passing through the state, (5) RNs working for the Red Cross during a disaster, and (6) RNs practicing in a federal agency such as a military hospital. Some states also exempt attendants working under the supervision of licensed nurses and physicians, although this is opposed by organized nursing.

Interim and Temporary Permits

An *interim permit* is a full and unrestricted license to practice professional nursing in the state issuing the permit, pending some specified condition. It is available to new graduates who have completed educational requirements and whose application for a license has been approved pending results of the first licensing examination. Interim permits are also available to RNs who are licensed in other states and some foreign countries and who meet licensure requirements of the state, pending verification of some detail. Interim permits are not renewable and are in effect until the results of the next scheduled examination are mailed or verification is received. They require payment of a fee.

Persons with interim permits may not call themselves registered nurse (RN) but may identify themselves as an interim permittee (IP). Persons who possess interim permits are subject to the same disciplinary action of the law as registered nurses.

A *temporary permit (license)* is issued to registered nurses for special circumstances, such as excusable delays in completing license renewal applications or in meeting license requirements.

Endorsement and Reciprocity

Endorsement is the granting of a license without requiring re-examination. Because boards of nursing cooperate with one another and use the same standardized examination, nurses in the United States have greater mobility than other licensed health professionals. With few exceptions, nurses must be licensed in the state in which they practice. But if they fulfill requirements for licensure, submit proof that the license they possess in another state is in good standing, and pay an endorsement fee, they are granted a license without having to retake the examination. Endorsement is not the same as reciprocity.

Reciprocity means acceptance of a licensee by one state only if another state does likewise. It results from reciprocal agreements between states.

Foreign Nursing School Graduates

Nurses who have graduated from nursing schools in foreign countries and want to practice nursing in the United States must meet requirements of the state in which they reside and must pass the NCLEX-RN to become licensed RNs. To prevent exploitation of foreign graduates who come to the United States to practice nursing but fail to pass the licensing examination, the ANA and NLN sponsor an independent organization called the Committee on Graduates of Foreign Nursing Schools (CGFNS). The organization administers an examination to foreign-educated nurses in various locations throughout the US and the world. The examination tests proficiency in both English and nursing and helps foreign nurses assess their chances of passing the NCLEX-RN, which they must pass in order to become licensed. There is no such examination for LPNs. Foreign nurses must pass the CGFNS examination before they can obtain a work permit from the US Labor Department or a nonimmigrant preference visa from the US Immigration and Naturalization Service. Most states require that foreign-educated nurses submit CGFNS test results with their NCLEX-RN applications.

Disciplinary Action

CAUSES AND CONSEQUENCES.   Every licensee and holder of a certificate awarded by a board of nursing may be disciplined for unprofessional conduct. State laws vary. The ANA lists the following acts as unprofessional: (1) fraud in gaining a license, (2) conviction of a felony, (3) addiction to drugs, (4) harming or defrauding the public, and (5) willfully violating a nurse practice act (LeBar 1984).

Disciplinary action may take the form of revocation, suspension for a period of time, or restriction on licenses or certificates. It must respect individual constitutional rights and be based on criteria stated in the law.

The process begins with a report filed with the board of nursing charging a nurse with an unlawful act. After investigating the charge, the board notifies the nurse of the charges, giving the nurse time to prepare a defense. A hearing is set and subpoena issued. The nurse has the right to appear personally or be represented by counsel, who may cross-examine witnesses. The board then decides what disciplinary action, if any, is appropriate.

REHABILITATION PROGRAMS.   Some states have programs that identify and rehabilitate nurses whose competency may be impaired due to substance abuse or mental illness, yet still function to protect public health and safety. Called diversion programs, they are board-recognized, independent agencies that specialize in treating substance abuse and mental illness. Nurses who enroll in these programs are assured that all information is confidential and not available to the licensing boards nor subject to discovery or subpoena.

No nurse is forced to enter a diversion program, but any nurse may enter, whether or not charges have been filed. If charges have been filed and the nurse decides to enter the program, the board is notified only if the nurse fails to complete the program. Programs include assessment, development of a rehabilitation plan, referral for treatment, monitoring of participation and compliance, and referral to a support network (*Registered Nurses in Recovery* 1989).

Educational Programs in Nursing

An important function of nurse practice acts is to regulate educational programs, assuring the public that programs meet certain standards. Only graduates of accredited programs may take the examination to become a licensed nurse. When the board examines a program and finds that it meets their standards the board then issues a certificate of accreditation. This process is further discussed later in this chapter.

Expanded Roles for Nursing Practice

Some nurse practice acts provide for expanded roles for nurses such as nurse anesthetists, nurse practitioners, and nurse midwives. Often these laws require that the person be certified for advance practice by a professional organization such as the ANA. In some states no mention is made of expanded roles, but the board approves specialty practice based on provisions in the NPA. In other states expanded roles are not legally sanctioned.

The inclusion of expanded roles for nurses in licensure laws is not universally approved. It is opposed by the professional nursing organizations. They believe that licensure laws should regulate minimum safe practice, but that professional specialty boards should regulate advanced practice, just as they do in medicine. These organizations point out that nurse practice acts, as laws, are rigid and less responsive to evolving roles of nursing practice. They also note that in some states, boards of nursing include persons from occupations other than nursing. By placing advanced nursing practice under nonnurse control, the power of nursing to regulate its own practice is diminished.

Continuing Education

Many states make continuing education mandatory for renewal of a license to practice nursing. The board of nursing stipulates the number of required education units, the process for verifying units, and standards for educational offerings. Since each state is different, nurses need to learn the continuing education requirements in their state well before it is time to renew their license. They can obtain that information from their board of nursing. (See Chapter 2 for a more detailed discussion of continuing education.)

Certification

Certification is a form of credentialing that has both professional and legal status. Generally, it indicates a level of competence above the minimum standard required for licensure. The essence of certification is evaluation, a process of determining the extent to which individuals and organizations meet certain standards of preparation and performance. Certificates are issued to individuals and groups by private (nongovernmental) and public (governmental) agencies.

Certification of Individuals

Certification, according to the American Nurses' Association Interdivisional Council on Certification, is the "documented validation of specific qualification demonstrated by the individual registered nurse in the provision of professional nursing care in a defined area of practice" (*The Study of Credentialing* 1978). On the basis of specific criteria, certificates are awarded to individuals who then may use the designated title of the certificate, such as family nurse practitioner (FNP). Many nursing organizations offer certification, but the ANA offers the largest number and widest variety of certificates to individuals.

Nongovernmental Certification

AMERICAN NURSES' ASSOCIATION CERTIFICATION. The ANA certification program was established in 1973 to provide tangible recognition of professional achievement in a defined functional or clinical area of nursing. The program is administered by the Center for Credentialing Services and is based on assessment of knowledge, demonstration of professional achievement, and recognition by peers (*The Career Credentials* 1990). Four categories of certificates are offered: generalist, nurse practitioner, clinical specialist, and nursing administrator (see Table 3-2). Applicants take a national examination and submit evidence of education and nursing practice in a specific clinical area. Certificates are valid for five years. Renewal requires evidence of continued education and related clinical practice. Information about the program is published annually in *The Certification Catalog,* American Nurses' Association, 2450 Pershing Road, Kansas City, MO 64108.

SPECIALTY NURSING ORGANIZATION CERTIFICATION.   A number of specialty nursing organizations offer certification to individuals. (See Table 3-3 for a sampling of educational programs from which individuals must graduate to qualify for certification.) When such a dual function occurs, a closely related, but separately titled and funded organization certifies nurses, thus protecting the specialty organization from what the Federal Trade Commission ruled was an illegal restraint of trade. This ruling prevents organizations from monopolizing credentials by requiring membership of all candidates.

Governmental Certification

Some states award certificates for expanded roles in nursing on the basis of specific educational and practice criteria set up by state boards of nursing. They also may recognize certificates awarded by private specialty organizations. Certificates issued by governmental agencies assume legal status because they are enforced by the police power of the state. For example, state law may include a scope of practice for nurse-midwives and restrict use of the title certified nurse-midwife (CNM) to persons who meet criteria for that certificate. The states authorize a variety of titles for expanded roles of nurses, including advanced registered nurse (ARN), nurse practitioner (NP), specialized registered nurse (SRN), advanced registered nurse practitioner (ARNP), independent nurse practitioner (INP), and certified registered nurse (CRN). (See the discussion of expanded roles for nursing practice earlier in this chapter.)

American Nurses' Association Certification Practice Areas

Generalist Certification
(Requirement: clinical experience)

General nursing practice
Medical-surgical nurse
Gerontologic nurse
Pediatric nurse (plus continuing education in pediatric nursing)
Perinatal nurse (plus continuing education in perinatal nursing)
Psychiatric and mental health nurse (plus letter of reference)
School nurse (plus academic course work and practicum)
College health nurse (plus academic course work and a practicum)
Community health nurse (plus baccalaureate degree)

Nurse Practitioner Certification
(Requirement: master's degree or bachelor's degree and one academic year in a
specialty program)

Pediatric nurse practitioner (plus practicum)
Adult nurse practitioner
Family nurse practitioner
School nurse practitioner
Gerontologic nurse practitioner

Clinical Specialist Certification
(Requirement: master's degree in area of specialty plus clinical experience)

Clinical specialist in gerontologic nursing
Clinical specialist in adult psychiatric and mental health nursing
Clinical specialist in child and adolescent psychiatric and mental health
nursing
Clinical specialist in medical-surgical nursing
Clinical specialist in community health nursing

Nursing Administration Certification
(Requirements as stated)

Nursing administration (baccalaureate degree and experience in middle
management or on executive level)
Nursing administration advanced (master's degree and experience on
executive level)

From: *The Certification Catalog.* ANA, 1990.

A Sampling of Specialty Organization Certification*

American Association of Critical Care Nurses (AACN)
  Certified critical care nurse (CCRN)
American Association of Occupational Health Nurses (AAOHN)
  Certified occupational health nurse (COHN)
American Association of Nurse Anesthetists (AANA)
  Certified registered nurse anesthetist (CRNA)
American College of Nurse-Midwives (ACNM)
  Certified nurse-midwife (CNM)
American Heart Association (AHA)
  Cardiopulmonary resuscitation (CPR certified) also called
  Basic life support (BLS certified)
  Advanced cardiac life support (ACLS certified)
American Society of Post-Anesthesia Nurses
  Certified post-anesthesia nurse (CPAN)
Association of Operating Room Nurses (AORN)
  Certified nurse operating room (CNOR)
Association for Practitioners in Infection Control (APIC)
  Certified in infection control (CIC)
Association of Rehabilitation Nurses (ARN)
  Certified rehabilitation registered nurse (CRRN)
Emergency Nurses' Association (ENA)
  Certified emergency nurse (CEN)
International Association for Enterostomal Therapy (IAET)
  Certified enterostomal therapy nurse (CETN)
National Association of Pediatric Nurse Associates/Practitioners (NAPNAP)
  Certified pediatric nurse practitioner (CPNP)
National Association of School Nurses (NASN)
  Certified school nurse (CSN)
Oncology Nursing Society (ONS)
  Oncology certified nurse (OCN)
The Organization for Obstetric, Gynocologic, and Neonatal Nurses (NAACOG)
  Reproductive nurse certified (RNC):
    Inpatient obstetric nurse
    Low-risk neonatal nurse
    Neonatal intensive care nurse
    Neonatal nurse clinician/practitioner
    Ob/gyn nurse practitioner
    Reproductive endocrinology/infertility nurse

* Certificates may be awarded by closely related, but separate and independent organizations.

A Uniform Credentialing System

Ideally, a system of credentialing for individuals communicates qualifications clearly and concisely. By 1975, numerous certificates were being awarded by sundry specialty organizations. It became apparent to nursing leaders that the system lacked uniformity and consistency. To address the problem the ANA funded a major research study on credentialing in cooperation with 47 specialty groups. Researchers at the University of Wisconsin, Milwaukee School of Nursing conducted the study, guided by an ANA-appointed committee. The study assessed all types of credentialing mechanisms, including licensure, certification, and granting of degrees. In its conclusion in the 1978 final report, the researchers suggested various ways to increase the effectiveness of credentialing and a means to implement the proposed changes (*The Study of Credentialing* 1978).

The major recommendation of the study was that nursing establish an independent center for nurse credentialing. The authors of the study believed such an independent center would provide the checks and balances necessary to preserve equity for every part of the system. It would be an efficient, cost-effective service that would avoid duplication of efforts and provide geographic mobility for nurses. The committee recommended that the profession of nursing move toward supporting a centralized, independent credentialing center. Although further discussion followed the study, the organizations involved in the study have not yet implemented its recommendations.

Certification of Organizations

Certification of organizations is called *accreditation*. Like certification of individuals, accreditation is a documented validation of specific qualifications demonstrated by the organization in carrying out its goals and objectives. Certificates of accreditation are awarded to organizations on the basis of specific criteria, usually after they have engaged in a self-study process. As with certification of individuals, certificates of accreditation are awarded by both nongovernmental (private) and governmental (public) agencies.

Nongovernmental Accreditation

EDUCATIONAL INSTITUTION ACCREDITATION. Nongovernmental accreditation of educational institutions is provided by both institutional and specialized accrediting agencies. *Institutional accrediting agencies* evaluate entire educational institutions such as colleges and universities. There are six such regional agencies in the United States: (1) New England Association of Schools and Colleges, (2) Middle States Association of Schools and Colleges, (3) North Central Association of Colleges and Secondary Schools, (4) Southern Association of Colleges and Schools, (5) Western Association of Schools and Colleges, and (6) Northwestern Association of Secondary and Higher Schools.

The accreditation process begins with intensive self-evaluation followed by an on-site visit of a team of peer educators. Accreditation is awarded for varying periods of time. When schools are accredited, students can transfer credits more easily and their degrees are honored when graduates wish to pursue advanced study.

Specialized accrediting agencies evaluate particular programs within educational institutions. The National League for Nursing is the designated accrediting agency that sets standards for all educational programs in nursing. It is recognized as such by the US Office of Education.

Specific NLN evaluation criteria for nursing programs are revised continually. They include five areas: (1) organization and administration, (2) students, (3) faculty, (4) curriculum, and (5) resources, facilities, and services. The process of accreditation consists of a self-study report, an on-site visit by two or more peers, and scrutiny by a board of review that grants or denies accreditation, with or without recommendations. Because most graduate programs in nursing require a BSN from an NLN-accredited program, BSN programs seek NLN accreditation.

HEALTH-CARE INSTITUTION ACCREDITATION. Nongovernmental accreditation of health-care institutions is provided by the Joint Commission on Accreditation of Healthcare Organizations (JCAHCO) and by state medical associations. The accreditation process begins with an intensive self-evaluation followed by an on-site visit of an evaluation team. Accredited hospitals are eligible to receive funds from state and federal sources and from insurance companies.

Governmental Accreditation

Governmental accreditation of institutions of higher learning is unusual. However, accreditation of specialized programs within educational institutions is common. For example, boards of nursing are responsible to the public for minimum competency in nursing. Therefore they closely monitor basic nursing programs, stipulating that only graduates of accredited programs may take the licensure examination.

The accreditation process by state boards of nursing is patterned after the NLN model. The board distributes criteria in specific areas, such as (1) philosophy, (2) policies and procedures, (3) physical space, budget, and personnel, (4) faculty qualifications and roles, (5) curriculum, (6) evaluation plan, (7) clinical facilities, (8) student involvement, and (9) cooperation with the licensing board of nursing. Prior to expiration of their accreditation, programs engage in intensive self-evaluation, writing a detailed report. Board-appointed evaluators then visit the school to verify the information. They report their findings to the board, which grants or denies accreditation with or without recommendations, for a specific period of time, usually up to five years.

Governmental accreditation of health-care institutions varies considerably from state to state. In many states hospitals are accredited or licensed by state agencies such as the department of health. In other states, accreditation by JCAHCO is recognized as adequate protection for the public and the state does not conduct it own accrediting evaluation. Nurses would do well to find out if prospective hospital employers meet accreditation standards.

Summary

Credentials, as proof of the qualifications of individuals and groups, take many forms: individual registration, licenses and certificates, and institutional accreditation. The first licensure laws of nurses were really registration acts with permissive rather than mandatory licensure. Today, all states have nurse practice acts and administrative boards that regulate both registered and practical nursing practice. All state boards of nursing are members of the Council of State Boards of Nursing, which oversees the licensing examinations (NCLEX-RN and NCLEX-PN) used by all states. Professional nursing organizations and licensing boards offer certification of nurses for expanded roles and accreditation of institutions.

Learning Activities

1. Obtain a copy of the nurse practice act and rules and regulations in your state, noting the definition of nursing, licensure requirements, interim permits, and disciplinary action.

2. Find out if there is a rehabilitation program for nurses with mental illness or chemical dependency in your state. If so, interview the consultant who oversees the program, asking how it is administered and its success rate.

3. Attend a public meeting of your state board of nursing. Write a paper stating the number of members on the board and their occupations, the role of the executive director and consultants, the issues discussed, and your reactions to the experience.

4. In a group, discuss the advantages and disadvantages of including expanded roles for nurses in nurse practice acts.

5. Interview someone in the personnel department of a hospital in your community regarding requirements for certification. Write a report stating what positions require certificates and if there is a pay differential for certified nurses.

6. In a group, discuss the advantages and disadvantages of a single certifying agency for nurses.

Annotated Reading List

Lagerquist S: *Addison-Wesley's Nursing Examination Review,* 4th ed. Addison-Wesley, 1991.

This is an excellent review text for graduates preparing to take the NCLEX-RN. This review book is organized completely around the nursing process. It has a straightforward outline format and includes a simulated NCLEX-RN mail-in prep-test exam to help students tailor their own study. This book emphasizes transcultural diversity, and is readable and current. It also includes a pretest and posttest; new material on AIDS, universal precautions, and Kawasaki's disease; appendices on client needs and categories of human function. The principles of anatomy and physiology are integrated throughout the book to stimulate and promote recall, relevance, and application of information in the clinical setting.

Sullivan E, Bissel L, Williams E: *Chemical Dependency in Nursing: The Deadly Diversion.* Addison-Wesley, 1988.

This timely, informative book explores the nature and extent of chemical dependency in the nursing profession, identifying its destructiveness to nurses and patients. The book describes characteristic behaviors of dependent nurses and tells how nurse managers and others can intervene appropriately. Guidelines for effective re-entry programs are offered. The authors stress that rehabilitation is based on personal responsibility and that "most affected nurses can be helped to overcome their problems and return to work." Excellent references and guidelines for effective rehabilitation are provided.

References

Bullough BL: *The Law and the Expanded Nursing Role,* 2nd ed. Appleton-Croft, 1980.

The Career Credentials: Professional Certification, 1990 Certification Catalog. Center for Credentialing Services, ANA, 1990.

Kelly LY: Danger: Creeping institutional licensure. *Nurs Outlook* Sept 1979; 27:624.

LeBar C: *Statutory Requirements for Licensing of Nurses.* ANA, 1984.

The Model Nurse Practice Act. NCSBN, 1982.

New computer formats forseen for NCLEX. (Newscaps.) *Am J Nurs* May 1988; 88:747.

The Nursing Practice Act: Suggested State Legislation. ANA, 1990.

Registered Nurses in Recovery. Diversion Program, California Board of Registered Nursing, 1989.

State board council eyes computerized NCLEX test. (Newscaps.) *Am J Nurs* Nov 1988; 88:1566.

State board failure rate shoots up to 16.4%; higher standard, lower "ability level" blamed. (Newscaps.) *Am J Nurs* 1988; 88:1566, 1582, 1584.

The Study of Credentialing in Nursing: A New Approach. Vol 1, The Report of the Committee. ANA, 1978.

Test Plan of the National Council Licensure Examination for Registered Nurses. NCSBN, 1987.

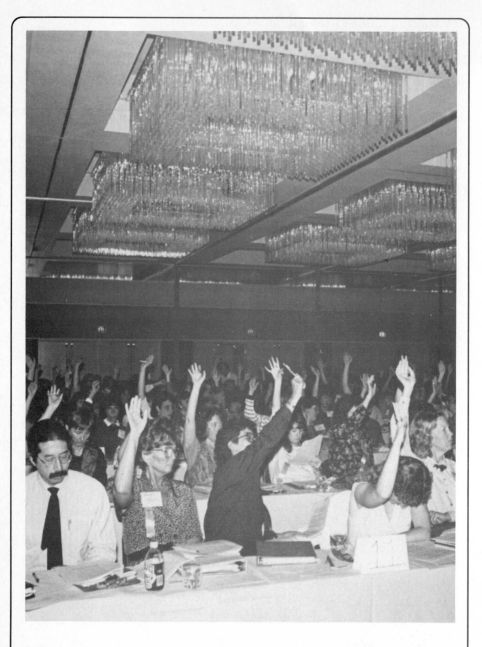

State Nurses' Association delegates set the agenda of the organization when they meet, discuss, and vote on resolutions and bylaws. (Courtesy California Nurses Association)

CHAPTER 4

⟨❦⟩

Nursing Organizations

LEARNING OBJECTIVES

1. Describe the origin, membership requirements, organizational structure, purposes, and activities of an alumni association.

2. Discuss the origin, membership provisions, organizational structure, and activities of the American Nurses' Association (ANA).

3. Describe the National Student Nurses' Association (NSNA), its membership requirements, organizational structure, and major activities.

4. Describe the origins of the National League for Nursing (NLN) and relate them to its stated purposes and functions.

5. Compare the membership requirements and organizational structure of the ANA and NLN.

6. State the purposes, functions, and membership of the International Council of Nurses (ICN).

7. State the frequency of and next scheduled year of the conventions/congress of the ANA, NLN, NSNA, and ICN.

8. Describe types of specialty organizations and list ten such organizations.

9. Explain the increasing membership and popularity of specialty organizations over the past 20 years.

10. Discuss the importance of governmental and health-related organizations to the nursing profession.

11. Name the official publications of the ANA, NLN, NSNA, and ICN.   103

" **I'll tell** you right up front, Joan, I do things for love, money, or to stay out of trouble. You tell me why I should join your nursing organization, and I'll decide if it's worth it to me." Joan swallowed whole the piece of bagel she had just bitten off. Jim's pronouncement took her by surprise. She had always thought he was a real marshmallow . . . sweet and soft. She suddenly saw Jim as a no-nonsense, take-care-of-yourself hermit crab.

Joan sputtered something about getting back to him with the answer. . . . She'd better get back to the ward right away. Joan nearly tripped over a chair rushing to leave the cafeteria.

As she walked back to her unit Joan thought about what Jim had said. He was right, of course. People join organizations for personal support, for professional advantage, or because it is a requirement of their job. She had never before thought of membership in an organization in such a pragmatic way. Maybe it wasn't such a bad idea to ask, "What's in it for me and my profession? What can this organization do to make my life better or to improve the image of nursing, and by extension, me? Will the benefits of joining outweigh the costs in time and money? If I don't join, will I lose my job? Is there another organization that would give me more for my efforts than this one?"

By the time Joan got back to the unit she knew what she had to do. She needed to gather a great deal of information about the different professional organizations before she talked to Jim again, before she got too involved in the current membership campaign. Maybe there was a better one for her . . .

Activities of Professional Organizations

Although Joan did not understand it, both she and Jim recognized that an important function of a professional organization is to enhance the personal identity of its members, their "professionalhood," as Styles (1982) put it. In fact, through their many activities, these organizations benefit both individual nurses and the profession as a whole. These activities include: (1) giving professional information and education, (2) supporting economic and general welfare, (3) setting standards, (4) granting scholarships, (5) giving recognition, (6) providing opportunities for networking, (7) supporting research, (8) taking political action, (9) providing public education and information, and (10) working with other organizations to solve health problems.

Joan will find that there are a great many nursing organizations. Each year the *American Journal of Nursing* publishes a directory of them, part of which is in Appendix B. Although the number and variety of these organizations may seem bewildering, they can be divided into five categories: alumni, general, special interest, government, and health-related.

Alumni Organizations

Description and History

Alumnae organizations were the first professional nursing associations. *Alumna* is the female form of the word; *alumnae* is the plural form. Those early organizations were called alumna because nursing schools were not coeducational and schools for men were rare. Now that nursing programs are coeducational, the correct name is the plural form of *alumnus,* or *alumni.*

The oldest alumni organization in the United States was organized in 1889 by graduates of the Bellevue Hospital Training School in New York (Notter, Spaulding 1976). Others followed, including Illinois Training School in 1891, Johns Hopkins Hospital Training School in 1892, and Massachusetts General Hospital School in 1895. In 1897, representatives of ten alumnae associations established the National Associated Alumnae (NAA) of the United States and Canada. When the association sought incorporation, it found that New York law prohibited foreign membership. "And Canada" was removed from the name. In 1911 it was changed to the American Nurses' Association (ANA). In 1908 Canadian nurses formed the Provisional Organization of the Canadian National Association of Trained Nurses, and in 1924 changed the name to Canadian Nurses' Association (CNA) (Donahue 1985). Although the ANA in the US and the CNA in Canada became the consolidated voice for nursing, individual alumni organizations across the United States and Canada continued to prosper.

Membership and Organizational Structure

Membership in alumni associations is traditionally open to graduates, faculty, and specially honored individuals. The organizational structure of alumni associations varies greatly from school to school. Many schools maintain independent associations with relatively uncomplicated arrangements. Others have more complex structures. Often alumni of university nursing schools form subgroups within larger university alumni associations.

Purpose and Activities

Regardless of their organizational structure, alumni associations provide a lifelong link between the school and its graduates. These groups provide many mutual benefits. They give schools a source of committed graduates to whom they look for advice on current nursing practice, assistance with recruitment, fund-raising for scholarships and research, and service to students and new graduates as mentors and role models.

Alumni associations help graduates maintain a personal commitment to and identification with the ideals they first encountered as students. They provide continuing education programs and a channel for networking with others in the nursing profession. Alumni organizations offer a means for maintaining a special personal and professional bond between members. They furnish a focus for membership pride and an opportunity to display loyalty for the nursing profession. Usually dues to alumni organizations are minimal and time commitments are optional. Regardless of other organizations Joan and Jim join, membership in the alumni association will give them lifelong benefits.

General Interest Organizations

General interest organizations serve a wide spectrum of nurses and have a variety of activities. Some of the most notable of these organizations are the American Nurses' Association, Student Nurses' Association, National League for Nursing, and International Council for Nursing.

American Nurses' Association

Description and History

The American Nurses' Association is the primary professional organization for registered nurses in the United States. It is composed of 54 constituent associations in the 50 states, District of Columbia, Virgin Islands, Guam, and Puerto Rico. These constituents, called state nurses' associations (SNAs), have over 900 regional associations that serve nurses at the local level.

The American Nurses' Association grew out of the Nurses' Associated Alumnae of the United States and Canada, as described earlier. Since its founding in 1897 and subsequent renaming in 1911, the American Nurses' Association has undergone many changes. Through them all it has remained the leading voice for professional nursing.

Membership and Organizational Structure

Membership is open to registered nurses and new graduates of RN programs who have not yet passed the licensing examination. Individual nurses become members of an SNA through a local region; the SNA is a constituent part of the ANA. (Figure 4-1 shows the organizational structure of the ANA according to the bylaws in 1985.)

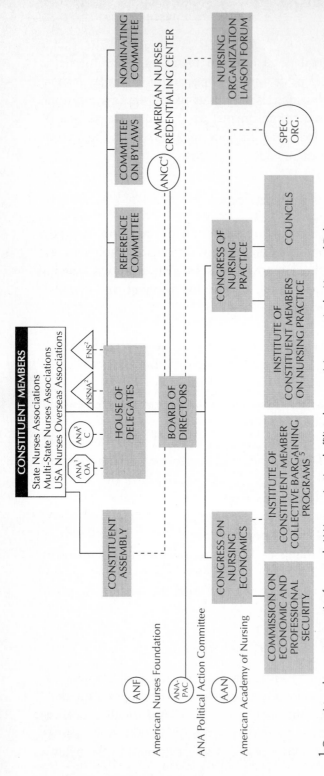

CONSTITUENT MEMBERS
State Nurses Associations
Multi-State Nurses Associations
USA Nurses Overseas Associations

ANF — American Nurses Foundation

ANA-PAC — ANA Political Action Committee

AAN — American Academy of Nursing

CONSTITUENT ASSEMBLY

HOUSE OF DELEGATES

NOMINATING COMMITTEE

COMMITTEE ON BYLAWS

REFERENCE COMMITTEE

AMERICAN NURSES CREDENTIALING CENTER

ANCC[4]

NURSING ORGANIZATION LIAISON FORUM

SPEC. ORG.

BOARD OF DIRECTORS

CONGRESS OF NURSING PRACTICE

COUNCILS

INSTITUTE OF CONSTITUENT MEMBERS ON NURSING PRACTICE

CONGRESS ON NURSING ECONOMICS

INSTITUTE OF CONSTITUENT MEMBER COLLECTIVE BARGAINING PROGRAMS[5]

COMMISSION ON ECONOMIC AND PROFESSIONAL SECURITY

ANA[1] OA

ANA[3] C

NSNA[2]

FNS[2]

1 One registered nurse representive from each ANA organizational affiliate has a participant seat in the House of Delegates.

2 One representative each from the Federal Nursing Services and the National Student Nurses Association has a courtesy seat in the House of Delegates.

3 One representative from each ANA council has a participant seat in the House of Delegates.

4 The American Nurses Credentialing Center is autonomous with respect to development and implementation of credentialing operational policies and procedures; is accountable ANA's administrative structure in other aspects. ANA retains the authority to set standards for nursing education, nursing practice and nursing service.

5 Institute is autonomous with respect to development of operational standards, positions, policies, practices, and all other matters related to constituent member collective bargaining programs; provides informational reports to Congress on Nursing Economics.

© 1990 by American Nurses Association, Kansas City, MO. Reprinted with permission.

Figure 4-1 *American Nurses' Association Organizational Structure*

At the national level the organization is managed by an executive director and a professional staff, headquartered in Kansas City, Missouri. The executive director is hired by the Board of Directors, who are elected by the House of Delegates to carry out their policies. The House of Delegates is made up of representatives from state associations. It meets annually and is the top policy-making body of the ANA. Elections occur at national conventions, held in even-numbered years in various cities throughout the United States.

The ANA Board appoints members to various committees and cabinets, maintains a relationship with the National Student Nurses' Association, holds official membership in the International Council of Nurses, is sole stockholder of the American Journal of Nursing Company, constitutes the membership of the American Nurses' Foundation, and is the ANA liaison with other health-related agencies.

Cabinets are seven-member deliberative bodies that are accountable to the board and report to the house. The six cabinets are: nursing education, practice, research, services, economic and general welfare, and human rights. Each evaluates trends, developments, and issues in their area of responsibility and recommends policies and positions to the board and House of Delegates. They report their findings to the house and are accountable to the board.

Councils are organizational units through which members advance the profession in specialized areas of nursing practice or interest. These councils are designed to meet the same needs of practitioners that independent specialty organizations meet. Membership in a council is open to ANA members by paying an additional fee. Currently there are 12 councils: continuing education, nurse researchers, computer applications in nursing, nursing administration, clinical nurse specialists, psychiatric and mental health nursing, medical-surgical nursing practice, gerontologic nursing, community health nurses, primary health care nurse practitioners, maternal-child nursing, and cultural diversity in nursing. Councils are accountable to the board through the appropriate cabinet.

Purposes and Functions

The purposes of the ANA are to: (1) work for the improvement of health standards and the availability of health-care services for all people, (2) foster high standards of nursing, and (3) stimulate and promote the professional development of nurses and advance their economic and general welfare . . . unrestricted by considerations of nationality, race, creed, lifestyle, color, sex, or age (*ANA Bylaws* 1985).

The functions of the ANA are to: (1) establish standards of nursing practice, education, and services; (2) establish a code of ethical conduct for nurses; (3) ensure a system of credentialing in nursing; (4) initiate and influence legislation, governmental programs, national health policy, and international health policy; (5) support systematic study, evaluation, and research in nursing; (6) serve as the central agency for the collection, analysis and dissemination of information relevant to nursing; (7) promote and protect the economic and general welfare of nurses; (8) provide for the professional development of nurses; (9) conduct an affirmative action program; (10) ensure a collective bargaining program for nurses; (11) provide services to constituent SNAs; (12) maintain communication with constituent SNAs through official publications; (13) assume an active role as consumer advocate; (14) represent and speak for the nursing profession with allied health groups, national and international organizations, governmental bodies, and the public (*ANA Bylaws* 1985).

Activities

The ANA carries on a great many activities that help fulfill their stated functions, including certification, political action, publishing, research, collective bargaining, giving recognition, and international participation.

CERTIFICATION.   Certification of advanced nursing practice is a way for the public and other health-care providers to recognize quality in specialized fields. It is offered by ANA in 175 clinical specialties. Applicants must meet education and practice requirements and pass a written examination. Through the certification process nurses demonstrate ability in leadership, judgment, and decision making, and specialized knowledge in a clinical field of nursing (*Credentialing in Nursing* 1985). (See Chapter 3 for more information about certification.)

POLITICAL ACTION.   The ANA is actively involved in political action through its ANA Political Action Committee (ANA-PAC). The ANA-PAC is a voluntary, nonpartisan organization that works to meet the ANA's legislative objectives. Its major functions are education and political action. The ANA maintains an office in Washington, DC. Its registered lobbyists work with legislators on health and welfare issues. At the state level, SNAs maintain lobbyists in state capitals to speak for nursing on state and local issues.

PUBLICATIONS.   The *American Journal of Nursing* (AJN) is the official journal of the ANA. It is published monthly by the American Journal of Nursing Company in New York City, a company that is wholly owned and controlled by the ANA. In 1900 the *AJN* became the first nursing journal in the United States to be owned, operated, and published by nurses. Later the company added *Nursing Research, Nursing Outlook, MCN: American Journal of Maternal-Child Nursing, Geriatric Nursing: American Journal of Care for the Aging* and *International Nursing Index.*

The *American Nurse* is the official organ of the association. Published every other month, it contains official announcements of the association and news relevant to nursing and other health-care providers.

Each year the ANA publishes *Facts About Nursing* and many pamphlets and informational resources for nurses. A complete list of these is available from the association (*American Nurses' Association Publications Catalog*).

RESEARCH SUPPORT.   In 1955, the American Nurses' Foundation (ANF) was established as a tax-exempt, nonprofit corporation for the purpose of supporting research related to nursing. The members of ANF are the board of directors of the ANA. The stated purpose of this organization is to "conduct analyses of specific problems, to provide information needed in order to make policy decisions, to develop a group of nurse scholars who engage in such areas as journalism and public policy, and to support the research and educational activities of ANA" (*Bylaws* 1980).

COLLECTIVE BARGAINING.   As part of its goal to promote economic welfare for nurses, an important activity of ANA is its support for collective bargaining. Carried out at the state level, these negotiations focus not only on financial gains for individual nurses, but also on participation in patient care decisions and working conditions (*Representing Nurses is Our Business* 1987). (See Chapter 10: Collective Bargaining.)

RECOGNITION GIVING.   In 1966, in order to recognize significant contributions of individuals to the nursing profession, the House of Delegates voted to establish the American Academy of Nursing (AAN). Its members are called Fellows of the American Academy of Nursing (FAAN) and may place the initials FAAN after their name. The original members were chosen by the board in 1973. In a self-perpetuating system of membership, additional nominations are made by active fellows. Criteria for selection is ANA membership, evidence of outstanding contributions to nursing, and potential for continuing contributions to nursing and the Academy.

NATIONAL PARTICIPATION.   Through its Nursing Organization Liaison Forum (NOLF) the ANA maintains working relationships with many organizations in the United States on issues of concern to the nursing profession. In addition, the ANA actively collaborates and has an ongoing relationship with the National Student Nurses' Association.

INTERNATIONAL PARTICIPATION.   The ANA is the official United States representative to the International Council of Nursing (ICN). As such, the ANA speaks for all the nurses in the United States to the nurses of the world. ANA delegates participate in ICN activities and attend its quadrennial congress.

Joan and Jim should consider membership in the ANA. It is the official voice of nursing, both in the United States and the world. As members they can influence its positions and actions.

National Student Nurses' Association

Description and History

The National Student Nurses' Association (NSNA) is the largest independent health professional student organization in the United

States, and the only one for nursing students. Founded in 1953 and incorporated in New York in 1959, NSNA is composed of constituent associations made up of school chapters or state associations. While it is an independent organization, it works closely with the ANA, providing a student viewpoint on matters of common interest.

Membership and Organizational Structure

Membership is open to all students in nursing programs for registered nurses. It is also open to students taking prenursing course work in colleges where there are nursing programs. Categories of membership are: active, associate (prenursing majors), sustaining (nonstudent, interested individuals or organizations), and honorary. Individual membership in the national organization is open to eligible students when it is not available through constituent organizations.

At the national level, the NSNA is managed by an executive director and a staff, headquartered in New York City. The executive director is hired by the Board of Directors, who are elected by the House of Delegates to carry out their policies.

The House of Delegates is made up of representatives of school chapters and state associations. It meets annually in various cities across the United States and is the top policy-making body of the NSNA. The Council of State Presidents meets twice a year to share ideas, set priorities, and plan activities.

The Board of Directors maintains liaison with the ANA, state licensing boards of nursing, and legislative bodies. It makes up the membership of the NSNA Foundation, a separate corporation devoted to providing scholarships for nursing students.

Purposes and Functions

The purposes of the NSNA are to: assume responsibility for contributing to nursing education in order to provide for the highest quality health care, provide programs representative of fundamental and current professional interests and concerns, and aid in the development of the whole person, his/her professional role, and his/her responsibility for the health care of people in all walks of life (*Getting the Pieces to Fit* 1987, pp 10–15).

The NSNA fulfills its purposes by influencing the educational process; promoting and encouraging participation in community affairs and activities; representing students to the consumer, institutions, and other organizations; promoting and encouraging student participation in interdisciplinary activities and promoting recruitment efforts regardless of a person's race, color, creed, lifestyle, sex, national origin, age or economic status; and promoting collaborative relationships with other nursing and health organizations.

Activities

Some of the most significant activities of the NSNA include networking with other students at the local, state, and national level, taking political action, publishing, scholarship granting, and serving local communities.

NETWORKING. Local, state, and national meetings of the NSNA provide members the opportunity to meet nursing students from many geographic areas and backgrounds. The resulting collegial network continues long after graduation, serving both individuals and institutions.

POLITICAL ACTION. One of the important activities of the NSNA is political action, by which it takes positions on such diverse issues as toxic waste disposal, voter registration, abortion, educational preparation for the practice of professional nursing, and national health insurance. When the House of Delegates votes to take a position on some issue, officers and members are free to do what they can to implement it in the name of the NSNA, including making public statements, taking action, and serving on advisory committees to advocate that position.

PUBLICATIONS. *Imprint* is the official journal of the NSNA, published five times an academic year and sent to members. The *NSNA News* contains organizational news and is published six times a year. It is sent to state officers and school presidents. *Dean's Notes* is published for faculty members and deans and contains news about the NSNA. In addition to these periodicals, the NSNA publishes many useful pamphlets on such topics as guidelines for planning meetings, career planning, and surviving as a student.

SCHOLARSHIPS.   The Foundation of the NSNA, Inc. administers scholarships to nursing students on the basis of criteria set up by the foundation. Funds for these scholarships are tax deductible and donated by both individuals and organizations.

PROJECT BREAKTHROUGH TO NURSING.   Since 1965, the NSNA has actively supported *Project Breakthrough*. The aim of this project is to increase the number of nurses from minority groups, such as men, African-Americans, Hispanics, and Native Americans. Involved members gather information about nursing programs in their geographic area. Then they go out to speak with minority groups to encourage individuals from those groups to consider a career in nursing.

COMMUNITY SERVICE.   Members of the NSNA participate in many community service activities at the local level. These include participation in health fairs, hypertension screening and education, child abuse education and prevention programs, immunization drives, drug abuse education campaigns, and working with elderly people (Preparing for technology, titling, and licensure 1985).

Joan and Jim may want to consider working with the local NSNA, especially in community service activities. In addition to the service they would render they would gain great personal satisfaction and make long-term professional and personal contacts with future colleagues.

National League for Nursing

Description and History

The National League for Nursing (NLN) was formed in 1952 from the merger of seven national organizations and committees concerned with nursing. These organizations and their founding dates were the National League of Nursing Education, 1893; National Association of Collegiate Schools of Nursing, 1918; Association of Collegiate Schools of Nursing, 1933; Joint Committee on Practical Nurses and Auxiliary Workers on Nursing Service, 1945; Joint Committee on Careers in Nursing, 1948; National Committee for the Improvement of Nursing Services, 1949; and National Nursing Accrediting Services, 1949 (*Bylaws, June* 1985).

With the formation of the NLN, two large nursing organizations became a reality, the ANA focusing on the needs of individual nurses, and the NLN focusing on community health, education, and nursing service.

Membership and Organizational Structure

There are five types of members in the NLN: individual, forum, agency, allied agency, and honorary. *Individual membership* is open to anyone interested in fostering the development and improvement of nursing services and education. *Forum membership* is open to individual members who wish to belong to a forum, a special interest group sponsored by the NLN. *Agency membership* is open to any organization that provides a nursing service or conducts an educational program in nursing. *Allied agency membership* is open to any interested organization not engaged in providing nursing service or an educational program in nursing. *Honorary membership* is conferred on individuals by the board of directors (*Proposed Amendments* 1987).

Figure 4-2 shows the organizational structure of the NLN. At the national level the NLN is managed by an executive director and staff, headquartered in New York City. The executive director is hired by the Board of Directors.

The 32-member Board of Directors is made up of elected and appointed representatives of the Division of Individual Members and Division of Agency Members. It meets annually just before and after the national convention and is the top policy-making body of the NLN. Elections are held before biennial conventions in odd-numbered years throughout the United States.

The Division of Individual Members is made up of individual members who work through constituent leagues, forums, and the Assembly of Constituent Leagues for Nursing (ACLN). Constitu-

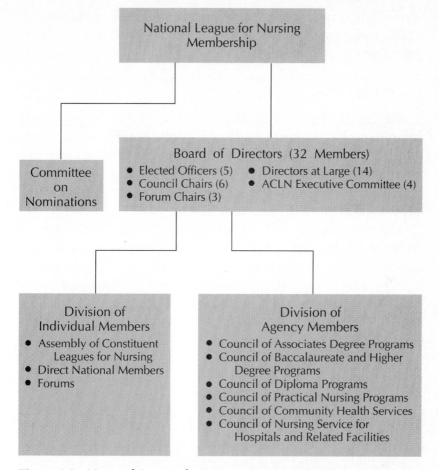

Figure 4-2   *National League for Nursing Organizational Structure, 1991*

ent leagues work at the community level and may be associated with others in a regional assembly of constituent leagues. Forums are interest groups for individual members. The assembly meets biennially or more often and is composed of the president of each constituent league and other designated persons.

The Division of Agency Members is made up of agency members that work through six councils: associate degree programs, baccalaureate and higher degree programs, diploma programs, practical nursing programs, community health services, and nursing practice (*Proposed Amendments* 1987). Each council meets biennially or more often as needed.

The 13 standing committees of the NLN are composed of various individual and agency representatives. They draft policy proposals and suggest programs to the Board of Directors and carry out other essential functions.

Purposes and Functions

The stated purpose of the NLN is to foster the development and improvement of hospital, industrial, public health, and other organized nursing services and of nursing education through the coordinated action of nurses, allied professional groups, citizens, agencies, and schools to the end that the nursing needs of the people will be met (*Bylaws, June* 1985).

The stated functions of the NLN are to: (1) identify the nursing needs of society and to foster programs designed to meet these needs; (2) develop and support services for the improvement of nursing service and nursing education through consultation, continuing education, testing, accreditation, evaluation, and other activities; (3) to work with voluntary, governmental, and other agencies, groups, and organizations for the advancement of nursing and toward the achievement of comprehensive health care; and (4) to respond in appropriate ways to universal nursing needs (*Proposed Amendments* 1987).

Activities

The NLN engages in many activities that help fulfill its stated functions, including consultation and accreditation, testing and evaluation, information and continuing education, publishing, and research.

CONSULTATION AND ACCREDITATION.   Consultation is offered by the NLN to schools and agencies that are initiating new programs and services or seeking to improve existing ones. It is provided by on-site visits and written and oral communication by representatives of the NLN, usually associated with the accreditation process.

Accreditation is a voluntary self-study process whereby a school or agency measures various aspects of their program or service against a set of criteria. When the self-study is complete, NLN representatives visit and verify its findings and issue a certificate of accreditation for a period of time. (Chapter 3 describes this process in greater detail.) The NLN is the official accrediting body for nursing programs, designated by the US Office of Education and the Council on Postsecondary Education.

TESTING AND EVALUATION.   The NLN has been a pioneer in testing and evaluation services. They provide a wide variety of examinations, including pre-entrance, achievement, and proficiency tests for practical, registered, graduate, and practicing nurses.

INFORMATION AND CONTINUING EDUCATION.   The NLN Career Information Service publishes lists of accredited schools, scholarships, and loans for prospective students and others. The NLN Office of Public Affairs provides information about a wide area of nursing concerns and is sometimes asked to testify at legislative hearings. The NLN's tax status, however, prohibits it from engaging in lobbying efforts.

The NLN offers continuing education workshops and conferences from time to time throughout the nation. Topics are selected in consultation with forums and councils to meet current needs.

PUBLICATIONS AND AUDIOVISUALS.   The official organ of the NLN is the monthly magazine *Nursing and Health Care*. Its focus is on educational and administrative concepts, theories, methods of health care delivery, research, and other broad issues affecting nursing rather than on direct patient care.

The NLN publishes a great many pamphlets, books, and audiovisuals on many topics at nominal cost. They are described in the annual *Book and Video Catalog*, available from the National League for Nursing, 350 Hudson Street, New York, NY 10014.

RESEARCH.   The Division of Research collects statistical data about nurses, nursing education, and service, publishing it in the annual *Nursing DataSource*. It publishes annual "blue books" about state-accredited schools of nursing and conducts other studies of areas of concern to nursing.

Jim and Joan may want to consider individual membership in the NLN, particularly if they become educators or administrators in hospitals or community health agencies.

International Council of Nurses

Description and History

The International Council of Nurses (ICN) is the oldest international organization for professional workers (Donahue 1985). It is a federation of nurses' associations from around the world, banded together to improve nursing service, education, and professional ethics. Through its member associations the ICN represents nearly a million nurses. It was one of the first organizations to adopt a policy of nondiscrimination due to nationality, race, creed, color, politics, sex, or social status.

The ICN began as an idea among nursing leaders at the Columbia Exposition in Chicago in 1893. A provisional committee laid the groundwork. In 1899, at a meeting of the International Council of Women in London, the ICN was founded. In 1900, the constitution was adopted, with nurses from England, the United States, Canada, New Zealand, Australia, and Denmark listed as founding members (Bridges 1967). By 1985, there were 88 national nurses' organization members of the ICN with others soon to join.

Membership and Organizational Structure

The membership of the ICN is composed of one national nurses' association from each country. The ANA is the constituent member for the United States, the Canadian Nurses' Association for Canada.

The governing body of the ICN is the Council of National Representatives (CNR), composed of the president of each member association. It meets every two years and operates on the principle of one country, one vote. Every four years the council meeting is held in conjunction with the Quadrennial Congress.

The Board of Directors is responsible for making decisions between meetings of the CNR, recommending action, appointing committees, and governing the Florence Nightingale International Foundation, an endowed trust established to advance nursing education.

The Board of Directors consists of the president, three vice-presidents, seven area representatives, and four members-at-large.

Representatives are elected from seven regions of the world: Africa, Eastern Mediterranean, Europe, North America, South and Central America, Southeast Asia, and Western Pacific.

The ICN has two standing committees that make recommendations to the Board of Directors: professional services and socioeconomic welfare. They consider trends and problems relative to nursing education, practice, service, and socioeconomic welfare of nurses.

The ICN is managed by an executive director and staff headquartered in Geneva, Switzerland. It maintains an official relationship with many international organizations, including the World Health Organization (WHO), United Nations Educational, Scientific, and Cultural Organization (UNESCO), International Labour Organization, United Nations International Children's Emergency Fund (UNICEF), Economic and Social Council (ECOSOC), and International Committee of the Red Cross (*Introducing the ICN* 1984).

Purposes

The stated purposes of the ICN are to: (1) promote the development of strong national nurses' associations, (2) assist national nurses' associations to improve standards of nursing and competence of nurses, (3) assist national nurses' associations to improve the status of nurses within each country, and (4) serve as the authoritative international voice for nurses and nursing.

Activities

The activities of the ICN reflect the wide range of interests and needs of its international membership. These interests include education, nursing practice and service, economics and welfare of nurses, research, legislation, and cooperation with other health professions. At any given time the ICN is involved in 30 to 40 projects, such as:

- Regulating nursing practice
- Revising and updating the ethical code for nurses (see Chapter 6)

- Staging the Quadrennial Congress and conducting educational programs in various cities throughout the world
- Making policy statements on health and social issues such as family planning, equal pay for equal work, and the role of nurses in caring for prisoners and detainees
- Offering legislative seminars for member associations
- Annually administering the 3M Nursing Fellowship Programme awards for recipients
- Publishing a bimonthly official journal, *International Nursing Review* (ICN 1985)

As individual nurses, Joan and Jim are not eligible for membership in the ICN. As members of the ANA they would participate in this organization, be kept informed of scholarships, international opportunities for nurses, educational programs, and the Quadrennial Congress. Such contacts could be of great personal and professional benefit.

Special Interest Organizations

Description and History

Special interest nursing organizations began as a result of a need felt by nurses to associate with others with similar concerns for personal and professional support. The first groups began before there were large, general interest nursing organizations to which nurses could turn. Later, specialty organizations were formed by nurses who felt their needs were not being addressed by existing organizations.

The earliest groups began with informal meetings of nurses of like interests. As these groups sought recognition they formed into local clubs, such as the Industrial Nurses' Club established in 1915, and the Nurses' Christian Fellowship begun in 1936. As nurses with other interests heard of these clubs they formed their own groups and then combined into larger groups. As a consequence, from 1965 to 1985 the number of special interest nursing organizations increased dramatically and the number of nurses actively supporting the ANA decreased.

In an effort to stem the tide and better meet the needs of individual nurses, the ANA instituted councils in areas such as maternal-child nursing, gerontologic nursing, and nursing administration. In addition, the ANA formed the Nursing Organization Liaison Forum as a means to increase communication between itself and specialty organizations.

In 1973, a group of specialty organizations formed the Federation of Specialty Nursing Organizations to provide a formal network between their organizations. In 1981, the name was changed to the National Federation for Specialty Nursing Organizations. Its stated purpose is to foster excellence in specialty nursing practice by providing a forum for communication and collaboration and to support activities that contribute to the recognition of specialty nursing practice (Kelly 1987).

Types

Special interest nursing organizations can be divided into five groups: clinically related, educational, political action, honorary, and minority. Clinically related organizations make up the largest group of specialty organizations by far. These include the American Association of Occupational Health Nurses, the Association of Operating Room Nurses, and the National Flight Nurses' Association. Educational groups include such organizations as the American Association of Colleges of Nursing and the National Association for Practical Nurse Education and Service. Honorary organizations include such organizations as the Sigma Theta Tau and Alpha Tau Delta National Fraternity for Professional Nurses. Ethnic-cultural-religious organizations include such groups as the National Black Nurses' Association, the Transcultural Nursing Society, and the Catholic Health Association of the United States.

Purposes and Activities

The purposes of special interest organizations vary from group to group. In general, they promote the personal and professional growth of members and support their collective concerns. To carry out their purposes, specialty organizations engage in a wide variety of activities, including sharing information; providing educational seminars, workshops, and conferences; publishing; lobbying; and networking. Many of these organizations are run primarily by volunteers. They do not support large headquarters and staff, or engage in the expensive process of collective bargaining. As a result, dues are relatively small and participation of members in activities is high. No doubt these factors contribute to the success of specialty organizations.

Jim and Joan may want to join a specialty organization in the area of their interest because it will give them personal and professional satisfaction. Membership in such a group would not prevent them from belonging to and participating in ANA or NLN activities.

Government Agencies

Nurses are interested in agencies of the United States government, not only because someday they may seek employment in those agencies, but because those agencies have so much power and influence on nursing. Some governmental agencies are directly involved in delivery of health care, such as the US Public Health Service and the Navy Nurse Corps. Others influence nursing and health care indirectly, such as the Office of Personnel Management.

Government agencies are included in this chapter because of their importance to nursing. However, because of the large number of organizations and the volume of information about them, they are not described in detail in this chapter. However, complete information about any or all of them is available on request by writing directly to the specific agency. Addresses of some of the most important ones are included in the directory in Appendix B.

Health-related Organizations

There are many health-related organizations of particular interest to nurses, such as the American Heart Association, American Cancer Society, Planned Parenthood, and the like. The activities of these organizations have great influence on health care and nursing. These organizations provide direct patient care, fund research, and offer professional education and public information. Often they are not-for-profit corporations.

Nurses can contribute a great deal to such organizations and can gain much in return. Their contributions may be to raise funds, lobby, give direct patient care, teach, hold office, serve as spokespersons, serve on committees, and lend reputation and expertise. Their benefit may be to develop new skills, obtain additional education, participate in research projects, gain a network of personal and professional colleagues, and find especially satisfying employment working in an area of intense personal interest.

As Jim and Joan weigh membership in the various organizations, they may want to consider the benefits of involvement with health-related organizations, not as a substitute, but as an adjunct to other professional activities.

Summary

One of the criteria of a profession is that it have its own professional organizations. One of the ways nurses experience their "professionalhood" is to become officially identified with one or more professional organizations. These groups perform many important activities, educating, setting standards, giving recognition, supporting economic welfare, and contributing to research. Professional organizations can be classified into five categories: alumni, general, special interest, government, and health-related. Nurses benefit both personally and professionally when they learn about, belong to, and work with these organizations.

Learning Activities

1. To a group of beginning nursing students, present the history, organizational structure, primary activities, and reasons for belonging to a nursing school alumni association.

2. Attend a meeting of the members of a regional state nurses' association and visit the regional office.

3. Participate in a debate in which the resolve is: Membership in the American Nurses' Association is the mark of a true professional.

4. Write a comparison of the ANA with the NLN regarding the following: membership, purposes, policy-making body, activities, publications, and national convention dates.

5. To a group of students, present the organizational structure, primary activities, and benefits of membership in the National Student Nurses' Association.

6. Assign a different specialty organization to each of a group of students. Ask each one to present a summary of the purposes, membership requirements, and benefits of membership.

7. Write a list of government and health-related agencies whose services might be helpful to the following people: sexually active teenagers, homeless schizophrenics, refugees from a famine, and elderly cancer victims.

8. Review copies of each of the official publications of the ANA, NLN, and NSNA. Note the type of article, editorial slant, special features, and subscription price.

Annotated Reading List

American Nurses' Association Bylaws, as Amended July 23, 1985. ANA, 1985.

The actual bylaws of an organization provide uncluttered, factual information. These bylaws make surprisingly interesting reading.

Bylaws, June 1985. National League for Nursing, 1985.

Especially interesting when compared to the ANA bylaws, NLN's philosophy is revealed by the writing style and plan of their organization. Worthwhile reading.

Moloney MM: *Professionalization of Nursing, Current Issues and Trends.* Lippincott, 1986.

An examination of the concept of professionalism and "nursing's journey toward its current state of professionalism" is comprehensive, realistic, and fact-filled, yet highly readable.

References

American Nurses' Association Bylaws, as Amended July 23, 1985. ANA, 1985.

Bridges DC: *History of the International Council of Nurses, 1899–1964, the First 65 Years.* Lippincott, 1967.

Bylaws, American Nurses' Foundation, 1980.

Bylaws, June 1985. NLN, 1985.

Credentialing in Nursing: Contemporary Developments and Trends. ANA, 1985.

Donahue MP: *Nursing, The Finest Art.* Mosby, 1985.

Getting the Pieces to Fit 85/86: A Handbook for State Associations and School Chapters. NSNA, 1987.

ICN '85. (Newscaps.) *Am J Nurs* 1985; 85:918–920.

Introducing the ICN. ICN, 1984.

Kelly LY: *The Nursing Experience: Trends, Challenges, and Transitions,* p 160. Macmillan, 1987.

1990 directory of nursing organizations. *Am J Nurs* 1990; 90:143–151.

Notter LE, Spalding ED: *Professional Nursing: Foundations, Perspectives, and Relationships,* 9th ed. Lippincott, 1976.

Preparing for technology, titling and licensure, tackling world health problems. . . . All contenders in the bid for attention at student convention. (Newscaps.) *Am J Nurs* 1985; 85:730–731.

Proposed Amendments to NLN Bylaws. NLN, 1987.

Representing Nurses is Our Business. ANA, 1987.

Styles M: *On Nursing: Toward a New Endowment,* p 19. Mosby 1982.

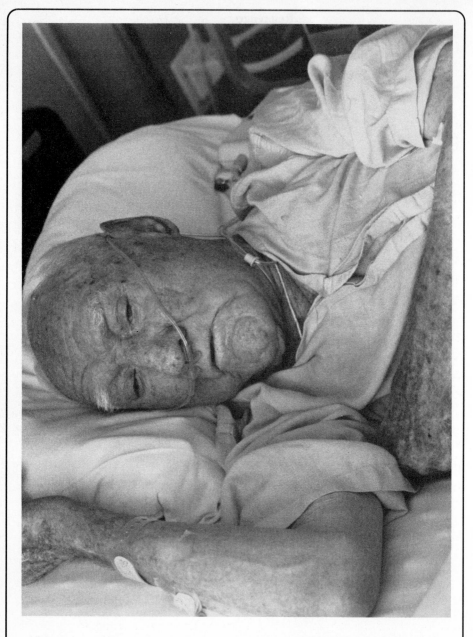

Alone and ill, this old man stares blankly from his nursing home bed. He misses his home and wife, but she is no longer able to care for him and home health care is not covered by his insurance policy.

CHAPTER 5

Health Care Systems

LEARNING OBJECTIVES

1. Discuss the influence of political and economic forces on health-care systems.

2. Describe the purpose and composition of health systems.

3. Discuss effects of standards and regulations on health care.

4. Discuss how the principles of shared sovereignty between the states and federal government and separation of powers among the branches of government affect the United States health-care system.

5. Trace the history of the United States health-care system.

6. Explain the importance of the Social Security Act of 1935 to US health care.

7. Describe the involvement of the federal government in health care following World War II.

8. Compare and contrast categorical programs with block grants.

9. Discuss methods of financing health care in the United States.

10. Describe and compare Medicare, Part A and B, with Medicaid.

11. Describe some special programs that provide essential health services.

12. Discuss the role of policy in a health-care system, giving an example of how health policy affects services.

13. Describe some of the major indicators of health status.

14. Discuss the current status of personal health services in the United States and changes that may occur in the future.

Nellie Greer

hung up the phone and stared into space. The discharge planner at the extended care facility had just called to tell her that the three weeks allowed by Medicare and the health maintenance organization (HMO) would end in two days and her husband would have to be discharged.

John was 73 years old. He had a stroke a month ago, was incontinent and paralyzed. Nellie could not care for him at home. After his stroke he had been transferred to the extended care facility from the hospital. As a result of conscientious nursing care and daily physical therapy he had no pressure sores or contractures. Before the stroke, when the transient ischemic attacks had made him increasingly helpless, the HMO had provided home health care, nursing supervision, and even a hospital bed. Maybe they would help her now.

Nellie dialed their number. They were sorry, but John's policy did not provide for any more care; perhaps the hospital discharge planner could find an inexpensive nursing home. The only one with a vacancy cost $2400 per month.

In the nursing home John was no longer eligible for physical therapy. He developed contractures and bedsores and was readmitted to the hospital. Since bedsores count as "an acute episode of an illness," Medicare paid the bill. John returned to the nursing home, but died ten months later, leaving a $14,500 bill. To pay the debt Nellie sold their home and went on welfare. Ironically, through a combination of Medicare and Medicaid, Nellie now has full medical insurance.

How could such a sequence of events occur? In a democracy with a free market economy, is comprehensive health care possible?

Health-care Systems

Purpose and Influences

The purpose of health-care systems is to promote the health and well-being of the people for whom they are created. However, these systems are affected by powerful forces within the country where they develop.

Political and Economic Philosophy

The social organization of a health-care system is greatly influenced by the political and economic philosophy of a country. Roemer (1986) identified three organizational types: permissive, as found in the United States; cooperative, as organized in the United Kingdom; and socialist, as established in the Union of Soviet Socialist Republics and People's Republic of China. Since this chapter focuses on US health care we will only discuss the permissive system.

In a permissive system, found in the United States with its free market economy, the health-care system is expected to make a profit or at least balance income with expenditures. This philosophy of freedom includes not only the economy, but every aspect of life for both individuals and sovereign states. Thus, individuals have the right to choose any lifestyle they wish, whether or not it is healthy, as long as it does not interfere with the rights of others.

States have the right to regulate delivery of health care within their political jurisdictions without regard to the needs of the residents. Such personal and public freedom is a deeply held value. However, it has produced a health-care system marked by tension and compromise between the private, for-profit health-care sector serving individuals and the tax-supported health-care sector serving the public. The permissive approach has created a system where health-care services are unevenly distributed among the people.

Definition of Health and Illness

While the political and economic system of a country influences the distribution of health care, the prevailing definition of health and illness influences the type of care and who provides it. Traditionally, biomedical science has defined health and medical care in terms of diseases that afflict the human body. It does not address factors that promote individual and community health, such as safe housing and neighborhoods, opportunities for education and employment, and adequate waste disposal. These factors are concerns of social science and social policy planners. However, if the health of individuals and communities is to be improved, social science must begin to influence the health-care system, at least to the same degree that biomedical science influences it.

Composition

Health-care systems are composed of the resources, functions, controls, and organization needed to deliver health care to populations (Roemer 1986). As an integral part of all health-care systems, nurses work to promote health, prevent and treat injury and disease, and foster rehabilitation. By gaining an understanding of the composition of a system and how it works nurses can support broader psychosocial aspects of health, using the system to benefit the population.

Resources

Resources of health-care systems are made up of the facilities and personnel that provide health care.

FACILITIES.   Facilities are the settings where health care providers work. These settings are centers of authority, service, and training where services for initial health care, prevention of complications of disease, and rehabilitation and terminal care are given (see Table 5-1). Myers (1986) reports that in the United States there are about 7000 acute care hospitals, 14,000 extended care facilities, 3000 home health agencies, 3000 local health departments, and thousands of clinics, mental health centers, laboratories, phar-

5 *Table 5-1*

Types of Health Service Facilities

Primary Care (initial health care)

Ambulatory care centers
Community health centers
Crisis centers
Day-care centers
Employee health centers
Health maintenance organizations
Neighborhood health centers
Physicians' offices
Preferred provider organizations
Prison health services
School of health services
Self-help support groups (Alcoholics Anonymous, etc)

Secondary Care (care to prevent disease complications)

Ambulatory care centers
Home health-care agencies
Hospitals:
    acute, short-stay (less than 30 days)
    long-term (more than 30 days)
Physicians' offices

Tertiary Care (supportive and rehabilitative care)

Hospice services
Long-term care facilities (extended care, intermediate care, nursing homes)
Rehabilitation

macies, and the like. There is also a network of emergency vehicles and specially equipped vans and taxis to transport disabled persons.

The type, number, and location of health-care facilities depends on the method of payment for health care and degree to which the system is centralized under government control or localized in the private sector.

Even in a permissive health-care system there are programs so crucial to the well-being of the population that some central planning is required. For example, most governments provide funds, research, and consultation to maintain pure food, air, and water; waste disposal; and immunization against infectious disease. The number and extent of these programs depends on the wealth of the country and its political will to allocate a portion of the budget for the health of citizens.

In health systems based on a free market economy, health-care facilities are built to compete for health-care dollars available through private insurance or programs funded by federal and state governments. In these systems, populations are served on the basis of ability to pay, not on need. The existence of a program to pay for medical care is not a guarantee that health care is available. For example, in the United States physicians may refuse to accept patients sponsored by programs such as Medicaid.

Availability of health care that is based on ability to pay is reflected in the health of the people. A sensitive indicator of such health is the infant mortality rate (number of infant deaths during the first year of life per 1000 infants born in a given year). This indicator reflects access to a number of vital health services such as prenatal care, intrapartal care, pure food and water, nutrition, education, immunizations, and well-child care. Table 5-2 gives infant mortality rates in four countries. It shows that the political and social organization of a health-care system is a more important factor in reducing infant mortality than is the relative wealth of the country.

It is important to remember that availability of health-care resources is influenced by cultural values, institutional racism, opportunities for employment, standards of housing, and literacy. Table 5-3 shows how these issues affect infant mortality rates in several states in the United States. Regardless of the state, African-American infants are more likely to die in their first year of life. These birth outcomes cannot be attributed to biologic differences. They are due to more social and economic barriers to health care for African-American citizens of the United States than for other citizens.

⟩⟩ *Table 5-2*

Infant Mortality Rate by Economic Level and Political Control of Health Care in 1986

Country	Per capita gross national product in US dollars[1]	Political control of health care[2]	Economic status	Infant mortality rate[3,4]
United States	$14,080	Permissive	Affluent	10.5
United Kingdom	$ 9,180	Cooperative	Affluent	9.6
Nigeria	$ 770	Cooperative	Poor	127.0
China	$ 300	Socialist	Poor	50.0

[1]An indicator of economic development, determined by the total number of hours worked by a nation's labor force and the average value of goods and services produced per hour of work.
[2]Roemer MI: Comparative health care systems. In: *Maxcy-Rosenau Public Health and Preventive Medicine,* 12th ed. Last JM (editor). Appleton-Century-Crofts, 1986.
[3]Infant deaths under 1 year of age per 1000 live births.
[4]Population Reference Bureau: *World Population Data Sheet.* 1986.

⟩⟩ *Table 5-3*

Infant Mortality Rate[1] by Selected States and Race in the United States in 1981[2]

	African-American	Other	Total
California	15.5	9.9	10.2
Illinois	24.4	11.2	13.9
New York	19.9	10.6	12.4
Kansas	20.9	10.6	11.4
Mississippi	20.6	10.5	15.4
Georgia	19.9	10.3	13.8

[1]Infant deaths under 1 year of age per 1000 live births.
[2]US Census Bureau: *Statistical Abstract of the United States,* 105th ed. 1985.

PERSONNEL.   All countries have similar categories of health personnel such as physicians, nurses, and allied health professionals. However, the number, type, distribution, and use of health professionals vary with the degree of government control and the wealth of the country.

In the United States, there are about 700 categories of health workers, including those who provide support services for health-care facilities such as janitorial and food service personnel. About 7% of workers are physicians, or about 200 per 100,000 population. The private sector employs about 96% of physicians, two-thirds of whom are in office-based practice in urban areas. Less than 40% of physicians are in general or family practice, internal medicine, obstetrics, or pediatrics, services most likely to focus on health promotion and illness prevention (Myers 1986).

In developing countries the supply of all types of health personnel is lower than in affluent countries. For example, in Nigeria the physician-to-population ratio is 7.2 per 100,000; in Columbia it is 51 per 100,000 (Roemer 1986). Yet developing countries with centralized health-care systems have a higher ratio of all types of health workers-to-population than developing countries with private enterprise systems. In countries with centralized systems, ministries of health decide how many and which types of physicians, nurses, and other health professionals are needed, how many to educate, and where to send them when educated, thus assuring a balance of primary and specialty providers throughout the country (Roemer 1986). As a result, education and employment are maximized, costs reduced, and the return on educational dollars increased. For example, in Thailand, the cost of educating one physician is about $30,000 US dollars. For the same amount of money the government can educate 5 nurses, 19 auxiliaries, or 250 village health workers (Williams et al 1985). Professionals in these countries promote health through patient teaching, preventative health services such as immunization, recognition and treatment of common illnesses, and physician referral.

Although there is no centralized planning of health care in the United States, nurses are as crucial to the US health-care system as they are in centralized systems. In the United States there are three times more nurses than physicians, with about 600 registered nurses per 100,000 population. Over 66% are employed by hospitals, 8% in nursing homes, 6.6% in community health, 5.7% in offices of physicians and dentists, 3.7% in education, and the remainder in such settings as schools, prisons, and industry (McKibbon et al 1985). In recent years nurses have assumed expanded roles, providing health services to children, child-bearing women, and the aged. Several thousand nurses now work in areas of advanced clinical practice as nurse practitioners and clinical specialists, as described in Chapter 3.

Unfortunately, advanced nursing practice in the United States is restricted by two factors: numbers of physicians and liability insurance. Physician groups have pressured state legislators to pass laws requiring physician supervision in spite of extensive literature on patient safety, satisfaction, and cost containment attributed to nurse practitioners. Such pressure is exerted obstensibly to protect patient health. However, many observers believe the true reason is to protect physician control of health services, particularly the monies they generate. Liability limits the practice of advanced nurse practitioners because of the reluctance of insurance companies to provide coverage at a reasonable cost for self-employed nurses, especially nurse-midwives. Problems with liability insurance in the United States are severe, affecting the ability of all health-care providers to be protected from malpractice claims. Insurance problems are caused by a failure of the medical community to practice self-discipline, liberal laws that favor plaintiffs, profits gained by lawyers in malpractice litigation, and business practices of insurance companies. At the present time most nurses working in expanded roles do so in hospitals or other large practices where their insurance is paid for by the institution (Kendellen 1987).

Functions

Health-care functions are the services provided by a health system, ranging from health education to the treatment of disease. They are classified as primary care and specialty care.

PRIMARY CARE.   Primary care is the service patients receive at their first point of contact with the health-care system (ANA 1987). It includes health promotion, prevention, diagnosis, treatment of uncomplicated diseases, and referral to specialty care when required. Everyone needs access to a source of primary care. Providers may be physicians in general practice, family practice, internal medicine, pediatrics, and sometimes obstetrics; or nurses in family, pediatric, and school practice; midwives; and physician assistants. Because expanded roles for nurses and physician assistants have developed, more people now receive primary care.

Community-oriented primary care is a modification of personal primary care. This type of care links the techniques of individual primary care to public health practice such as epidemiology, demography, biostatistics, health services planning, and program evaluation. Individuals are viewed as members of a community. The practitioner uses demographic information to describe a community in terms of the age range of the population, sex distribution, access to health services, and payment for health services. The population of a community is further described by its need for health service. For example, health service needs of an elderly population are different from the needs of young families or single college students.

The World Health Organization (WHO) places particular emphasis on primary care as a means to achieve its goal of health for all by the year 2000. In 1978, at a conference in Alma Ata, USSR, member nations were urged to cooperate in allocating national health care resources to achieve a universally accessible, affordable, primary health-care system. These systems would rely on both health workers and traditional healers for routine health care and use a referral system for specialty services. They would establish relationships with national programs for agriculture and employment. By so doing they would foster economic prosperity, an important factor in the physical and mental health of individuals and communities.

SPECIALTY CARE.   Specialty care is given by health-care providers who specialize in a particular area of medicine. Except for emergency care, most specialty care is provided on referral after patients enter the health-care system by way of *primary care*. Specialty care is used for *secondary care* to prevent the complications of disease and injury, and for *tertiary care* to provide rehabilitation and support, as shown in Table 5-1. Specialty care developed as a result of the growth in medical knowledge to the point that no individual practitioner could master the knowledge and skill of every medical specialty. Beginning in 1913 with the founding of the American College of Surgeons, specialty societies were formed to verify the competence of members practicing in these areas.

Nurses patterned their practice after medical societies, but in areas appropriate to nursing. In 1955 nurse-midwives organized a professional certifying body, the American College of Nurse-Midwives. In the 1970s the ANA established a program to certify other nursing specialties, as described in Chapter 3.

Specialty services in countries with centralized health systems usually are found in hospital settings. In localized systems, specialty care is available in private and public settings affiliated with medical schools, teaching hospitals, or private charitable institutions. Such care is offered by private providers on a fee-for-service basis. Free market forces are believed to balance the supply of specialists with the demand for service by patients. Where similar institutions compete for patients, uneconomical duplication of services may occur.

Controls

The controls of the health-care system are the standards and regulations created to assure that resources are used safely and effectively.

STANDARDS.   Standards for the health-care system specify the scope and depth of professional practice. They guide health professionals toward optimal procedures and activities for specific clinical services and settings. They do not have force of law, but serve to protect the health of people indirectly. Standards influence what the community expects from a health-care system in areas of scientific excellence and humanitarian practice. They fulfill the obligation of professional societies to improve quality of care and are used as the basis for job descriptions, educational programs, and certification. Standards reflect the current state of knowledge in specific fields and characterize, measure, and provide guidance for achievement of excellence in various health services (McKibbon et al 1985).

In the United States, the Cabinet on Nursing Practice of the ANA sets standards for the nursing profession. To date the cabinet, through its councils and specialty task forces, has published standards for 23 areas of nursing practice. These include medical-surgical, geriatrics, maternal and child health, and psychiatric-mental health, with their subspecialties (ANA 1987). The cabinet also has established standards for hospital nursing practice areas, primary health care, and health services in home, school, and correctional facilities. Other professional groups publish standards to guide individual practitioners in specific health-care settings. The American Public Health Association (APHA) has several sets of standards for water, food, and dairy products; ambulatory, maternal, and child health; family planning services; and health services in correctional institutions (APHA 1985). The federal government has established standards in an array of areas for the protection of public health (Jonas 1986).

REGULATIONS. The laws that license health-care providers and practice settings are intended to protect the population from unsafe practices by regulating such things as the education of health professionals, drugs, treatments, products, and the environment of health-care settings. Governmental regulations impose controls on rates and quality. They place restrictions on entry into practice with licensure laws to ensure safe practices that promote health.

Rate controls are fee schedules used by Medicaid and Medicare. These federal health-care payment programs reimburse physicians, hospitals, and other providers. Such controls are maintained by means of the Professional Standards Review Organizations (PSRO) and accreditation of providers, hospitals, and other institutions, allowing reimbursement for care of patients on Medicare and Medicaid.

Certification signifying expertise in a specialty area of medicine or nursing is another type of restriction on entry into practice. While certification is not a requirement for basic licensure, prospective employers may specify certification for advanced clinical practice as a prerequisite for a specific position (LoGerfo and Brook 1984). Control is also exerted over entry into practice by specialty boards and professional societies who accredit educational programs and postgraduate education for individual specialty practice.

In other countries of the world, licensure examinations for health professionals are not uniformly required. Graduation from a government-approved educational program is sufficient for licensure without additional examination. In nations with cooperative or socialist health-care systems, individuals are registered by a ministry of health or its equivalent on completion of the prescribed education. Professional societies in these countries have less influence on both licensure and certification than they have in the United States.

In a study conducted by the International Council of Nurses (ICN), researchers found that credentialing of nursing is difficult because "nursing" has no universal meaning, definition of functions, or standards of education and practice. Laws regulating the professions differ widely. "A common finding for all countries is that the legal definition of the scope of nursing practice is generally more restrictive than the performance ability of nurses and the public's need for services" (Styles 1986). In response to these findings ICN adopted several principles for professional regulation. Among these is the principle that two categories of nursing personnel should be designated: nurse and nurse auxiliary. They should be licensed and regulated as all other professionals in the country.

Organization

The organization of health care involves planning and administration. Planning is required to assure appropriate allocation of human and material resources in meeting priorities. Administration is necessary to monitor activities and evaluate outcomes, including use of services, cost of care, and client health status. Planning and administration of health programs is an attempt to make the best use of facilities, personnel, and funds for the purpose of achieving an equitable and cost effective system of health care.

Blum (1981) points out, however, that planning may be reduced to a technical exercise. Without a balanced view of what health is (a biologic, social, and psychologic state of well-being), the allocation of resources may promote only special interests of powerful business and professional groups.

PLANNING.   Health planning requires several steps, beginning with *assessment*. The country, state, or local region may be divided into units. Data are collected on a particular health index, such as children injured and killed in motor vehicle accidents. The planning agency may want to know the ages of children most affected, availability and accessibility of emergency services, design of automobiles and highways, and preparation of emergency medical personnel. The first level of assessment regards relevance. It asks, "Is there a problem? If so, how reliable is the data? Is a solution needed?" This is called a *needs assessment*.

Following the careful definition of a health problem, overall goals and specific objectives are identified to give direction. A program is then designed and implemented to correct the problem. Measures of evaluation are identified, such as counting the number of deaths or days of hospitalization during a time period, and procedures for data collection are designed. When a program is implemented and shown to be working well, planners then ask if the program is efficient. Evaluation of efficiency gives information about relative benefits compared to costs of the program. Since health-care resources are limited and programs compete for available funds, administrators must know if benefits can be obtained for less cost. They study the records to answer the question. Unfortunately, such study may not demonstrate a relationship between lower costs and improved health, because often only short-term benefits are assessed.

ADMINISTRATION.   Administration of the health-care system in the United States is influenced by two constitutional principles: shared sovereignty between the states and federal government, and separation of powers among the executive, legislative, and judicial branches of government (Jonas 1986).

The states have primary responsibility for planning and administering health-care services. This responsibility is based on their authority to enact and enforce laws to promote and protect public safety. Table 5-4 lists typical program areas within state health agencies (Jonas 1986). Agencies responsible for health services vary from state to state and may be shared by more than one branch of government. The legislative branch enacts the legal framework for public and private health services, allocating funds for these services. The judiciary protects the rights of individuals, settling controversial issues in the courts such as access to abortion. The executive branch of state governments implements health legislation, provides for education and professional licensure, and supports research. Health administration at the federal level is also subject to the checks and balances of the legislative, judicial, and executive branches of government. The federal government, acting through its health planning and administrative agencies, gives money to the states for health care and professional education. These funds are administered by a variety of federal programs that set reporting requirements and standards for the states. The states are free to participate in federally recommended health programs

⚕ Table 5-4

Program Areas of State Health Agencies

Alcohol and drug abuse
Chronic disease screening
Communicable disease control
Dental health
Environmental health
Health education
Health professions licensure
Health resources management
Laboratory
Maternal and child health
Mental health
Mental retardation
Services for children with special health-care needs

---

and may or may not accept federal funding to supplement state health care budgets. This same process of setting policy, recommending programs, and funding them goes on between state and local health jurisdictions.

Selected planning and administrative agencies of the federal government are listed in Table 5-5. The Department of Health and Human Services is the principal health agency. It was founded in 1979. Its functions were formerly in the Department of Health, Education, and Welfare, which began in 1953. The two major fi-

⟶ Table 5-5

Selected Health Administration and Planning Agencies of the United States Government

Department of Agriculture
Concerned with animal, human, and plant health; establishes minimum daily food requirements and food safety regulations; Women, Infants, and Children feeding program (WIC); National School Lunch Program; food stamp program

Department of Commerce
Conducts the decennial census; provides a wide variety of US population and statistical data on people and the economy

Department of Defense
Concerned with comprehensive health planning, education, and medical care of military personnel and their dependents

Department of Health and Human Services
Principal federal agency concerned with health, includes:
1. *Health Care Financing Administration:* Responsible for financing the two major treatment service programs: Medicare and Medicaid
2. *United States Public Health Service:*
   a) Office for the Assistant Secretary of Health: Responsible for programs in disease prevention and health promotion, smoking and health, international health, President's Council of Physical Fitness and Sports, National Center for Health Statistics, and National Center for Health Services Research
   b) Centers for Disease Control
   c) Food and Drug Administration
   d) Agency for Toxic Substances and Disease Registry
   e) Alcohol, Drug Abuse, and Mental Health Administration
   f) National Institutes of Health, the major national force in biomedical research
   g) Health Resources and Service Administration responsible for direct health care and program support in Native American health, federal prisoner health care,

nancing programs for health-care services, Medicare and Medicaid, are located in this agency under the Health Care Financing Administration. Within the Department of Health and Human Services is the United States Public Health Service, the administrative center for major policy decisions and reseach for public health in the United States. Federal agencies are linked to both private and public health-care sectors by revenue-sharing and grants for health training, health-care demonstration projects, and research.

Planning and administration for health in the United States is

Table 5-5 (continued)

Selected Health Administration and Planning Agencies of the United States Government

   health science education, and community health center programs, National
   Health Service Corps, and development of health maintenance organizations
3. *Administration on Aging*
4. *Social Security Administration:* Administers Social Security program
5. *Administration for Children and Families*
   a) Family Support Administration
      1) Administers Aid to Families with Dependent Children (AFDC)
      2) Assists states in enforcement of child support obligations owed by absent parents
      3) Administers the community service block grants and refugee resettlement program
      3) Administers adoption assistance, foster care, and child welfare services
      5) Administers the Social Services Block Grant
   b) Office of Human Development
   c) Maternal and Child Health Block Grant

Department of Interior
   Bureau of Indian Affairs

Department of Labor
   Occupational Safety and Health Administration

Department of Transportation
   Provides for safe and efficient transportation through the US Coast Guard and maritime, aviation, highways, and railroad

Environmental Protection Agency
   Concerned with air and water quality, radiation hazards, pollution and toxic substances control, solid waste disposal, and pesticide regulation

Source: Office of the Federal Register, National Archives and Record Administration: *The United States Government Manual 1990/91.* US Government Printing Office, 1991.

decentralized to the states and local communities, but with continued support by the federal government in the form of funds and technical expertise. In this decentralized system people have the right to demand accountability for the way their health-care dollars are spent. Citizen activity greatly influences what kinds of programs are supported by state legislatures and the United States Congress. The Children's Defense Fund is an example of a citizen lobby. It continually monitors the needs of poor, handicapped, and minority children and attempts to influence United States policy for child health.

Planning and administration in other countries varies with the degree of centralization of the health-care system. When planning is centralized in the government, a potential for a more equitable distribution of health services exists. However, Roemer (1986) notes that administrative officials who plan health care are not necessarily appointed because of technical expertise. Political considerations and favoritism play a strong role, with voluntary health groups and citizens playing a relatively minor part in planning. The Soviet Union, with a highly centralized health-care system, permitted data to be released on some failures of central planning (Schultz and Rafferty 1990). This data revealed that both male and female life expectancy is about 10 years less than in the United States and has been declining over the past 20 years. Infant mortality has risen to 2.5 times that of the United States and ranks 50th in the world. Soviet leadership has made a commitment to increase the share of gross national product going to health care, from 3.9% to 6.0% by the year 2000. They also expect gradually to introduce private enterprise in the form of staff-owned, cooperative clinics that will rely on patient fees for operating expenses.

United States Health-care System

Historical and Cultural Influences

General Health-care

Health care in the United States began as a private business. In the 1700s and 1800s, physicians were viewed as tradesmen, relying entirely on patients to pay for service. Private philanthropies provided for the poor in ambulatory settings, which became out-patient departments of teaching hositals. Medical schools operated as commercial enterprises, charging tuition and conferring diplomas. Some schools offered only lectures with no clinical experience. Although New York City passed the first licensing law in 1760, it did not mandate licensure or require graduation from medical school (Myers 1986). Licensing of physicians was not widely accepted until after 1900.

The Flexner Report of 1910 was a turning point in medical education. It exposed a serious lack of uniformity and standards in specific schools. Subsequently, schools with higher standards, such as those found in colleges and universities, received financial grants and schools with lower standards closed. Admission criteria rose and curricula began to reflect the scientific discipline that characterizes medical education today.

During the years medicine was developing into a regulated, scientific discipline, nursing was also undergoing change. Curricula of nursing schools were modeled after the Nightingale school in England. By the turn of the century, the precursor organizations of the American Nurses' Association and National League for Nursing were formed. By 1923, 48 states had licensure laws (Henderson and Nite 1978). Just as medical and nursing education were self-regulated, so too was the health-care industry. Prior to 1900, the only health service provided by the federal government was for seamen and members of the armed forces. After that time, especially following the flu epidemic of 1917, the government became increasingly involved in health care.

Mental Health-care

Care of the mentally ill followed a different path from that of general health care. Whereas general health care was built on private practice, mental health care began as a state government responsibility. Private psychiatric practice and its teaching in medical schools was not well established until the 1930s (Gruenberg 1986). Before state mental hospitals began in the 1840s, mentally ill people were cared for by their families, in poorhouses, or in jails.

Government involvement in mental health care preceded government involvement in general health care by 50 years. State hospital systems were alternatives to the abusive or nonexistent ones of local communities. However, these systems isolated psychiatry from mainstream medicine.

Conditions in state mental hospitals were far from ideal. The reform movement of the early 1900s was sparked by the publication of *A Mind that Found Itself,* an account of the experience of Clifford Beers, a patient in a mental hospital. In 1909, Beers founded a voluntary association, the Association of Mental Hygiene, initiating interest in preventative mental health and improved care for the mentally ill. During World War II, the federal government became involved in the treatment and research of psychiatric disorders among military personnel. Federal funds were made available to states in 1946, under the National Mental Health Act. This act continues to provide funds for mental health research, training, and community service centers.

Community Responsibility for Health

Health as a community concern came about as a result of the increasing knowledge of bacteriology and communicable disease of the late nineteenth century. Provision of clean milk at "milk stations" in metropolitan areas and physical examination of school children were early efforts to promote public health. Nurses actively participated in these programs, providing care and education in clinics, schools, and homes.

Establishment of the Children's Bureau in the Department of Labor in 1912 was the first example of federal acceptance of some responsibility for child health. It may seem unusual to have an agency concerned for the well-being of children in the Department of Labor. The reason is that the major threat to child health was their employment in hazardous industries such as mines and mills. Ironically, child labor did not end in the United States until the economic depression of the 1930s. It ended then, not because society noticed that child labor was hazardous to health and deprived children of an education, but because children took the jobs of men who needed employment in a depressed economy.

Social Security Act of 1935

A survey conducted by the Children's Bureau contributed to passage of the Social Security Act of 1935. This act provided for income support and health care. Income supports were of two types: insurance (old age, survivor's, disability, and unemployment) and assistance (aid to families with dependent children). Health care, embodied in Title V of the act, consisted of maternal and child health and crippled children services. The act also included a provision for grants to state public welfare agencies to establish and extend services for homeless and neglected children.

The Social Security Act was landmark legislation. As never before, it involved the federal government in the health and welfare of individuals. Its passage represented a national desire to prevent a recurrence of the Great Depression and the culmination of efforts by humanitarian groups to promote the well-being of families and children. Federal assistance to states in specific areas of health and welfare became an established policy, even though this assistance meant some loss of control by states over health and welfare programs.

With the passage of the Social Security Act, some members of Congress considered a compulsory national health insurance program. However, it was not included because of the zeal with which the American Medical Association argued against any proposal that might take the practice of medicine out of private hands (Harris 1966). Even so, the act has served as a major vehicle for health and welfare legislative amendments ever since its passage.

Increasing Federal Involvement

Following World War II, the federal government increased its role in health care. As mentioned earlier, research and training in mental health was strengthened by the National Mental Health Act of 1946. That same year the Hill-Burton Act provided funds for the construction of hospitals, improving access to hospital care (Myers 1986). Government involvement with health care reached new heights with passage of the 1965 amendments to the Social

Security Act: Medicare and Medicaid. Discussed later in this chapter, these major programs provide care for the aged, indigent, and disabled.

Over time the original Medicaid legislation was modified to mandate states to increase benefits for designated recipients. In 1972, a program called the Early Periodic Screening Diagnosis and Treatment Program (EPSDT) was developed to provide preventative health services for children under Medicaid. In 1984, the states were required to cover single women who were pregnant for the first time and women who were pregnant in two-parent families with an unemployed breadwinner. In 1989 Congress raised income eligibility for Medicaid benefits for pregnant women and children under six years to 133% of the federal poverty index and mandated increased reimbursement by states for pediatric and obstetric care providers.

The *poverty index* is based on a determination by the Department of Agriculture that families spend approximately one-third of their incomes on food. The *poverty level* is therefore set at three times the cost of an economy food plan that includes specific amounts of meat, vegetables, and other commodities. As of March 1990, a family of four meets the family guidelines stated at 100% of poverty if their income is $12,700.

Regional Health Planning

As federal direct payment and revenue sharing programs for health care grew in the 1960s and 1970s, interest in monitoring programs and avoiding costly duplication of services increased. In 1974, the National Health Planning and Resource Development Act was passed. It enabled state planning boards to regulate health-care facilities, determining if new construction, programs, or modification of facilities were in the public interest (Shonick 1986). The act divided the nation into 212 local planning agencies that were to carry out population-based health planning. Opinions differed on the benefits of federally financed regional planning. Many saw this as interference in a free market system, stifling price competition. Others insisted that the market for health care is different from other markets. The general population is not necessarily motivated to purchase health care at the lowest possible cost nor can it be fully informed about such care. Therefore, to protect the public some regulation is needed, as provided by health planning districts.

At present, health planning by the federal government is directed more to containing cost than to meeting needs. The current executive branch supports market competition as the preferred mechanism to develop health resources (Shonick 1986).

Categorical Programs

The trend in federal-state relations from about 1945 to 1975 was for the federal government to play an increasing role in planning health services and in directing how states spent federal dollars. Such control required a large bureaucracy in Washington, DC. Some saw this bureaucracy as an unmatched source of technical assistance. Others viewed it as a costly and unwelcome interference in affairs rightfully belonging to the states.

Most controversial were the increasing numbers of *categorical programs* for distinct populations. Funds for such programs were limited to narrowly defined services and channeled through special grantees, usually universities. State and local health departments had no power to determine the need for a program or to alter use of the funds in any way. Limitation and duplication of services resulted. Examples of categorical programs authorized by 1965–1967 amendments to the Social Security Act included maternity and infant care projects, children and youth projects, neonatal intensive care, family planning, and dental care. While these programs were recognized as excellent, federal funds supporting them could not be used for any other purpose, even though another use might be more needful.

Block Grants

A profound change in federal health policy took place following the 1980 presidential election. The administration initiated a block grant method of funding. The Omnibus Reconciliation Act of 1981 consolidated more than 50 categorical grants for health promotion and care. Funds formerly allocated to categorical programs were given to the states in block grants, increasing state control and decreasing federal involvement. Such freedom from federal regulation seemed too good to be true. Indeed, it was. With program consolidation came funding reduction. For example, in 1981 the states received about 25% fewer federal health-care dollars for programs consolidated under the maternal and child health block grant (General Accounting Office, United States 1984). Lobbying for health programs moved to states and local communities where the decisions were made about use of block grant funds. The change in funding mechanisms had little effect on private health care providers and their clients. However, people who depended on publicly funded programs experienced uneven and inequitable health care as a result of political pressure at state and local levels. For example, funds for family planning services were cut in response to the action of certain conservative groups.

Financing Health Care

Methods of financing the health-care system in the United States are diverse and complicated, yet understanding them is crucial for nurses working in the system. Table 5-6 lists the principal sources of private funds and the major programs supported by public funds in the United States.

Private Funds

Private sources of funding for health care come from individuals, Blue Cross, Blue Shield, commercial insurance, self-insurance, health maintenance organizations, hospital and physician health plans, contributions to philanthropic health services, workers' compensation, and employee health services.

Although about 80% of the nonmilitary population has some type of private health insurance, that insurance pays for only 27% of the national expenditures on personal health care (Myers 1986). This gap occurs because covered services and liability (who-pays-for-what) vary so widely. For example, many insurance policies pay physician and hospital charges if a person is hospitalized, but they do not pay physician charges if that person seeks preventive care or treatment as an outpatient. Most third-party payment systems, including Blue Cross-Blue Shield, Medicare, and Medicaid, discriminate against mental health services as compared to other

Table 5-6

Sources of Private Funds for Health Care and Programs Supported by Public Funds in the United States

Sources of Private Funds

1. Individuals
2. Blue Cross–Blue Shield
3. Commercial insurance
4. Self-insurance (corporations)
5. Health maintenance organizations
6. Contributions of philanthropic organizations
7. Workers' compensation insurance
8. Employee health services

Programs Supported by Public Funds

1. Federal health programs
   a. Medicare
   b. Native Americans
   c. Federal employees
   d. Merchant marines
   e. Members of armed forces
   f. Veterans
2. Federal-state revenue-sharing programs
   a. Medicaid
   b. Other programs
      1) Family planning
      2) Food assistance
      3) Immunization
      4) Injury control
      5) Children with special health-care needs

types of care (Gruenberg 1986). Blue Cross-Blue shield is the oldest type of health insurance, originating in a hospital prepayment plan for school teachers in Dallas, Texas in 1929 (Fein 1986). These plans cover 30% to 39% of privately insured persons (Myers 1986). They are run by nonprofit organizations, usually controlled by hospitals and physicians. Often, payment is made to a provider for covered benefits, with policy holders given free choice of physicians. Recently, subscribers have had the option of paying a lower premium in return for choosing a physician or hospital that agrees to fixed rates for services (Arnett et al 1986).

Commercial insurance companies entered the health-care market in the 1940s (Fein 1986). These for-profit businesses sell many types of insurance. Subscribers have free choice of physicians, and they, not physicians or hospitals, receive reimbursement. Insurance payments cover only part of the total cost and require an additional deductible or coinsurance payment by subscribers. Since 1950, commercial health insurance has covered about 49% of privately insured individuals (Myers 1986).

Independent plans include both profit and nonprofit organizations. Companies may self-insure for health benefits under the Employee Retirement Income Security Act of 1974. They establish a self-funded, nonprofit health plan, escaping the taxes and regulations of state insurance laws.

Health maintenance organizations (HMOs) are another type of independent insurance. HMOs contract with an enrolled population to provide comprehensive health care as either for-profit or nonprofit agencies. They emphasize prevention and provide both inpatient and outpatient care. Services are guaranteed and prepaid, usually by employers or by employees through payroll deductions. Choice of providers is limited to those working for the plan. Since 1974, HMOs have become increasingly popular, currently enrolling about 15% of privately insured people (Myers 1986). With the soaring cost of health care, many HMOs have raised premiums, limited benefits, and increased restrictions. A new version of the HMO model, a *preferred provider organization* (PPO) restricts the choice of physicians to those who agree to a reduced fee schedule.

Contributions to philanthropic organizations support a wide variety of health-related services. Some philanthropies, such as the United Way, give funds to direct care agencies. Others provide direct services themselves, such as community hospitals and women's clinics. Without these philanthropies, many people would have no health care at all.

Workers' compensation insurance provides health care and income replacement for workers who suffer work-related injury, disability, or death. Employers are liable for the cost of this insurance and must purchase a policy from a state-operated insurance fund, offer proof of self-insurance, or contract with a commercial insurance provider. Compensation and amounts awarded to workers are related to the degree and permanence of injuries and number of dependents. Amounts workers receive are usually less than the wages they earned before their injury.

Employee health services began in 1887, when the Homestake Mining Company sponsored the first industrial medical department in the United States. In 1895, Ada Stewart was hired by the Vermont Marble Company as the first occupational health nurse. About that time Dr. Alice Hamilton began her work, becoming the foremost proponent of occupational safety and health of her day. The labor movement gained strength and the Department of Labor was formed. In 1911, New Jersey passed the first workers' compensation act upheld by the courts. By 1948, all states had similar laws. In 1970, the Occupational Safety and Health Act made the health of workers a public concern. By 1990, employee health services offered education, direct services, referral, rehabilitation, counseling, and environmental surveillance.

Publicly Funded Programs

Voluntary health insurance does not help people who are unemployed or otherwise unable to purchase insurance. In the free market system of the United States, the government has been unable and unwilling to provide a national health insurance plan for all its citizens or a tax-supported system of health care (Fein 1986). In spite of this the government pays 42% of all health-care expenditures (Myers 1986). It provides comprehensive health care for Native Americans, members of the armed forces and their dependents, veterans, merchant marines, members of Congress and various other federal employees and their dependents, victims of Hansen's disease, and Medicare recipients. Federal grants enable states to provide health care for medically indigent persons through Medicaid. Other federal programs fund services for children with special needs, immunizations, injury control, and food assistance.

MEDICARE. Medicare is a compulsory federal health insurance program providing health insurance for eligible persons age 65 and over and certain disabled individuals. It was created by 1965 amendments to the Social Security Act. Medicare is paid for by currently employed people through payroll deductions under the Federal Insurance Contributions Act (FICA). It is administered by the Bureau of Health Insurance within the Social Security Administration. Medicare has two parts: A and B.

Part A covers inpatient hospital services for 90 days per illness episode. Each year patients pay deductible costs equal to about one hospital day and a copayment cost of 25% of the cost of care for days 61 through 90. Other covered expenses include outpatient diagnostic services and 100 posthospital days of skilled nursing services. The Omnibus Budget Reconciliation Act of 1981 added home health nursing and hospice services.

Part B covers physician's fees and other services such as diagnostic tests, rental of medical equipment for home use, and physical therapy in and out of the hospital. Medicare recipients pay monthly premiums, an annual deductible amount, 20% of an approved fee, and any amount above that fee. General tax revenues pay 80% of the approved fee (Myers 1986). Providers who agree not to charge more than approved fees are said to "accept assignment." Those who do not accept assignment charge patients their normal fees and patients pay the difference or find other physicians. "Intermediaries," such as Blue Cross, process the claims. About 95% of the elderly are enrolled in Medicare as well as some younger persons who are disabled or have end-stage renal disease.

The cost of Medicare has increased about 18% per year since 1970. A major effort to control this cost is now underway in the form of a prospective payment system (PPS). This system is based on the average cost of care for a person of a given age with a given medical diagnosis, called a diagnosis-related group (DRG). Hospitals are reimbursed according to DRGs. Provision is made for transfer of patients between hospitals and for a limited number of extended hospital days. The Health Care Financing Administration controls quality of care by sampling volume of admissions, case mix, and discharge status. Peer review organizations (PROs) validate diagnoses and monitor quality of care and appropriateness of admissions. Regardless of length of stay or complications, hospitals must agree to accept a set fee as full payment. Thus, prospective payment provides an incentive to discharge patients. The long-range effects of this system as compared to retrospective billing for ordinary and customary fees are not yet known.

Medicare legislation increased access to home care for the elderly by providing reimbursement for acute convalescent needs. However, it has not met the need for long-term care. For example, Nellie Greer's husband was not eligible for long-term care even though his condition was deteriorating. When he could no longer manage at home and needed nursing home care, Medicare would not pay the bill. Nellie had to sell the home to pay for his care. Mundinger (1983) studied problems associated with home care and recommended that reimbursement be based on nursing diagnoses concerning functional status and living arrangements rather than medical diagnoses. McKibbon et al (1985) noted that even in acute-care settings, DRGs were developed without considering nursing care needs.

MEDICAID.   Medicaid is a health assistance program providing medical services for the poor. Both federal and state funds pay for Medicaid, with the ratio of federal funding varying from 50% to 83%. Medicaid differs from Medicare in that the federal government does not entitle individual recipients. Instead, it gives money to the states. The states decide who is eligible for Medicaid. The primary criterion for eligibility is to be in a welfare category, that is, to receive Aid to Families with Dependent Children (AFDC), or Supplemental Security Income (SSI) due to old age, blindness, or disability (Myers 1986). In 1988, state income eligibility for these programs ranged from a low of 14.6% of the federal poverty level to 85.8%, with an average of 48.8%. Therefore Medicaid covers about 40% of persons defined as living in poverty (Myers 1986). In two-thirds of the states, people with incomes above these amounts up to slightly above the poverty level—the *medically needy*—are also eligible for Medicaid. As previously described, the 1989 amendments to Medicaid law raised income eligibility for pregnant women and children under six years of age to 133% of poverty. Even with these changes in eligibility, medical care may be unavailable because physicians may refuse Medicaid patients, citing low levels of reimbursement, burdensome record-keeping, and delays in payment. States may provide additional benefits if they wish, such as inpatient psychiatric care, home health visits, eye glasses, dental care, and drugs.

In 1972, the Early Periodic Screening Diagnosis and Treatment Program (EPSDT) was added to Medicaid services. It provides health screening and follow-up diagnostic services for infants, children, and adolescents who are classified as medically indigent or medically needy. The program provides outreach, health screening, and referral services, linking poor children with permanent sources of medical care.

Medicaid is the chief source of funds for long-term care of the elderly (Myers 1986). Medicare requires that covered services be related to an acute illness. When long-term care is needed because of functional disabilities, Medicare will not pay the bill. Personal resources must be used. When patients have used up all their resources, in a process called *spending down,* they may be eligible for Medicaid. Such forced impoverishment puts a critical hardship on the living spouse. It requires that a spouse either divorce the disabled spouse, or become indigent by giving the property away or allowing it to be debt-ridden in order to qualify for medical assistance.

SPECIAL PROGRAMS.   Although Medicare and Medicaid are the most expensive and best known of federal and state programs, tax revenues support many others. These programs are of special interest because of the populations they serve and the impact they have on the health and quality of life of recipients. Family planning services are provided by both federal and state governments. Federal funds come from Title X of the Public Health Service Act, Title XIX (Medicaid) of the Social Security Act, and maternal and child health and social services block grants. Among patients served, 80% are below or slightly above the poverty level (Children's Defense Fund 1987).

Food assistance is provided through federal food stamp, school food, and Women, Infant, and Children (WIC) programs. The food stamp program helps about 19 million people. Eligible families are given or purchase food stamps at a fraction of their value and use them to purchase food in grocery stores. School food programs provide free or low-cost meals for poor children. The WIC food-supplement program provides nutrition counseling and food supplements such as milk for pregnant women and mothers with children up to five years of age (Children's Defense Fund 1987).

Immunization grants from the federal government are used by the states to purchase vaccines. These federal-state programs, along with improved social and environmental conditions, have achieved a 99% reduction in diphtheria, pertussis, rubella, and polio. As a result of an internationally coordinated program by the World Health Organization, smallpox has been eradicated from the Western World. The rising cost of vaccines (from $6 in 1980 to $30 in 1986) and liability for reactions to immunizations cause great concern. Western Europe has passed national compensation laws to limit liability of agencies administering vaccines. However, there are no such laws in the United States at this time.

Injury control is a serious concern throughout the world. Intentional injuries (homicides, suicides, and nonfatal assaults) and unintentional injuries (automobile crashes, falls, fires, and drowning) are the leading causes of death in people ages 1 to 44 years. The term accident is no longer used to describe these events because the word implies that little can be done to control the problem. Epidemiologic studies reveal that many personal and environmental interactions resulting in injury are preventable. The Center for Disease Control (CDC) and Center for Environmental Health (CEH) support a number of injury control activities. In 1986, they provided $7.8 million for injury prevention research, working with the National Highway Traffic Safety Administration (Center for Disease Control 1986).

The Program for Children with Special Health Care Needs (CSHCN), formerly the Crippled Children's Service, was begun by the Social Security Act of 1935 and retained in the Omnibus Reconciliation Act of 1981. Funds are provided by maternal-child health block grants. Federal funds, together with state matching funds, pay for treatment and rehabilitation for certain categories of disabilities. The states decide what they will cover and the amount of money they will spend. Many states overmatch federal funds. CSHCN has been very successful, providing specialized medical care for children not otherwise assisted. It is supported by the private health sector, recruits qualified specialists, and promotes the treatment team concept, requiring the inclusion of nursing, social work, and other therapies. Case managers control expenditures, act as advocates for the family, obtain appropriate specialty care, and conserve funds by developing interagency agreements with other programs such as Medicaid. Unfortunately, CSHCN offers only specialty care, not overall health supervision (primary care). As a result, basic health needs such as immunizations, treatment of minor illnesses, and vision and hearing testing are not covered services. The policy to limit CSHCN to specialty care was made to avoid the appearance of government interference in the business relationship of primary care physicians to their patients.

Controlling Health-care Costs

Public and private expenditures for health care in the United States are enormous, and growing. In 1986, the cost of health care was estimated at $540 billion, about 42% paid from public and 58% from private funds (Arnett et al 1986). The development of cost controlling measures is of utmost concern.

In the private sector cost-saving measures include: (1) offering new forms and conditions for insurance such as preferred provider organizations, coinsurance, and deductibles; (2) requiring "second opinions" before surgery; (3) instituting a case management system similar to that used by CSHCN to limit choice of providers to those charging the most reasonable fees; (4) offering incentives for less expensive services such as outpatient care; and (5) educating about healthful life-styles.

In the public sector, with the number of people over age 65 growing, measures to reduce Medicare costs are urgently needed. Such measures include limiting hospital payments by using a prospective payment system and shifting more of the cost to recipients. Measures to reduce Medicaid costs include: (1) negotiating prospective payment contracts with hospitals; (2) limiting the choice of hospitals and providers; (3) permitting insurance companies to negotiate preferred provider agreements; (4) reducing the scope of coverage; (5) limiting the number of eligible people; and (6) returning the care of medically indigent adults to counties.

The present method of controlling health-care costs leaves the poor with few choices. Social legislation of the 1930s and 1960s attempted to provide a system of health care for the poor that was equal to the private sector system. However, many forces have caused a return to the two-tiered system that prevailed when health care was paid out-of-pocket. Some of these forces include (1) inflation, (2) wasteful expansion of medical technology, (3) physician and insurance barriers to expanded practice by nonphysician health professionals, (4) failure of the health-care system to respond to free market forces, and (5) growth of for-profit health-care corporations. Many believe that federally-based comprehensive health insurance would achieve more equitable distribution of care. Much has been learned about responsible cost control since national health insurance was first proposed. Perhaps these lessons will serve as the basis for a more complete, equitable health-care system (Fein 1986).

Health-care Policy

A health-care system develops from health policy decisions. These decisions reflect the economic constraints, cultural beliefs, and political ideology of a nation. They are made on the basis of *policy research*, a process by which information pertinent to an area of concern is gathered, tested, and made available to policy makers.

Data Collection

Collection of appropriate data is essential to policy research. It is carried out by federal, state, and local agencies. Federal agencies that collect and disseminate data about health in the United States are listed in Table 5-7. The National Center for Health Statistics (NCHS) is the primary data collection agency. It uses census data collected every ten years by the Bureau of Census to formulate the total population at risk for various vital rates. The NCHS also conducts special surveys and publishes a wide range of health information. Its data is available on computer discs for research purposes and its publications are listed in the *Catalog of Publications,* US Department of Health and Human Services.

The National Health Interview Survey (NHIS) is especially important to health policy research. This household survey of a prob-

Selected Sources of Data on Health	

Sources of data	Type of data
United States Department of Health and Human Services	
National Center for Health Statistics	Only federal agency specifically established for collection and dissemination of health data
National Vital Statistics System	Collects and publishes data on births, deaths, marriages, and divorces
National Natality Survey	Conducted periodically since 1963; collects data about the nature of live births
National Health Interview Survey	A nationwide, continuing, sample survey; data collected by personal household interviews on personal and demographic characteristics, use of health resources, illnesses, chronic conditions, injuries, impairments
National Health and Nutrition Examination	A nationwide sample survey; data obtained by direct physical examination, clinical and laboratory tests, in order to measure and monitor indicators of nutritional status
National Master Facility Inventory	A comprehensive file of inpatient health facilities such as hospitals and nursing homes
National Hospital Discharge Survey	A nationwide sample survey that collects data about discharges from short-stay hospitals
National Ambulatory Medical Care Survey	A national probability sample of ambulatory medical encounters in the offices of nonfederally-employed MDs
National Medical Care Utilization and Expenditure Survey	A national sample survey of health expenditures for personal health services and individual family insurance coverage during 1980; checking eligibility status of respondents of Medicare and Medicaid
Health Resources and Services Administration	
Bureau of Health Professions	Evaluates both current and future supply of health-care personnel in various occupations, designating shortage areas for National Health Service Corps, loan repayment and scholarship programs
Centers for Disease Control	
Center for Infectious Diseases	Maintains a national morbidity reporting system with national surveillance of infectious diseases; publishes *Morbidity & Mortality Weekly Report,* which provides information about public health issues and current statistics on infectious diseases

Table 5-7 *(continued)*

Selected Sources of Data on Health

Center for Preventive Services	Conducts the US Immunization Survey, used to estimate immunization level of child population against vaccine-preventable diseases; periodically collects data on adult population
Alcohol, Drug Abuse, and Mental Health Administration	
National Institute on Alcohol Abuse/Alcoholism	Funds national surveys on drinking; provides data on trends in alcohol consumption
National Institute of Mental Health	Conducts surveys of inpatient and outpatient psychiatric facilities; studies characteristics of patients served by these facilities
Health Care Financing Administration	
Bureau of Data Management Strategy	Compiles annual estimates of public and private expenditures for health by type of expenditure and source of funds; maintains a Medicare statistical program tracking eligibility of employees, benefits they use, certification status of institutional providers, and payments made for covered services
Department of Commerce	
Bureau of Census	Beginning in 1790, the Bureau has taken census of population every 10 years; conducts a monthly current population survey
Department of Labor	
Bureau of Labor	Prepares a monthly *Consumer Price Statistics Index,* a measure of changes in the average prices of goods and services purchased by urban wage earners and their families, showing trends in medical care prices by using specific indicators of hospital, medical, dental, and drug prices
Environmental Protection Agency	Collects data on pollutants for which national ambient air quality standards have been set; maintains Aerometric Data Bank
United Nations	
Statistical Office	Prepares *Demographic Yearbook,* a collection of comprehensive international demographic statistics

Source: *Health and Prevention Profile.* US National Center for Health Services, HHS Publ. No. 84-1232, 207–216, 1984. In: Clemen-Stone S, et al: *Comprehensive Family and Community Health Nursing,* 2nd ed. McGraw-Hill, 1987.

ability sample of the population is particularly valuable because it represents the perceptions people hold of their health status and needs. Respondents are asked questions concerning their health, illness, and medical care. Data is classified by age and sex and used to predict the incidence of acute illness, injury, disability, limitation of activity due to chronic illness, and use of health-care services. In 1981, a special supplement of NHIS focused on children in families. It asked questions about child development and health, breast-feeding practices, and use of child-care services.

Unfortunately, the federal data collection and reporting process is slow, sometimes taking three to five years to compile and publish. Such delay complicates health planning, but emphasizes the importance of state and local data collection functions.

All states have an office of vital statistics that collects health information. Data from local communities is sent to the state office and on to federal agencies. This information is used for health planning and policy development at all levels of government. Vital events such as births and deaths are routinely collected and reported. Other data is collected periodically by health professionals carrying out small surveys in their work settings and local communities.

Major Indicators of Health Status

Major indicators of health status are *vital events*, such as births, deaths (mortality), and sickness (morbidity). *Demographic data* describes the size, distribution, structure, and change of a population over time. Vital events and demographics are usually expressed as proportions, called *rates*, with the vital event or descriptive feature the numerator and a total population at risk the denominator.

The *crude death rate* is an expression of all deaths for a given year as a proportion of the total population.

The *neonatal mortality rate* (deaths of infants in the first 28 days of life) reflects health system problems in caring for pregnant women, such as nutritional status and prevention of anemia. It also may demonstrate problems that exist in preventing infant infection or trauma during labor and delivery.

The *postneonatal mortality rate* (deaths of infants from age 29 days to one year) reflects unsafe feeding techniques and unintentional home injuries such as burns and falls. It also reflects environmental health issues such as unsafe water, improper sewage disposal, and inadequate food distribution. This kind of data is especially important in developing countries of the world, where enteric and respiratory infections are a leading cause of infant death.

The *perinatal mortality rate* (fetal deaths and deaths of infants under 28 days) is of special concern in the United States. It is a relatively accurate measure of the impact of (1) prenatal care on a mother's health and (2) technology in the management of labor and delivery and support of fragile neonates. The perinatal mortality rate in the United States reveals that technology is only reducing birthweight-specific neonatal mortality. Providers of health care are able to save more very small babies, but the system is failing to prevent births of low birthweight badies, particularly African-American ones. Low birthweight accounts for the greatest proportion of perinatal deaths.

Total fertility rate is based on the number of births per woman of childbearing age (15 to 49 years). It represents the average number of children that would be born alive to a woman during her lifetime if she were to pass through all her childbearing years conforming to age-specific fertility rates of a given year. In 1986, the total fertility rate for the United States was 1.8; that is, women in the United States, on average, were having less than two children throughout their childbearing years. During the same year the total fertility rate for Mexico was 4.4; that is, women in Mexico, on average, could expect to have over four children throughout their childbearing years (World Population Data Sheet 1986). Given such a rapid growth in population, it is easy to understand why Mexico might have different priorities for health planning than the United States.

Health Policy Research

As with other types of research, the first step in policy research is to formulate goals. These are expressions of values held by health professional and citizen groups. For example, a value identified by these organizations might be to make prenatal care available to all pregnant women regardless of ability to pay. That value might then become a policy goal. The next step is to review the history of a setting or situation relative to the goal and develop a methodology, identifying research objectives, significant vital events, and affected people. The research is conducted, data collected and analyzed, and findings presented to policy makers.

For example, in 1983, Public Advocates, a group of lawyers in San Francisco and the School of Public Health at the University of California, Berkeley, conducted a survey on the incidence of low birthweight and infant mortality in the United States (Public Advocates 1983). The focus of the survey was the incidence of African-American infant mortality. Data were collected on the relationship of low birthweight to infant morbidity and mortality and the impact of prenatal care on birth outcomes. The failure of current federal policies was identified. Recommendations were to (1) coordinate the fragmented financing system and (2) implement reforms, thus assuring a national commitment to comprehensive prenatal services.

At the same time, the Alameda County Health Care Services Agency was testing a program of comprehensive prenatal care in a community with one of the highest perinatal mortality rates in the nation. With a special grant from the State of California, low income pregnant women were served by 19 public and private prenatal services, including health education, nutrition, nurse midwifery, social work, physician assistant, public health nursing, and traditional physician-directed obstetric care. An important feature of the program was community outreach to bring the women into care. After three years, the high-risk infants served by the program had a lower rate of low birthweight than other high-risk infants in the general county population. The findings showed that low income women will complete prenatal care if given sufficient economic and social support. Cost to Medicaid was only 5% higher than usual prenatal service (Alameda County Health Care Services Agency 1982).

Results of this program were reported to the California State Legislature. Subsequently, legislation was passed funding statewide comprehensive prenatal-to-one-month postpartum services for Medicaid recipients (California State Assembly 1984). The study demonstrates how social policy research can influence services.

Personal Health Services and the Health-care System

Personal health services consist of activities that promote the health of individuals, such as disease detection, treatment, rehabilitation, immunization, and teaching. These activities, together with environmental concerns and health education, make up the broad spectrum of services needed for a healthy population. These services are offered in both public and private settings where federal and state health policies exert influence.

Traditionally, personal health services have been offered by private medical practice in offices and hospitals. In recent years local community health agencies have been called on to provide more and more of these services to an increasing number of individuals. There are several reasons for this change. Many temporarily unemployed persons have too many assets to be eligible for Medicaid, yet they cannot afford private health care. Physicians are not obliged to accept patients, even if the cost is paid by public programs. Underserved and unserved people have no place to turn for personal health care except local agencies. Only people with communicable conditions, such as tuberculosis and sexually transmitted diseases (STDs) receive tax-supported health care.

In an effort to provide personal health services, local health agencies follow varied patterns. Some offer comprehensive care, some provide primary care with referral to specialty care, and some limit services to categorical programs (Miller and Moos 1981). *Comprehensive care* offers a broad range of personal health services, including primary and specialty care, access to consultation, and hospitalization. Costs are covered by public and private funding. *Primary care with referral* to private and public agencies is offered in some rural areas using mobile clinics. In some large cities, storefront clinics provide primary care and patients with further needs are referred to medical centers for specialty care. *Categorical programs* are the only personal health services available in some communities. Such programs include health screening, dental care, special services to children, family planning, and treatment for STDs. People who do not have insurance or private funds may have to rely on tax-supported emergency care for minor illnesses. In these communities health agencies develop relationships with other providers to supplement their limited services.

The financing of personal health service has significantly affected community-health nursing services. Prospective payment DRGs severely limit hospital stays, mandating early discharge. Home visits by nurses focus on secondary prevention rather than primary prevention, because Medicare will not pay for traditional, comprehensive, family-centered health promotion and assessment visits. However, it will pay for in-home services to acutely ill or terminally ill patients and their families.

Financing of personal health services has greatly affected care of hospital patients. Fewer people are hospitalized as a result of cost containment efforts such as prospective payment, peer review, second opinions, increased deductibles, and coinsurance (Arnett et al 1986). Patients who do reach the hospital are acutely ill and in need of sophisticated treatment. Such treatment is expensive, using up scarce health-care dollars. A process for making ethical decisions about who should receive such care has not been developed. Thus, unequal care continues.

In order to increase the availability and affordability of personal health services, legislation has been passed to pay for community health nurses and nurse-sponsored ambulatory care centers with Medicare Part B reimbursement. The American Medical Association opposed this measure, but beginning in 1989, certified nurse anesthetists were paid for their services. Other services soon may qualify for reimbursement (Inglehart 1987).

Future Trends

In the vignette that began this chapter we asked if comprehensive health care was possible in a free market economy. Indeed, the future of the United States health-care system depends on the political and economic climate. The growth of for-profit health care is an important change. Profit-making corporations must have customers to stay in business. Physicians in private practice must have patients. Yet, the number of persons who can afford insurance or pay for private care out-of-pocket is decreasing. Those who are not insured cannot obtain care, except for those receiving government subsidies. The present system is incremental, fragmented, and inequitable. The immediate future for the Nellie Greers of the country is bleak. A social and political consensus to enact a national health-care system has not yet been achieved. However, when the people and the profit-making corporations see a benefit from a comprehensive health-care system, they will exert political pressure and a system will be adopted.

Summary

Health-care systems reflect the political and economic philosophy of the country in which they exist. These systems consist of the resources, functions, controls, and organization necessary to deliver health care. The United States health-care system reflects a free market economy philosophy. Its source of funding is diverse and complicated, made up of both public and private monies. Medicare, a federal-private program, and Medicaid, a federal-state program, are of particular interest to nurses. Large segments of the population are underserved or unserved by the US health-care system. By making policy research findings available to policymakers, some change can be effected.

Learning Activities

1. Obtain a description of the population of your community and identify at least eight health-care resources. In a small group discuss the extent to which the health-care resources in your community appear to be adequate for the population.

2. Obtain a description of a local health department program designed to serve a particular population, such as mothers and infants or the elderly of your community. Evaluate the program asking the following questions: What is the purpose? What data was used to show a need for it? Was the source of the data valid? Are the goals and objectives clearly stated? How does the health department plan to evaluate results of the program?

3. Interview a financial officer of a health facility such as a hospital or ambulatory care center, obtaining the following information: How does the facility implement the DRG method of reimbursement for Medicare patients? What impact have DRGs had on length of stay and cost of care of Medicare patients in your community?

4. Interview a member of the Gray Panthers, an advocacy group for the elderly, asking him or her to discuss access to health care for the elderly in your community.

Annotated Reading List

Arnett RH, McKusick DR, Sonnefeld ST, Cowell CS: Projections of health care spending to 1990. *Health Care Financing Review* 1986; 7: 1–36.

This article explains economic, population, and health profession factors contributing to national health expenditures. It provides a discussion of the way the government projects the cost of health care and explains the growth or decline of various resources such as physicians, dentists, other health professions, drugs, medical supplies, hospitals, nursing homes, health insurance, and public health services.

Fein R: *Medical Care, Medical Costs: The Search for a Health Insurance Policy.* Harvard University Press, 1986.

This leading health economist reviews the history of health care payment systems in the United States from the growth of private and government health insurance to the present. The strengths and limitations of each payment scheme are clearly presented. This report helps readers understand more about the inequities in access to appropriate health care among the citizens.

Harris R: *A Sacred Trust.* New American Library, 1983.

In this work, Richard Harris, a distinguished writer and reporter, traces the progress of Medicare through Congress. It is an excellent introduction to political lobbying and the influence of special interest groups on the health-care policy of the United States. He presents the American Medical Association position on national health insurance.

Last JM (editor): *Maxcy-Rosenau Public Health and Preventive Medicine,* 12th ed. Appleton-Century-Croft, 1986.

This classic text on the maintenance of health and prevention of disease was first published in 1913. The twelfth edition is noteworthy for its expanded coverage of health care planning, organization, and evaluation, co-edited by Joyce C. Lashof, MD, MPH, Dean and Professor of Public Health, University of California, School of Public Health, Berkeley. The book gives a history of the development of the United States health-care system. Social and political forces influencing the system are presented and compared to health-care systems in other countries.

Mundinger MO: *Home Care Controversy.* Aspen Systems, 1983.

The focus of this excellent policy analysis is the impact of Medicare on community health nursing in the home. Vignettes of nurse-patient-family interactions are used to convey the complexities of planning care of the elderly under Medicare and the DRG cost-reduction plan. The history of Medicare legislation is reviewed. This analysis is especially useful for nurses preparing to observe or deliver health care in the home.

References

Alameda County Health Care Services Agency: *Report of Prenatal Women and Infants Enrolled in the Oakland Perinatal Health Project and the Obstetrical Access Program,* 1982.

American Nurses' Association: *Standards of Practice for the Primary Health Care Nurse Practitioner.* ANA, 1987.

American Public Health Association: Publications '85. APHA, 1985.

Arnett RH, McKusick DR, Sonnefeld ST, Cowell CS: Projections of health care spending to 1990. *Health Care Financing Review* 1986; 7:1–36.

Blum HC: *Planning for Health.* Human Science Press, 1981.

California State Assembly: Bill 3021, 1984.

Center for Disease Control Division of Injury Epidemiology and Control, Center for Environmental Health: *1986 Annual Report*. Department of Health and Human Services, 1986.

Children's Defense Fund: *A Children's Defense Budget: FY 1988,* p 71. The Children's Defense Fund, 1987.

Clemen-Stone S, Eigsti DG, McGuire SL: *Comprehensive Family and Community Health Nursing,* 2nd ed. McGraw-Hill, 1987.

Fein R: *Medical Care, Medical Costs: The Search for a Health Insurance Policy.* Harvard University Press, 1986.

General Accounting Office, United States: *Maternal and Child Health Block Grant: Program Changes Emerging Under State Administration.* GAO/HRD-84-35, May 7, 1984.

Gruenberg EM: Mental disorders. In: *Maxcy-Rosenau Public Health and Preventive Medicine,* 12th ed., Last JM (editor), pp 1341–1384. Appleton-Century-Croft, 1986.

Harris R: *A Sacred Trust.* The New American Library, 1966.

Henderson V, Nite G (editors): *Principles and Practice of Nursing.* Mac-Millan, 1978.

Inglehart JK: Problems facing the nursing profession. *N Engl J Med* 1987; 317:646–651.

Jonas S: Provision of public health services. In: *Maxcy-Rosenau Public Health and Preventive Medicine,* 12th ed., Last JM (editor), pp 1621–1638. Appleton-Century-Croft, 1986.

Kendellen R: The medical malpractice insurance crisis: An overview of the issues. *Journal of Nurse Midwifery* 1987; 32:4–10.

LoGerfo JP, Brook RH: The quality of health care. In: *Introduction to Health Services,* 2nd ed., Williams SJ, Torrens PR (editors), pp 403–432. Wiley, 1984.

McKibbon RC, Brimmer PF, Clinton JF, Galliher LM, Hartley S: *DRG's and Nursing.* ANA, 1985.

Miller CA, Moos MK: *Local Health Departments: 15 Case Studies.* The American Public Health Association, 1981.

Mundinger MO: *Home Care Controversy.* Aspen Systems, 1983.

Myers BA: Social policy and the organization of health care. In: *Maxcy-Rosenau Public Health and Preventive Medicine,* 12th ed., Last JM (editor), pp 1639–1667. Appleton-Century-Croft, 1986.

National Center for Health Statistics Services, Public Health Service:

Health and Prevention Profile, United States, 1984. (DHHS Publication No. PHS 84-1232), pp 207–216. US Government Printing Office, Dec 1983.

Office of the Federal Register, National Archives and Records Administration: *The United States Government Manual, 1988/1989.* US Government Printing Office, 1989.

Public Advocates: *Administrative Petition to Reduce the Incidence of Low Birth Weight and Resultant Infant Mortality.* Public Advocates, San Francisco, CA, 1983.

Roemer MI: Comparative health care systems. In: *Maxcy-Rosenau Public Health and Preventive Medicine,* 12th ed., Last JM (editor), pp 1747–1792. Appleton-Century-Croft, 1986.

Schultz DS, Rafferty MP: Soviet health care and perestroika. *American Journal of Public Health* 1990; 80 : 193–195.

Shonick W: Health planning. In: *Maxcy-Rosenau Public Health and Preventive Medicine,* 12th ed., Last JM (editor), pp 1669–1688. Appleton-Century-Croft, 1986.

Styles MM: *Credentialing in Nursing: U.S.A. within a World View.* ANA, 1986.

US Census Bureau: *Statistical Abstract of the United States,* 105th ed. US Government Printing Office, 1985.

Williams CD, Baumslag N, Jelliffe D: *Mother and Child Health: Delivering the Services,* 2nd ed. Oxford University Press, 1985.

World Population Data Sheet of the Population Reference Bureau, Inc. Population Reference Bureau, 1980.

World Population Data Sheet of the Population Reference Bureau, Inc. Population Reference Bureau, 1986.

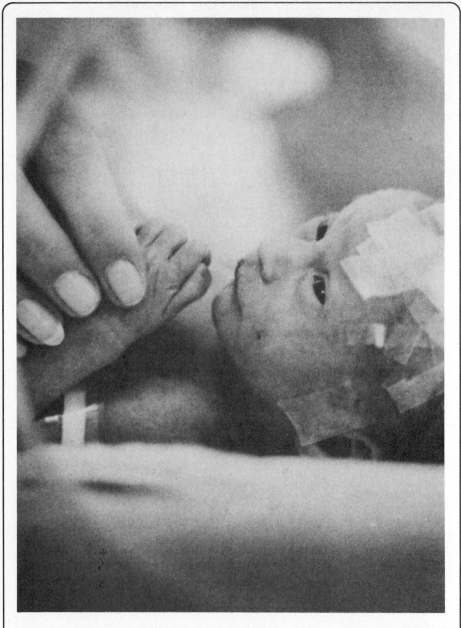

Born at the gestational age of 23 weeks, this baby has less than a 50% chance for survival. Even so, the medical costs will be more than most people earn in a life-time. Can society justify these costs? (Copyright San Francisco Examiner)

CHAPTER 6

―――――― ∾ ――――――

Ethical Concerns

LEARNING OBJECTIVES

1. Discuss the types, functions, acquisition, and importance of values.

2. Describe some value clarification strategies and apply the process to a nursing situation.

3. Explain how belief systems develop and how they influence health care.

4. Compare the Piaget and Kohlberg stages of moral development.

5. Discuss the Kohlberg stages of moral development as they apply to the behavior of nurses.

6. Compare deontological and teleological ethical theories and give real-life examples of how they may affect the ethical decisions of nurses.

7. Discuss the difference between personal ethics and ethical codes.

8. Explain the ethical principles of autonomy, nonmaleficence, beneficence, veracity, confidentiality, accountability, and justice, giving examples of how each applies in nursing practice.

9. Apply the decision-making process to a real-life ethical dilemma, showing how the dilemma can be resolved.

Jamie *was a beautiful 3-year-old. She was bright, well-behaved, and much loved by her parents and 11-year-old brother. She delighted in going to the ocean, wading along the shore, and feeling the sand move under her toes as the waves rolled in and out on the beach. Her brother was permitted to go out to where the waves were high and the current swift because he knew how to swim. One afternoon, when her mother was distracted by a conversation, Jamie followed her brother out into the deeper water. A huge wave caught her and swept her under, but no one missed her for some time. When they did, it took nearly 30 minutes to find her. The EMTs finally got Jamie's heart started, connected her to a mechanical ventilator, started intravenous fluids and took her to the emergency room. Jamie never regained consciousness. Eventually, she was weaned from the ventilator. The intravenous tubes were replaced by a feeding tube and she was transferred to a long-term care facility.*

Now Jamie lies in a bed on the total care unit, unresponsive except to painful stimuli. Her care costs $1200/month. When she develops penumonia, which is often, Jamie is taken to the acute hospital where the cost is $800/day. Her parents have exhausted their financial resources. Unable to "give up hope," they remain in a constant state of grief and guilt.

In the same community homeless children live in squalor, inadequately clothed and fed and chronically ill. Is Jamie's care an appropriate use of public money? Should her life be maintained at all costs? If not, how much cost? Who should decide?

A few years ago, medicine knew no way to prolong life. The primary task of nurses and physicians was to support the sick until they healed or to comfort them until they died. There were no weighty decisions about who should live and who should die. Even when they desperately wanted to, no one had the power to change the course of nature.

Gradually at first, and then at an ever-increasing rate, scientific knowledge expanded. Medicine gained greater and greater control over disease and death. Treatments and drugs were discovered that changed the course of nature. Where once it was impossible to sustain life functions for even brief periods, now it was possible to maintain them for years. These advances have brought hope and life, but they have created profound problems. Is the mere presence of a heart beat the sole criterion for sustaining it? What about the person in whom that heart beats? What about the *quality* of life as opposed to its mere presence, the *quantity* of life? What criteria should be used when resources are scarce and needs are great?

To help resolve some of these questions health professionals turn to *ethics,* that branch of philosophy that deals with the evaluation of human behavior. The result is a field of study called *bioethics,* the moral and social implications of medicine and science upon human life. Some of the concepts encompassed in bioethics are values, belief systems, and ethics.

Values

Values are perceptions of worth that people place on objects, attitudes, ideas, and attributes. They are part of a person's innermost being. They are general guides to behavior or standards of conduct that people hold and demonstrate by the choices they make. Values provide a frame of reference through which people integrate, explain, and appraise ideas, events, and personal relationships.

A *value system* is a set of values such as autonomy and accountability, even though the system may not be internally consistent. For example, a father of adult children may value autonomy for himself, but deny it to his children by insisting they conform to his standards of conduct.

Types of Values

Values have been categorized in many ways according to the way they are viewed or used. *Intrinsic values,* according to Steele and Harmon (1983), are related to the maintenance of life. Food and water are intrinsically valuable because they are essential for life. *Extrinsic values* originate outside the individual and are not essential for life. People, things, and concepts, such as loyalty, kindness, health, family, and personal possessions, are extrinsically valuable and not vital to life.

Personal values are attributes that individuals hold valuable in their private lives, such as independence and recognition. *Professional values* are attributes that are prized by a professional group. For example, creativity is highly valued by architects, obedience by military officers, and empathy by nurses. *Cultural-societal-religious values* are values that are unique to a culture, society, or religion. For example, stoicism, or the ability to bear pain without complaint, was a cultural-societal value of the Stoics of ancient Greece. Altruism is a value of the Jewish, Christian, and Muslim religions. *Terminal values* are concerned with end states or goals such as world peace, happiness, and career success. *Instrumental values* involve desirable modes of conduct such as honesty, kindness, and loyalty (Rokeach 1973).

Functions of Values

Values serve many useful functions. They provide standards by which people judge others. For example, when people who value kindness see a parent hurting a helpless child, they appraise that parent as cruel, a perpetrator of child abuse.

Values reflect personal identity. People incorporate the values of those with whom they identify. For example, student nurses assimilate the professional values of cleanliness and efficiency and incorporate those values into themselves.

Values furnish a basis on which to make decisions. For example, a 92-year-old woman refused to move into a residential care facility even though she was nearly blind from glaucoma and crippled with arthritis. She valued independence highly and insisted she would not live in an "old people's home." Her decision was based on her value of personal independence. Her granddaughter visited her daily, although it was a great burden. When the home health nurse explained how difficult it was for the granddaughter to visit so often, the woman agreed to move to a residential care facility. Her second decision was based on another value: consideration of others.

Values give meaning to life. They fulfill the need for self-esteem and promote self-actualization. Values involve a search for meaning and a desire for understanding of the universe and one's place in it. People find fulfillment in acting to promote the things they value, such as world peace and great music. When people promote such values they experience personal satisfaction.

Values motivate behavior. Because of their values, people make sacrifices, take risks, and generate extraordinary effort. Parents may sacrifice to provide children with private schooling because they value education. Athletes may risk serious injury because they value fame. Disabled persons may overcome great obstacles because they value the mobility or recognition such attainment represents.

Values lead people to make "ought" and "should" demands on themselves, no matter what the cost. For example, Martha grew up in a professional family of high achievers and incorporated that value into her life, even though she was not gifted. As a result Martha worked exceptionally hard at school and studied more than others. When she earned less than perfect scores she felt she had failed. By the time she was 25 years old Martha had developed an ulcer from her constant effort to meet inner demands.

Acquisition of Values

Values are not inherited. They are acquired by observation, reasoning, and experience. They are taught by modeling and moralizing and they are influenced by intellectual development.

Initially, values are learned in childhood as boys and girls are socialized into the family, school, church, and other social groups. Values are demonstrated (modeled) by parents and others and are deliberately taught (moralized about). As children observe such modeling and listen to such admonitions, they internalize values, claiming them as their own. Karen's father was a military officer who valued self-discipline and respect for authority. He both modeled and taught those values to his children. As a result, Karen incorporated her father's values into her own value system. She now is quite comfortable working in a position of authority within a rigid corporate structure.

The values of children are influenced by their intellectual and emotional development. Young children value concrete objects such as toys or favorite blankets. Older children value activities and objects appropriate to their development. Adolescents value peer approval more than family approval or personal comfort. Young adults value idealized abstractions such as dedication and loyalty. The values of adults are more likely influenced by life experiences and reasoned choices.

Importance of Values

While the number of values a person holds may be relatively small, their importance is great. Values influence the choices people make, the way they use their time, spend their money, expend their energy, who they choose as friends, what they aspire to become, and what gives them pleasure and self-actualization. Verbal and nonverbal behaviors reveal values, even though those values may not be recognized or acknowledged by the individual.

Values Clarification

Because values are so important, nurses in particular need to become aware of their own values. The process of gaining this knowledge is called *values clarification*. Values clarification helps nurses act in ways that are consistent with their values. It helps them make decisions, solve problems, and establish more effective relationships with patients and peers. Values clarification helps nurses integrate personal values and professional nursing values.

A variety of strategies have been developed to help people identify values, including voting, sentence completion, and rank ordering (see Tables 6-1, 6-2, and 6-3).

⚄ *Table 6-1*

Values Clarification Strategy: Voting

Indicate if you: (1) strongly agree, (2) agree, (3) don't care, (4) disagree, (5) strongly disagree

1. _____ Women should have the right to have an abortion on demand.
2. _____ Parents should have the right to discipline their children in any way they see fit.
3. _____ Euthanasia is wrong in all circumstances.
4. _____ Mentally retarded people should be sterilized.
5. _____ People should have the right to purchase any drug without a prescription.
6. _____ Life should be sustained at all cost, regardless of mental status.
7. _____ The death penalty as a method of punishment is archaic and should be eliminated from all statute books.

⚄ *Table 6-2*

Values Clarification Strategy: Sentence Completion

1. If I had only six months to live I would . . .
2. If I won three million dollars I would . . .
3. If I had a twelve-month paid vacation I would . . .
4. If I were president of the United States I would . . .
5. If I wrote my epitaph it would say . . .

⁵⁾ *Table 6-3*

<hr>

Values Clarification Strategy: Rank Ordering

Within each group of questions, rank your choices from 1 to 4, with 1 the highest priority and 4 the lowest priority.

1. With limited medical resources, which of the following patients should be given care?

_____ Premature infants weighing less than 2 pounds at birth

_____ Antepartal patients with complications of pregnancy

_____ Men, ages 40–50, with acute myocardial infarcts

_____ Women, ages 75–85, with crippling osteoarthritis

2. You are assigned to a patient with cirrhosis of the liver. Rank the things you should do for her:

_____ Explain the effects her drinking has on her liver

_____ Make her as physically confortable as you can

_____ Encourage her to talk about her feelings

_____ Allow her to make decisions about her care

<hr>

The Valuing Process

Values clarification is concerned with the process of valuing. In 1966 Raths, Harmin, and Simmons (1979) proposed a process for values clarification. It provides a means for people to sort out, analyze, and set priorities for their own values. The seven-step process is divided into three elements, as follows:

I. Choosing
  1. Choosing freely
  2. Selecting from alternatives
  3. Choosing after consideration of the consequences of each alternative

II. Prizing
  4. Being proud of and happy with the choice
  5. Being willing to affirm the choice publicly

III. Acting
  6. Making the choice part of one's behavior
  7. Repeating the choice

Application of the Process

John had a secure position at the state hospital as a licensed psychiatric technician when he enrolled in an associate degree nursing program at the community college. He continued to work at the state hospital part time. When John graduated, the hospital offered him a charge position. His family lives nearby, as does his girlfriend, and he values their support and closeness. However, since he has become an RN many other career options have opened to him. He uses the values clarification process to make a choice about his career.

CHOOSING

(1) John considers the many values he holds, including: personal, financial, and professional security; carefreeness; independence; challenge; adventure; and educational achievement. He realizes he cannot have all of these things at this time and must choose between them.

(2) John selects those values he holds highest from among the many. He decides that he most values independence, challenge, educational achievement, and financial and professional security.

(3) John considers carefully the consequences of his choices. If he chooses security he will return to the state hospital where he will be professionally comfortable and financially secure. If he chooses challenge, adventure, and educational achievement he will go on for an advanced degree and become a nurse practitioner, but it will mean many years of hard work, financial sacrifice, moving to a large city away from his family and friends, and taking a part-time job in a new and unfamiliar hospital. John chooses challenge, adventure, and educational achievement.

PRIZING

(4) John is proud and happy about his choice. He feels a sense of joy as he considers his decision.

(5) John affirms his choice publicly by announcing his decision to his classmates and his supervisor at the state hospital.

ACTING

(6) John makes the choice part of his behavior by sending for information about various BSN and MSN nurse practitioner programs and by beginning to look for a nursing position in the city.

(7) John confirms his choice of action, or repeats it, by applying for entrance into a BSN/MSN program; he goes for job interviews and looks for an apartment near the university.

Belief Systems and Religions

Belief systems are organized schemes of thought regarding the origin, cause, purpose, and place of humans in the universe. They seek to explain the mysteries of life and death, good and evil, health and illness. Typically, these systems include ethical codes that prescribe correct conduct. People may have a personal belief system or they may subscribe to a religion that includes a belief system, devotional rituals, and organizational structure.

Many sociologists believe that religions develop because humans feel the need to control the forces of nature and bring order (cosmos) out of disorder (chaos). Durkheim (1915) said that religion is an effort of humans to "pass science and complete it prematurely in an effort to keep the experience of chaos within limits that humans can sustain." Joachim Wach (1944) noted that "all religions, despite their difference, are characterized by systems of worship, belief, and organization." Religions often include ethical codes to regulate social order, especially within families. Such codes regulate sexual behavior, socialization of children, sexual roles, support for weak or aged persons, ownership of property, inheritance, and commerce.

Belief systems are no less important to people now than they were before the advent of the scientific method. They give meaning to life and provide a framework by which people order their lives. They assist people to cope with feelings of powerlessness and meaninglessness in the face of injustice and suffering. Ethical codes of these systems provide people with standards of behavior by which they measure right and wrong conduct. Belief systems give identity and importance to people. They may provide comfort to believers who are ill or grieving. Thus, nurses need to acknowledge the significance and value of belief systems.

Ethics

Ethics is the branch of philosophy concerned with the rightness or wrongness of human behavior and the goodness or badness of the motives behind it. Ethics implies that a decision about behavior must be made. It is a subject that has fascinated people for centuries, one that has produced an enormous body of writing. From these writings, three general schools of thought have evolved: descriptive ethics, metaethics, and normative ethics.

Descriptive ethics concerns itself with descriptions of how people behave. *Metaethics* analyzes language about moral concepts, seeking to know the meaning of words. *Normative ethics* raises questions about what is good, what is right, and how to decide. It analyzes, evaluates, and develops standards for dealing with moral problems. Normative ethics affirms that ethical decisions about moral problems may be made from a mode of reasoning represented by two basic ethical theories: teleological and deontological.

Teleological theories are theories of end results or consequences (from the Greek *teleios,* meaning "end"). They assert that the rightness or wrongness of an action can be determined by its end results. Therefore, in order to determine if an action is ethically right, the probable results of one action are compared with the probable results of another action. The action that produces the greater good is chosen. The central proposition of these theories is "the greatest good" principle. Aristotle's teachings and Fletcher's situational ethics are teleological theories. They place love above law. Teleological theories reject fixed moral rules and principles. End results and context are key factors. They seek to foster morality by developing the capacity of people to make the best choice.

Deontological theories are theories of duty or obligation to fixed laws (from the Greek *deontos,* meaning "duty"). They assert that certain kinds of actions are inherently right or wrong as a matter of principle, regardless of end results. For example, they affirm that an act, such as divorce or birth control, is wrong because it is proscribed by civil or church law. Laws and rules are key factors. Deontological theories seek to foster morality by controlling the right of people to make choices.

For example, a woman has five children and is physically and emotionally exhausted. Her husband is unemployed and a heavy drinker. Following end results (situational) ethics, she may decide for the sake of her children and herself to have a tubal ligation to prevent further pregnancies. If she follows duty (legalistic) ethics, she may decide for the sake of obedience to church teachings to do nothing, hoping she will not become pregnant again and that if she does she will be able to cope.

Bioethics

Bioethics is the application of morals to matters of life and death. Bioethics implies that a judgment should be made about the rightness or goodness of a given medical or scientific practice as it relates to human life. The term bioethics is used when life is involved. The term ethics is used when other areas, such as politics or economics are involved. Health professionals have concerns in both areas.

Ethics and Morals

Although some authors use the word "ethics" to refer to standardized codes and "morals" to refer to common practices, both words mean habits or customs (ethics from the greek word *ethos* and morals from the Latin word *mores*). They are used interchangeably to mean accepted standards of honorable behavior, goodness, and virtue.

The Nature of Virtue

Historical records tell that Socrates was asked how virtue was acquired. He replied, "You must think I am very fortunate to know how virtue is acquired. The fact is that, far from knowing whether it can be taught, I have no idea what virtue is." His reply makes clear that the fundamental question is not how to teach virtue, but to know what the nature of virtue or goodness might be. Philosophers and scholars have sought answers to this question for centuries.

Piaget

Perhaps the first scientific attempt to answer the question, "What is good?" was made by Piaget through his studies of human intellectual development. He deduced that, since an understanding of what is "good" requires the intellect, then an understanding will develop and change as the intellect develops. Piaget postulated that there were two stages of moral development that must follow the initial stage of concrete action in young children. They are: (1) rigid judgment based on edicts of external authority and (2) relativistic agreement to principles obtained from social contacts (Piaget 1985). The first is characterized by a mother saying, "You are a bad girl because you disobeyed me." The second stage is characterized by a child saying, "He is a bad boy because he is a tattletale."

Kohlberg

Kohlberg and his associates at Harvard University built on the work of Piaget. They focused their research on the questions: "Does what is good continue to change with intellectual development? If so what are those stages?"

The Harvard study found that there is a parallel between the stages of intellectual development described by Piaget and the stages of moral development they identified. However, they found that some people attain much higher stages of moral development than Piaget described and some people never move beyond the lowest ones. They identified six stages of moral development, which they grouped under Piaget's preoperational, concrete operations, and formal operations stages of intellectual development (Kohlberg 1973). People who have reached the highest level of moral development base their conduct on abstract principles of right and wrong such as the Golden Rule rather than on concrete laws like the Ten Commandments. (See Table 6-4.)

Table 6-4

Kohlberg's Stages of Moral Development

Level I: Preconventional
(Piaget's stage of preoperational thought, in which a child begins to recognize relationships)

Person recognizes power of someone to enforce rules by physical force

Stage 1: Punishment and obedience
What is right: Actions that avoid punishment. Obedience for its own sake.
Reason for doing right: To avoid punishment.
Social perspective: Egocentric viewpoint. Actions are considered in physical rather than psychologic terms. Confuses perspective of authority with the self.

Stage 2: Individualism; instrumental-relativist
What is right: Actions that satisfy one's needs and sometimes the needs of others. What is fair or agreed upon.
Reason for doing right: To serve one's needs in a world where one may have to recognize the needs of others.
Social perspective: Concrete individualistic. Aware that people have their own interests to pursue.

Level II: Conventional
(Piaget's stage of concrete operations, in which a child begins to think logically, especially about concrete events)

Person maintains expectations of the self and the immediate group without regard for consequences. Conforms, and is loyal to, existing enforcers of social order.

Stage 3: Interpersonal conformity
What is right: Action that conforms to the society's expectations of person's given role, showing loyalty, gratitude, and trust.
Reason for doing right: To be a good person in one's own eyes and in the eyes of others.
Social perspective: Perspective of individual in relationship to others. Able to put the self in someone else's shoes, but not yet able to consider multiple relationships.

Stage 4: Social system and conscience; law and order
What is right: Actions that fulfill agreed upon duties and keep the system going. Laws are to be obeyed except in extreme cases where they conflict with other fixed social duties.
Reason for doing right: To keep the institutions going. To avoid breaking down the system by not meeting obligations. The imperative of conscience.
Social perspective: Viewpoint of a system that defines rules and roles. Considers individual relations in terms of their place in the system.

Level III: Postconventional, Principled
(Piaget's stage of formal operations, in which child is able to think abstractly)

Person tries to define moral values and principles apart from identity with the existing authority.

Table 6-4 (continued)

Kohlberg's Stages of Moral Development

Stage 5: Utility and individual rights; social contract, legalistic
What is right: Being aware that people hold a variety of values and that these are relative. Usually upholds these relative rules in the interest of impartiality because they are a social contract. However, holds nonrelative values, such as life and liberty, regardless of majority opinion.
Reason for doing right: To fulfill one's obligation to law because of the societal contract to do so for the welfare of all people's rights. To provide the "greatest good for the greatest number."
Social perspective: Viewpoint of a rational individual aware of values and rights prior to social attachments and contracts. Considers moral and legal points of view and recognizes that they sometimes conflict. Finds it difficult to integrate them.

Stage 6: Universal ethical principles
What is right: Following self-chosen ethical principles that are based on universality and consistency. Principles are abstract rather than concrete and include justice, reciprocity, equality of human rights, and respect for the dignity of humans as individuals.
Reason for doing right: To fulfill one's personal commitment and belief in the validity of universal moral principles.
Social perspective: Viewpoint of a rational individual who recognizes that persons are ends in themselves and must be treated as such, that social arrangements derive from a moral perspective.

Adapted from Kohlberg L: Implications of developmental psychology for education: Examples from moral development. *Educational Psychologist* 1973; 10:2–14.

Ethical Principles

Ethical principles are fundamental concepts by which behavior can be judged. They help people make ethical decisions because they serve as criteria with which to measure actions. Laws flow from ethical principles, but they are limited to exact circumstances. Laws are rules made by governing authorities that operate because the authority has power to enforce them. Ethical principles, on the other hand, operate at a much higher level than laws. They are not bound by detailed rules and they take into account specific conditions. Ethical principles speak to the "spirit" of a law, rather than the "letter." However, decisions are sometimes complicated by the existence of more than one ethical principle. Some of the important principles that form the basis for ethical decisions of health-care providers are autonomy, justice, nonmaleficence, beneficence, confidentiality, veracity, and accountability.

Autonomy

Autonomy is the right of self-determination, independence, and freedom. Smith (1985) said that autonomy is the "ability to absorb information, comprehend it, make a choice, and carry out that choice." The ethical principle of autonomy requires respect for the right of others to make decisions about themselves. Nurses implement this principle by providing information to patients, assisting them to understand information, and either carrying out patients' choices or making sure that no one interferes with their ability to carry out their decision.

The principle of autonomy requires that health-care providers respect a patient's choice even when they disagree with it. Nurses may not substitute their will for a patient's choice. However, they may interfere if they believe a person does not have sufficient information, capacity to understand, or is being coerced. Once it is determined that a patient's decision is informed and freely made, nurses must allow that person to carry out the decision. Nurses have no duty to assist people to carry out harmful decisions, nor are they required to allow patients to harm themselves in a health-care facility.

Mrs. Hansen, an 84-year-old woman, was diagnosed as having a stage II carcinoma of the breast. Her physician explained that treatment would consist of a lumpectomy followed by radiation and chemotherapy. On the day before her scheduled surgery Mrs. Hansen phoned the office nurse to say that she had decided to cancel the surgery, radiation, and chemotherapy. The nurse explained the need for the planned therapies and likely consequences if they were not carried out. Mrs. Hansen replied, "I understand, but I have decided I do not want to suffer all that misery and expense. I have lived a good life and I am ready to die." According to the ethical principle of autonomy, health-care providers cannot force Mrs. Hansen to submit to treatment. The nurse determined that Mrs. Hansen understood the consequences of her decision and that she was making it freely, without coercion. Health-care providers must respect her choice, even though it may not be the one they recommend.

Nonmaleficence

The principle of nonmaleficence requires that health-care providers not harm others intentionally or unintentionally, and further, that they protect from harm those who cannot protect themselves due to age, illness, or mental state.

Nurses care for many developmentally and mentally disabled persons who are vulnerable and unable to protect themselves, such as Jamie in the vignette. Because of the special trust placed in them, nurses are ethically bound to protect these patients from all kinds of harm, including personal illness, environmental hazards, chemical or emotional impairment, and any person who might hurt them.

Jan and Phillip worked evenings in the emergency room. The narcotic count had been short on several occasions during the prior two months. One evening Jan acted "spacey" and when Phillip commented about it she became defensive. He noticed that when Jan administered pain medications, often the pain was not relieved. Phillip did not want to think that Jan might be stealing narcotics from patients for herself, but on the basis of the ethical principle of nonmaleficence he decided he must take action. He watched Jan closely and observed that instead of giving the Demerol she signed out to patients, Jan pocketed it. Phillip reported the matter to his supervisor and they confronted Jan with the evidence. Jan admitted her narcotic dependency and agreed to enter a drug rehabilitation program.

Jan violated the principle of nonmaleficence by taking the pain-relieving medication of patients and by working when her judgment was impaired by drugs. She broke the law as well. Phillip could have remained silent, but he would have violated the principle of nonmaleficence by not taking action to stop the harm that was being done to patients.

Beneficence

The principle of beneficence requires that nurses do good to benefit others. This means more than providing technically competent care. It means meeting basic human needs for survival, security, belonging, recognition, and self-actualization to a degree that demonstrates caring. Beneficence means giving that extra nurturance that makes the difference, such as providing emotional support to Jamie's family.

Beneficence has been interpreted by some health-care providers as protecting competent persons who really could protect and care for themselves. In the name of beneficence these people withhold a diagnosis or the name or actions of a medication. By so doing, they violate the principle of autonomy.

José Perez, a Hispanic laborer, was hospitalized and isolated because of a staphylococcal infection in a leg wound. He spoke little English, seldom looked at television, and had no visitors. Sally noticed how lonely he seemed as he silently stared out the window day after day. She asked a Spanish-speaking nurse to explain the reason for isolation and the treatment plan. The next day she brought José some Spanish language magazines and asked the maintenance department for a portable radio so that he could listen to a Latino station. By doing these things Sally went beyond technical competency and demonstrated beneficence.

Justice

The ethical principle of justice requires that nurses treat every person equally, regardless of race, sex, marital status, diagnosis, social standing, economic status, religion, or anything else. Justice requires that supervisors apply the same criteria of performance for every member of the nursing team. It requires that work assignments, holidays, and opportunities for advancement are equal. Where management is concerned, perhaps no ethical principle is more important, because injustice undermines trust, creates hatred and disrespect, and destroys initiative.

All the beds in the intensive care unit were full. The emergency room called to report that a severely injured person was being sent to surgery and would need to be admitted to the intensive care unit after surgery. Manuel, the intensive care supervisor, had to make room for the patient. After consulting with the staff and considering the status of each patient, he decided to move a cardiac patient to the step-down unit. Justice demanded equal treatment for all patients. Nonmaleficence helped determine which patient might be least harmed by the transfer.

Confidentiality

The principle of confidentiality requires that nurses hold in strictest confidence information they have learned as a result of their special relationship to patients. The only exceptions are when patients give express permission to release confidential information or when the law dictates release of certain data, such as evidence of possible child abuse. Restricted information includes such data as names, diagnoses, ages, laboratory tests, and surgical procedures. The principle of confidentiality arises from the concepts of loyalty and respect for those who place their trust in caregivers. Revealing information is like stealing personal property and giving it away.

Larry, a manufacturer's representative, was admitted to the hospital with a diagnosis of pneumocystis carinii penumonia, an "opportunistic disease" common in persons with acquired immune deficiency syndrome (AIDS). Jean took care of Larry during the morning shift. In the evening she told her husband, Bill, that she cared for an AIDS patient with pneumonia who had just come back from Africa. She was careful not to mention the patient's name, thinking she was protecting his privacy. Bill was worried for his wife's safety and shared his concern with a co-worker. The co-worker had a neighbor who had just returned from Africa and was hospitalized for pneumonia. Before long, the employer learned of the diagnosis and fired Larry. Jean meant no harm. In fact, she had not mentioned the patient's name. Yet she damaged a man's reputation and violated the ethical principle of confidentiality. She also opened herself to a potential lawsuit for defamation of character.

Veracity (Truthfulness)

The principle of veracity requires that nurses tell the truth and not intentionally deceive or mislead. Deception can occur by deliberate lying or by omitting part or all of the truth. People who subscribe to the deontological theory of ethics say truthfulness is an absolute imperative and lying is always wrong. Those who follow the teleological theory of ethics say that deception is sometimes permissible if another ethical principle overrides that of truthfulness. The principles most often cited as justifying deception are nonmaleficence and beneficence. Then the lie is called "benevolent deception" because it is intended to prevent harm and promote good.

Tommy, age 9, was hospitalized for observation of a concussion following an auto accident in which both of his parents were killed. He kept asking for his mom and dad. The nurses were in a quandary as to what they should tell him. If they told him the truth they would risk an increase in intracranial pressure as a result of emotional distress. If they made up a story to explain why his parents did not come they would be violating the ethical principle of veracity in order to follow the principle of beneficence, a "benevolent deception." At a staff discussion they decided the benefits of temporary deceit outweighed the harm of truth. They told Tommy that his mom and dad were in another unit. After a while he could go to see them.

Accountability

The principle of accountability requires that nurses accept responsibility for their actions and be answerable to their patients for their professional conduct. From this ethical principle issues the concept of "standard of care," which provides criteria to measure nursing action and serves as a basis for establishing legal negligence. The ethical principle, however, goes beyond legal responsibility. It means that once people take responsibility to do something, they follow through, even though it is inconvenient.

The law does not require bystanders to rescue strangers, but once a rescue has begun, rescuers have a duty to continue to give aid as long as they can. Such a duty is required because others may leave the scene, thinking their help is no longer needed.

Cora had been working since 7:00 AM on a busy orthopedic unit. It was almost 3:30 PM and she was rushing to complete all the last-minute things that had to be done before reporting off. Suddenly, she remembered her promise to Mrs. Young to telephone her daughter to request that she bring a special robe. Cora could have "forgotten" her promise, but after she completed her work she made the call. She would not have been negligent in a legal sense had she failed to keep her commitment, but she would have violated the ethical principle of accountability.

Codes of Ethics

A code of ethics is a formal statement that sets standards of ethical behavior for a group of people. One of the hallmarks of a profession is that it has a code of ethics that spells out what constitutes ethical behavior for its members.

Codes of ethics emphasize ethical principles that particularly apply to the group of people who create them. For example, the code of ethics of manufacturers emphasizes the principle of confidentiality as it applies to respect for trade secrets of manufacturers. The code of ethics for nurses emphasizes the principle of confidentiality as it applies to respect for the privacy of patients.

Ever-changing and evolving, codes of ethics reflect the values of the profession and society at the time they are written. These changes are evidenced in the codes of physicians, nurses, and other health-care providers.

Physicians

An early effort to control ethical behavior among those who care for the sick is found in the Hippocratic Oath (470–360 BC). The American Medical Association adopted its first code of ethics in 1847. Since then, it has updated the code six times, most recently in 1980.

Nurses

The first generally accepted code of ethics for modern nurses was written in 1893 by Lystra Gretter, Superintendent of the Farrand Training School, Detroit, Michigan. She patterned the code after the Hippocratic Oath of medicine, and named it The Florence Nightingale Pledge (see Table 6-5). This pledge, or one of its many modified versions, is still heard at many nursing completion ceremonies.

⚑ Table 6-5

The Florence Nightingale Pledge

I solemnly pledge myself before God and in the presence of this assembly to pass my life in purity and to practice my profession faithfully.

I will abstain from whatever is deleterious and mischievous and will not take or knowingly administer any harmful drug.

I will do all in my power to maintain and elevate the standard of my profession and will hold in confidence all personal matters committed to my keeping and family affairs coming to my knowledge in the practice of my calling. With loyalty I will endeavor to aid the physician in his work, and devote myself to the welfare of those committed to my care.

Written in 1893, in honor of Florence Nightingale by Lystra Gretter, Superintendent of the Farrand Training School, Detroit, Michigan.

AMERICAN NURSES' ASSOCIATION.   In 1926, the American Nurses' Association (ANA) provisionally adopted and published a code of ethics entitled "A Suggested Code" in the *American Journal of Nursing*. Written in the nonspecific style of the nineteenth century, the code was not ratified by the membership. In 1940, the "Suggested Code" of 1926 was replaced by "A Tentative Code," reformulated in 1949, and adopted in 1950. It consists of a preamble and seventeen provisions. The first major revision of the 1950 code was ratified in 1960. In 1968, the term "professional" was omitted from the title to indicate it applied to both technical and professional nurses, the preamble was dropped, and the number of provisions reduced to ten. The 1968 version omitted reference to the "personal ethics" (moral character) of nurses, and focused on professional ethics.

The 1976 revision updated the wording, but maintained the same ethical principles of earlier codes. While the 1940 code disavowed discrimination on the basis of creed, nationality, or race, the 1976 version extended nondiscrimination to all personal attributes, socioeconomic status, and nature of health problems.

The most recent revision of the ANA code, entitled *Code for Nurses with Interpretive Statements,* was adopted in 1985 (ANA 1985). It revises and updates language, but does not substantially change any of the ethical principles affirmed in the prior version. The ANA describes the code as "more a collective expression of nursing conscience and philosophy than a set of external rules" (see Table 6-6).

INTERNATIONAL COUNCIL OF NURSES.   In 1933, the International Council of Nurses (ICN), headquartered in Geneva, Switzerland, formed an Ethics of Nursing Committee. In 1953, the ICN adopted its first *International Code of Nursing Ethics.* In 1965, minor revisions were made and the title was changed to *Code of Ethics as Applied to Nursing.* In 1973, during the Fifteenth Quadrennial Congress in Mexico City, a new code was approved by nurse representatives from around the world (ICN 1985). This code begins with a statement of the responsibilities of, needs for, and services rendered by nurses. Ethical behaviors of nurses are then described as they relate to people, practice, society, co-workers, and the profession (see Table 6-7).

Purpose of Ethical Codes

In the beginning of this section we said that codes of ethics are not static documents, but ever-evolving statements of values, reflecting social and professional change. The history of the ethical codes of nursing bears this out. However, while not static, neither are they altered by every current of thought. They are more constant, serving as foundations against which the enormous and sometimes chaotic forces of contemporary science exert pressure. On this point Fowler wrote, "Though it is not easy, ethical decision-making is not adrift in a rolling sea; it is anchored to the distinguished, distinctive, and definite moral and ethical tradition of the profession" (1985).

Ethics Committees

Because nurses, physicians, and other health-care providers must make bioethical decisions every day, hospitals have created

◰ Table 6-6

**American Nurses' Association, Code for Nurses
with Interpretive Statements, 1985**

1. The nurse provides services with respect for human dignity and the uniqueness of the client unrestricted by considerations of social or economic status, personal attributes, or nature of health problems.

2. The nurse safeguards the client's right to privacy by judiciously protecting information of a confidential nature.

3. The nurse acts to safeguard the client and the public when health care and safety are affected by the incompetent, unethical, or illegal practice of any person.

4. The nurse assumes responsibility and accountability for individual nursing judgments and actions.

5. The nurse maintains competence in nursing.

6. The nurse exercises informed judgment and uses individual competence and qualifications as criteria in seeking consultation, accepting responsibilities, and delegating nursing activities to others.

7. The nurse participates in activities that contribute to the ongoing development of the profession's body of knowledge.

8. The nurse participates in the profession's efforts to implement and improve standards of nursing.

9. The nurse participates in the profession's efforts to establish and maintain conditions of employment conducive to high quality nursing care.

10. The nurse participates in the profession's efforts to protect the public from misinformation and misrepresentation and to maintain the integrity of nursing.

11. The nurse collaborates with members of the health professions and other citizens in promoting community and national efforts to meet the health needs of the public.

Reprinted by permission from Code for Nurses with Interpretive Statements, Kansas City, MO, 1985.

Code for Nurses: Ethical Concepts Applied to Nursing, International Council of Nursing, 1985

The fundamental responsibility of the nurse is fourfold: to promote health, to prevent illness, to restore health, and to alleviate suffering.

The need for nursing is universal. Inherent in nursing is respect for life, dignity, and the rights of man. It is unrestricted by consideration of nationality, race, creed, color, age, sex, politics, or social status.

Nurses render health services to the individual, the family, and the community, and coordinate their services with those of related groups.

Nurses and People

The nurse's primary responsibility is to those people who require nursing care.

The nurse, in providing care, promotes an environment in which the values, customs, and spiritual beliefs of the individual are respected.

The nurse holds in confidence personal information and uses judgment in sharing this information.

Nurses and Practice

The nurse carries personal responsibility for nursing practice and for maintaining competence by continual learning.

The nurse maintains the highest standards of nursing care possible within the reality of specific situations.

The nurse uses judgment in relation to individual competence when accepting and delegating responsibilities.

The nurse when acting in a professional capacity should at all times maintain standards of personal conduct which reflect credit upon the profession.

Nurses and Society

The nurse sustains a cooperative relationship with co-workers in nursing and other fields.

The nurse takes appropriate action to safeguard the individual when his care is endangered by a co-worker or any other person.

Nurses and the Profession

The nurse plays the major role in determining and implementing desirable standards of nursing practice and nursing education.

The nurse is active in developing a core of professional knowledge.

The nurse, acting through the professional organization, participates in establishing and maintaining equitable social and economic working conditions in nursing.

Reprinted by permission of the International Council of Nurses, 1985.

ethics committees to share the responsibility. These committees are made up of health professionals, ethicists, clergy, and public members. A variety of court decisions and federal regulations give these committees an important role in making life and death decisions.

In addition, ethics committees have nonlegal functions. They provide education for health professionals on ethical issues and offer nonbinding consultation to families. Because life-and-death ethical decisions often are "tough calls," a committee approach involving family members and patient, when able, helps share the "guilt" and responsibility. A group decision, with family concurrence, gives assurance to the hospital, family, and legal representatives that a "right decision" has been made.

Ethical Dilemmas

A dilemma is a perplexing problem that offers a choice between equally unsatisfactory alternatives. An ethical dilemma is a moral problem that requires a choice between one or more ethical principles. Taking an action based on one principle, violates another. Each alternative has credibility, yet none will satisfy all of the ethical principles that apply. To further complicate the matter, ethical dilemmas often are charged with strong emotions such as anger and fear.

For example, if Jamie is allowed to die during one of her bouts of pneumonia, the cost of her care will end and Jamie's family will be free to complete their grieving and go on with their lives. However, to honor the principle of beneficence, her caregivers may believe they are violating the principle of nonmaleficence, since they will not have done all they could to keep her alive. Whichever action is chosen, the issue is charged with emotion.

Resolving Ethical Dilemmas

Ideally, resolution of an ethical dilemma requires clear, rational thought and knowledge of ethical principles and civil law. Knowledge of the ethical positions of decision-makers is also helpful, that is, whether they follow a teleological (end results, situational) tradition or a deontological (legalistic, duty) tradition. Although ethical dilemmas may be more emotional than most nursing problems, they require the same decision-making process that nurses use every day.

Decision-making Models

A number of decision-making models have been proposed to help nurses make ethical decisions. Purtilo and Cassel (1981) suggested a four-step process: (1) gather relevant data, (2) identify the dilemma, (3) decide what to do, and (4) complete the action.

Thompson and Thompson (1985) suggested a ten-step process: (1) review the situation to determine health problems, decision needed, ethical components, and key individuals; (2) gather additional information to clarify situation; (3) identify the ethical issues in the situation; (4) define personal and professional moral issues; (5) identify moral positions of key individuals involved; (6) identify value conflicts; if any, (7) determine who should make the decision; (8) identify range of actions with anticipated outcomes; (9) decide on a course of action and carry it out; and (10) review results of action.

We suggest a decision-making model similar to a crisis intervention process, taking into account legal as well as ethical issues. It is a seven-step process: (1) gather facts, including who the decision-makers are and whether they follow situational, end-result ethics or legalistic, duty ethics; (2) state the problem; (3) list alternative solutions; (4) for each solution state applicable ethical principles, laws, consequences, advantages, and disadvantages from the decision-maker's viewpoint; (5) assist decision-makers to choose a solution based on their ethical position; if the solution is illegal, assist them to decide if their belief is strong enough to accept the consequences of breaking the law; (6) provide emotional support for all affected persons; (7) evaluate the decision-making process and its results in order to provide anticipatory guidance for the future.

Case Studies

Ethical dilemmas occur in every area of human experience. Although each situation is different, ethical issues in nursing frequently arise around decisions about death, reproduction, scarce resources, behavior control, and professional relationships. Cases in each of these areas follow, with the decision-making model applied to the first dilemma.

DEATH

Quadriplegic Woman.   A 28-year-old quadriplegic woman with severe cerebral palsy had herself admitted to a hospital. She asked to be kept comfortable with medications and physical care but allowed to die by starvation because her life was unbearable. Instead, the hospital force-fed her. If the hospital had had an ethics committee, how might they have decided what to do?

(1) Gather the facts:

The woman is essentially alone and the state pays for her care. She has no religious or moral problems with voluntary euthanasia, but because of her helpless condition cannot end her own life. The woman is mentally competent and believes she has the right to die. The hospital is requested to take some action (administer pain-relieving drugs and provide care but to refrain from feeding her), so becomes the decision-maker. The hospital is run by a religion known for its legalistic/paternalistic interpretation of ethical principles (moral law).

(2) State the problem:

Should the hospital cooperate with the woman by allowing her to starve to death in their facility?

(3) List alternative solutions:
   a. Give humane care but allow the woman to starve to death
   b. Discharge the woman to her home with an attendant
   c. Force-feed the woman until she can be placed in another facility

(4) State applicable ethical principles, laws, and consequences; list advantages and disadvantages of each:
   a. Give humane care but allow woman to die
      Ethical principles: (From legalistic viewpoint of decision-maker) ultimate violation of nonmaleficence by allowing death; patient autonomy

Legal issues: Possible criminal charges of great bodily harm

Consequences: "Unbearable state" of woman would end; hospital might be charged with breaking laws; religious tenets would be violated

Advantages: Woman's misery would end

Disadvantages: Hospital might face civil and criminal legal action; religious tenets would be violated

b. Discharge woman to her home with an attendant

Ethical principles: (From legalistic point of view of decision-maker) nonmaleficence occurs because the hospital would not participate in assisting woman to die; (from paternalistic position of hospital) violation of autonomy is acceptable when it is required to "follow a higher law"

Legal issues: Possible charges of civil negligence by woman

Consequences: Misery of woman would continue; hospital would avoid criminal charges and violation of church doctrine

Advantages: Avoid legal charges and conflict with ethical tenets of church

Disadvantages: Almost none; possibly some negative publicity

c. Force-feed woman until she is transferred elsewhere

Ethical principles: (From legalistic viewpoint of hospital) beneficence occurs because the woman is being kept alive; (from paternalistic viewpoint) violation of autonomy of woman is acceptable under such circumstances

Legal issues: Possible charges of battery against hospital by woman

Consequences: Woman does not die from starvation in the hospital or at her home; her misery continues; hospital avoids criminal charges of great bodily harm but may be sued by the woman

Advantages: Moral position of paternalistic religion is upheld; probably no legal charges

Disadvantages: Possibly some negative publicity for the hospital

(5) Assist decision-maker to make a choice based on ethical
position:

The decision-maker is the hospital. The moral position of an ethics
committee of a hospital such as this one (legalistic, paternalistic)
would quickly eliminate the request of the woman to die in the
hospital. The decision to force-feed her and discharge her as quickly
as possible would be more acceptable. In another hospital, the decision might be different, depending on the interpretation of the
committee members of beneficence and their concern for patient
autonomy.

(6) Provide emotional support for those affected by the
decision:

In this case, the woman had to endure force-feeding and to continue to live in a condition she described as "unbearable." The ethics committee might refer the woman for counseling to the social
service department or chaplain.

(7) Evaluate the decision-making process and provide anticipatory guidance for the future:

The ethics committee of a hospital learns from each decision they
make. In this case they might recommend some method of screening admissions to avoid adverse publicity, or to publish their ethical religious tenets in the community so that physicians and prospective patients will know what to expect in the future.

Osteosarcoma in a Boy.   A 12-year-old boy has just been diagnosed as having osteosarcoma of the femur. The only hope of a
cure is radiation, chemotherapy, and amputation of the leg; however, a suspicious area in his lung indicates that metastasis already
may have occurred. Without treatment he will surely die. Even
with treatment his prognosis is poor. The treatment is painful, mu-
tilating, and traumatic. The parent must decide.

REPRODUCTION

Pregnant Janitor.   A 28-year-old part-time janitor has just found
out that she is pregnant for the fourth time. She has had three prior
abortions. She has just decided to leave the man with whom she
lives because he beats her. She is a new convert to a religion that is

strongly opposed to abortion and stresses the "place of woman" as subject to the rule of men. Her jobs pays too little to support her and a baby and she says that she is morally opposed to "going on welfare." Her only support system is her mother who lives in a nearby town. She has come to a health center. How might a nurse-counselor help her decide?

Older Mother.   A 42-year-old woman is pregnant for the first time. Her physician has recommended that she have an amniocentesis to find out if the baby has any birth defects such as Down's syndrome. Her church opposes this procedure and teaches that a woman is to obey her husband. Her husband is not religious and told her he wants the amniocentesis done. She has told the office nurse of her quandary. How might the nurse help her decide?

SCARCE RESOURCES

Multiple Defects in an Infant.   A baby is born with multiple defects. The mother is not able to care for the infant and he is placed in a state hospital. A legal guardian is assigned. The medical staff outlines a proposed treatment plan that involves numerous operations over a period of several years at enormous expense to the state. The guardian and the medical staff have asked the ethics committee of the hospital to advise them what to do. How might the committee advise them?

Two Men with Cardiac Arrests.   Two men on the same hospital unit have a cardiac arrest within moments of each other. The first to arrest is a bitter 80-year-old man with many health problems. The other is the 42-year-old editor of the local newspaper, a husband and father of five children. There is only one cardiopulmonary resuscitation cart. The physician who was present was asked to decide who to resuscitate first. How might he have reasoned out the answer?

BEHAVIOR CONTROL

Electroconvulsive Therapy.   A severely depressed woman was admitted as an involuntary patient to a psychiatric facility after she was found in a filthy room without food or water. When psychotherapy and medications failed to improve her condition she was asked to sign a permit for electroconvulsive therapy. She refused. Under the laws of that state, such treatment can be administered if it is recommended by three physicians. How might the physicians come to a decision?

Five-point Restraints.   A 7-year-old child was admitted to the psychiatric unit with a history of stabbing her sister to death with a scissors. The child was incredibly strong and had frequent violent temper tantrums during which she attacked other patients and staff members. When these tantrums occurred leather straps were placed around her waist, wrists, and ankles and she was tied to a bed in a seclusion room until she calmed down. The alternative to physical restraint was chemical restraint: large doses of sedatives. Members of the ethics committee were invited to a treatment team conference to help decide what should be done. How might they decide?

PROFESSIONAL RELATIONS

Assignment of Holiday Time.   The nursing supervisor is making the holiday time-off assignments. It is the custom for staff members to take turns having Thanksgiving, Christmas, and New Year's Day off. A staff nurse comes to the supervisor in private and asks for Christmas Day, even though she had it last year. The nurse explains that it is the last day before her brother is to enter a state penitentiary to serve a 20-year sentence for child molestation. None of the staff know of the brother's criminal history. How might the supervisor decide what to do?

Medication Error.   Two patients on the unit have the same last name and are in adjacent rooms. Seconal is prescribed for one and Nembutal for the other. The evening nurse switched their medications. She discovered her error after the second patient swallowed the capsule and remarked that he had had a yellow capsule the night before. The nurse had made two other medication errors in the past year and was warned that if another occurred she would be dismissed. She is the sole support of three children and needs to work. How should she decide what to do?

Summary

Advances in modern medicine create ethical dilemmas and make understanding of values, belief systems, and ethics vital to nurses. Values provide a frame of reference through which people integrate their lives. Values clarification helps people identify their values. Belief systems help explain the mystery of life and give comfort to believers. They exist independently or within religions that also have organizational structure and devotional rituals. Ethics are concerned with judging the goodness or badness of actions. Such judgment may be based on teleological theories that say the end result of an action determines its goodness, or deontological theories that say the action itself, judged by its obedience to law, determines its goodness. Ethical principles, or concepts of goodness, of special concern to nurses are autonomy, confidentiality, nonmaleficence, beneficence, justice, veracity, and accountability. Codes of ethics emphasize ethical principles of professional groups. Ethical dilemmas occur when a choice of action must be made between one or more ethical principles.

Learning Activities

1. Take the values clarification strategy tests found in Tables 6-1, 6-2, and 6-3. What did you discover about your values? How do they differ from those of your classmates and parents?

2. Discuss what Durkheim meant when he said religion was "an effort of humans to pass science and complete it prematurely."

3. Write a paper explaining the ethical theory to which you subscribe and why.

4. In small groups discuss the apparent moral development of fictional or historical characters such as Lucy of *Peanuts*, Scrooge

of *The Christmas Carol,* Ghandi of India, or Mandela of South Africa.

5. Write a paper explaining why the ICN's *Code for Nurses: Ethical Concepts Applied to Nursing* would be classified as "Stage 6" by Kohlberg (see Table 6-4).

6. Assign each of the seven ethical principles to a different person and ask each person to present a vignette that illustrates that principle.

7. Write a paper in which you compare the Florence Nightingale Pledge to the ANA code for nurses.

8. In a small group, resolve the initial vignette and other case studies in this chapter, using any decision-making model.

Annotated Reading List

Davis AJ, Aroskar MA: *Ethical Dilemmas and Nursing Practice,* 2nd ed. Appleton-Century-Crofts, 1983.

A second edition of a 1978 classic, has chapters on values clarification and moral development, moral principles, professional ethics, institutional constraints, rights, informed consent, and health-care ethics. Ethical dilemmas are clearly presented in fourteen case studies.

Ethics: Principles and Issues. California Nurses' Association, 1985.

A brief history of the evolution of the ANA Code of Ethics is followed by articles written by various ethicists. These present principles that form the basis for ethical decisions in nursing, with appropriate case studies. A bibliography of current books and articles on ethics concludes this excellent, concise presentation of essential concepts.

Fenner K: *Ethics and Law in Nursing: Professional Perspectives.* Van Nostrand, 1980.

This brief introductory text is divided in two parts, ethics and law. A variety of professional codes are compared; values clarification is discussed and several ethical dilemmas are described.

Fletcher J: *Situation Ethics: The New Morality.* Westminster Press, 1966.

A classic, this book clearly and simply presents the concept of "agape," or God-like love. Its thesis is that if the law of love that considers circumstances replaced the rigid laws of right and wrong our modern world would be a better place to live.

Jameton A: *Nursing Practice: The Ethical Issues.* Prentice-Hall, 1984.

The text is divided into three parts. Part I discusses professionalism, autonomy, and decision making. Part II discusses ethical implications of four moral principles inherent in nursing: competence, beneficence, non-exploitation, and loyalty. Part III explores several ethical issues in nursing practice.

References

American Nurses' Association: *Code for Nurses with Interpretive Statements.* ANA, 1985.

Durkheim E: *The Elementary Forms of the Religious Life.* Harvard Press, 1915.

Fowler MD: *The Evolution of the Code for Nurses in Ethics: Principles and Issues.* CNA, 1985.

International Council of Nurses: Code for Nurses: Ethical Concepts Applied to Nursing. ICN, 1985.

Kohlberg L: Implications of developmental psychology for education: Examples from moral development. *Educational Psychologist* 1973; 10:2–14.

Piaget J: *The Moral Judgment of the Child.* Free Press, 1985.

Purtilo RB, Cassel CK: *Ethical Dimensions in the Health Professions.* Saunders, 1981.

Raths LE, Harmin M, Simmons SB: *Values and Teaching,* 2nd ed. Charles E. Merrell, 1979.

Rokeach M: *The Nature of Human Values.* Free Press, 1973.

Smith SJ: The principle of autonomy. In: *Ethics: Principles and Issues.* CNA, 1985.

Steele SM, Harmon V: *Values Clarification in Nursing,* 2nd ed. Appleton-Century-Crofts, 1983.

Thompson J and Thompson H: *Bioethical Decision Making for Nurses.* Appleton-Century-Croft, 1985.

Wach J: *Sociology of Religion.* University of Chicago Press, 1944.

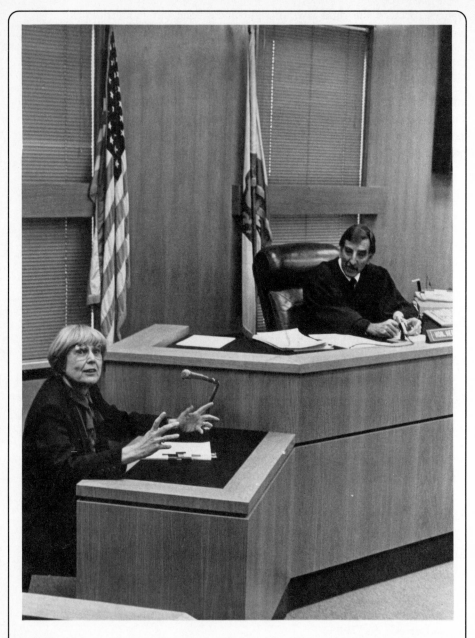

As an expert witness, a nurse testifies regarding the standard of care. She explains what could be expected of an ordinary, reasonable, and prudent nurse in a particular situation. (Photograph by David F. Singletary)

CHAPTER 7

Legal Issues

LEARNING OBJECTIVES

1. Discuss the origin of case law and the relationship between law and societal standards.

2. Compare constitutional, administrative, statutory, and common law as to source and how it is changed.

3. List some functions of the judicial system and give examples.

4. Compare civil with criminal law as to kinds and categories of offenses and requirements for determining liability or guilt.

5. Describe the civil and criminal trial process.

6. Compare four roles nurses play in trials.

7. Discuss the process and name some grounds for revoking a license to practice nursing.

8. Define negligence and professional negligence; state the four elements that must be proven in a negligence case.

9. Discuss the concept of standard of care as it relates to professional negligence.

10. Compare occurrence with claims-made insurance policies and state the meaning of tail-coverage.

11. Discuss various actions a nurse might take if served with a summons and complaint.

Mary stared at the official-looking envelope handed her by a stranger. The return address said: Superior Court. Fear swept through her body as she stiffly tore open the envelope. Two documents were inside: one entitled "Summons," the other "Complaint." Her name, Mary Jaffe, was listed as a defendant. So, too, was the Community Hospital and Simon Anslow, MD, an emergency room physician.

Shocked and confused, Mary shut the front door and walked to a chair. She felt numb. She tried to read the documents but the language was strange, its implications unclear. Only vaguely could she remember an incident that might have prompted the allegations. What did this mean? What should she do? To whom should she turn? Should she call her union representative? An attorney? The Emergency Department supervisor?

Mary started to call the hospital, then she remembered that she had paid premiums for professional liability insurance. Fearful that her policy might have expired, Mary rushed to her file and found the insurance folder. Yes, she was covered, and there were instructions about what to do and what not to do if she ever had a problem. There was also an 800-number to call.

Mary picked up the phone and dialed the number. As she waited for it to ring, Mary realized how vulnerable she was and how little she knew about the legal system.

Many nurses face the same situation as Mary. Although aware of some of the legal regulations in nursing practice, few have a working knowledge of the judicial system. Because nurses live in a litigious society and work in a profession fraught with risks, they need to know the history, structure, and function of the legal system. They need to understand the trial process and their responsibilities as professional nurses. Of course, if faced with a specific legal problem, nurses like Mary need advice from a competent attorney.

Historical Development of Law

Law in the United States is based on the old English system where the king had absolute power over his lands and people. He acted according to what he considered his "divine right." As a consequence, his decisions became the "law of the land" and were known as the *common* or *case law*. Creighton noted that the "practice of building a system of rules and sanctions by the accumulation of case-to-case decisions [remains a] . . . unique characteristic of Anglo-American jurisprudence" (1986).

The Magna Charta, granted by King John in 1215, is considered the foundation of English constitutional liberty and a landmark in the struggle for human freedom. It effectively limited the power of those who governed and protected individual rights and property. Thus, English law came to have two functions: to protect and enforce the rights and privileges of individuals and to provide an organized government with limited powers (Creighton 1986). Not surprisingly, US law incorporated those functions in its judicial system and in the Constitution, which governs all statutory, administrative, and case law.

In old England, when a law seemed too harsh or did not fully apply, people could appeal to the king for "equity." The appeal was made to the king's sense of justice. If he were convinced that an exception to common law should be made, he would so order. In time, the king established separate equity courts and appointed substitute chancellors to hear these cases. These courts became known as "courts of chancery" (Creighton 1986). In the US a separate equity court system has been mostly abolished, but the concept of equitable remedies remains.

The English and American legal systems grew out of the economic, political, and religious conditions of the people. Law, like ethics, is ever-changing, mirroring the society in which it is found. A very short time ago there were laws in the United States that prevented African-Americans from eating in the same restaurant with non-African-Americans. When society changed its beliefs, such laws were challenged in the courts and abolished.

Organization of Government

Separation and Balance of Powers

The US Constitution established three separate branches of government within the federal system: executive, legislative, and judicial. Likewise, state constitutions established three branches of government. In an attempt to ensure that no single branch became more powerful than another, this tripartite system authorized specific powers and responsibilities for each branch. This principle became known as the *doctrine of separation* and *balance of powers*.

The US Constitution also provides for a balance of power within the judicial branch. The Tenth Amendment of the Constitution grants specific powers to the federal government. All others are given to the states. Express powers given to the federal government include the power to promote and protect interstate commerce and to tax the citizens.

Executive Branch

The executive branch manages the government. Through Article II of the US Constitution and corresponding articles in state constitutions, the chief executive officer is granted specific powers and required to administer and enforce the laws of the land. The executive branch delegates its duties to various departments that enforce laws and promote regulations within their jurisdiction. For example, at the federal level, the Department of Health and Human Services and at the state level, a board of nursing are established under authority of the executive branch of government (Rhodes and Miller 1971). In both federal and state systems, the legislative and judicial branches of government keep close watch on the executive branch.

Legislative Branch

The legislative branch of the federal government is established in Article I of the US Constitution. Congress, the legislative body, is composed of a house and senate, as are many state legislatures. Its primary function is to enact laws. Table 7-1 indicates how a bill becomes a law. The legislative branch of government does not have unlimited ability to enact laws. Federal and state constitutions specify in what areas laws may be enacted. For example, at the federal level, Congress can coin money, provide for the general welfare, and amend the Constitution by a two-thirds vote (Northrop and Kelly 1987).

Judicial Branch

Federal Courts

The judicial branch of government is established by Article III of the Constitution, which states that judicial power shall reside in one supreme court and in inferior courts that Congress may establish. The judicial branch is empowered to *adjudicate* (judge or resolve) disputes in accordance with the law. The Constitution gives the Supreme Court exclusive *jurisdiction* (power to hear a case) when states are the *litigants* (parties) in a legal action and *appellate jurisdiction* (power to review and decide appeals) from lower federal and state appeal courts when cases from those courts involve federal law (Baum 1986).

United States district courts are the trial courts of the federal system. Circuit courts of appeal review cases decided by district courts. These courts, organized into geographic areas called *circuits*, may include several states. For example, Illinois, Michigan,

How a Bill Becomes a Law

Formation of Idea for a New Law:	By the president, members of congress, or citizen groups
Writing of Idea into Legal Form:	By legislative attorneys
Sponsorship by Member of House or Senate:	Up to 25 representatives and any number of senators may co-sponsor a bill; taxation bills originate in the House
Introduction of Bill, Assignment of Number, First Reading:	Sponsor introduces bill by handing it to the clerk or placing it in a box called a *hopper;* clerk gives bill a number and reads title into the *Congressional Record,* the *first reading*
Assignment to Committee:	Speaker of House or vice-president in Senate assigns bill to appropriate committee for study
Study by Committee:	Committee hears testimony from experts and interested persons; they can revise, pass and report out, or table the bill
Placement on Calendar:	In House, the Rules Committee can delay action, limit debate, limit or prohibit amendments; in Senate, bills are usually scheduled in order; leader of majority party may push bills ahead
Consideration by Full House:	In House, at *second reading,* entire bill is read; *third reading* is by title only after amendments have been added and before final vote; most bills pass by simple majority (one more than half the number of votes); then bill goes to Senate
Consideration by Full Senate:	In Senate, debate can last indefinitely unless there is an agreement to limit debate; when debate ends, vote is taken. Most bills require simple majority to pass; if bill passes, it goes to Conference Committee
Conferencing:	Conference Committee is made up of members of both houses. They work out differences between House and Senate versions of the bill; revised bill is sent back to both houses for final vote
Printing of Bill:	Bill is printed by Government Printing Office, a process called *enrolling*

Table 7-1 (*continued*)

How a Bill Becomes a Law	
Signing of Bill:	Speaker of House and vice-president sign enrolled bill, now called an *act of congress*
Consideration by President:	President can sign or veto act, or by waiting ten days, excluding Sunday, can allow act to become law without signature. If Congress adjourns before ten days are up, act dies, called a *pocket veto*
Reconsideration by Congress of Vetoed Act (Bill):	A two-thirds majority vote of both houses of Congress *overrides* a presidential veto; act, also called bill, becomes law
Becoming a Law:	When an act becomes a law it is given a number indicating the number of the Congress that passed it. A new Congress forms every two years after the election. For example, a law enacted by the 96th Congress might be designated 96-146

Indiana, and Wisconsin make up the Seventh Circuit. Federal courts have exclusive jurisdiction over cases about the US Constitution, disputes arising between two and more states or citizens of different states, and when the amount of money exceeds $50,000 (Twenty-eighth USC 1331, 1332 1982).

State Courts

The state court system is similar in organization to the federal system. Each state has its own trial, appellate (appeals), and supreme court, although they may be called by different names in different states. As with their federal counterparts, the constitution and laws of the states give state courts specific powers. Trial courts hear cases dealing with civil and criminal violations of the state's statutory and common laws. Many state court systems provide municipal courts to handle minor matters and divisions to handle cases of a specific nature, such as domestic relations.

Indeed, the judicial branch of government is complex. Perhaps that complexity is because there is not one judicial system, but many. Christoffel observed that in the United States there are 51 legal systems: those of the fifty states and the one of the federal government (1982).

Sources of Law

Laws arise from many sources. Constitutional law comes from the US Constitution, administrative law from the executive branch or governmental agencies, statutory law from laws passed by the legislature, and common law from decisions made in prior cases (Christoffel 1982).

Constitutional Law

The US Constitution is the *supreme law of the land.* It grants power to federal and state governments and ensures individual rights through its amendments. Constitutional law concerns itself with balancing the powers of government and protecting individual rights from unconstitutional infringement on those rights by federal or state governments.

The first ten amendments of the Constitution are termed the Bill of Rights (see Table 7-2). These, and various of the other 26 amendments, place restrictions on the power of government and establish specific individual freedoms, such as the right to free speech, assembly, and equal protection under the law. When individuals believe they have been denied any of these rights they can seek redress in federal courts. Similarly, state constitutions guarantee individual rights.

The rights granted individuals by the Bill of Rights are both substantive and procedural. *Substantive rights* give people the right to specific freedoms, such as speech. *Procedural rights* give people the right to due process. Likewise, the Constitution guarantees that all persons in the same situation must be treated equally under the law unless there is a "rational basis" for treating them differently, such as mental retardation. State constitutions may provide more protection to their citizens than the federal Constitution, but they cannot provide less.

Table 7-2

Amendments I to X of the US Constitution (the Bill of Rights), Amendment XIV, Section 1

I. Congress shall make no law respecting an establishment of religion, or prohibiting the free exercise thereof; or abridging the freedom of speech, or of the press; or the right of the people peaceably to assemble, and to petition the Government for a redress of grievances.

II. A well-regulated Militia, being necessary to the security of a free State, the right of the people to keep and bear Arms, shall not be infringed.

III. No Soldier shall, in time of peace be quartered in any house, without the consent of the Owner, nor in time of war, but in a manner to be prescribed by law.

IV. The right of the people to be secure in their persons, houses, papers, and effects, against unreasonable searches and seizures, shall not be violated, and no Warrants shall issue, but upon probable cause, supported by Oath or affirmation, and particularly describing the place to be searched, and the person or thing to be seized.

V. No person shall be held to answer for a capital, or otherwise infamous crime, unless on a presentment or indictment of a Grand Jury, except in cases arising in the land or naval forces, or in the Militia, when in actual service in time of War or public danger; nor shall any person be subject for the same offense to be twice put in jeopardy of life or limb; nor shall be compelled in any criminal case to be a witness against himself, nor be deprived of life, liberty, or property, without due process of law; nor shall private property be taken for public use, without just compensation.

VI. In all criminal prosecutions, the accused shall enjoy the right to a speedy and public trial, by an impartial jury of the State and district wherein the crime shall have been committed, which district shall have been previously ascertained by law, and to be informed of the nature and cause of the accusation; to be confronted with the witnesses against him; to have compulsory process for obtaining witnesses in his favor, and to have the Assistance of Counsel for his defense.

VII. In Suits at common law, where the value in controversy shall exceed twenty dollars, the right of trial by jury shall be preserved, and no fact tried by a jury, shall otherwise be re-examined in any Court of the United States, than according to the rules of the common law.

VIII. Excessive bail shall not be required, nor excessive fines imposed, nor cruel and unusual punishments inflicted.

IX. The enumeration in the Constitution, of certain rights, shall not be construed to deny or disparage others retained by the people.

X. The powers not delegated to the United States by the Constitution, nor prohibited by it to the States, are reserved to the States respectively, or to the people.

XIV. Section 1. All persons born or naturalized in the United States, and subject to the jurisdiction thereof, are citizens of the United States and of the State wherein they reside. No State shall make or enforce any law which shall abridge the privileges or immunities of citizens of the United States; nor shall any State deprive any persons of life, liberty, or property, without due process of law; nor deny to any person within its jurisdiction the equal protection of the laws.

Administrative Law

Administrative law is derived from the power of the legislative branch of government to regulate. The Congress or state legislatures delegate to administrative agencies the power and responsibility to create specific regulations to carry out their special functions. For example, state nurse practice acts create a regulatory board. The state legislature delegates responsibility to that board to enforce the nurse practice acts. The board then makes the rules and regulations it deems necessary to regulate nursing practice in the state.

Administrative agency rule-making does not go unchecked. Congress and state legislatures pass administrative procedure acts that spell out how rules and regulations are to be made and how the agency is to apply them to specific cases. Most often these acts require that agencies publish proposed rules in a central reporting publication. At the federal level, that publication is the *Federal Register*. At the state level, various media may be employed. For example, before a board of nursing may change a regulation, it may be required to send notices to all nursing schools and hospitals, publish proposed changes in newspapers, and hold public hearings throughout the state.

Rules and regulations passed by administrative agencies such as the board of nursing have the force of law. When interpreting regulations for specific situations, these agencies determine how they apply to particular cases. Thus, the functions of these agencies are *quasi-legislative* and *quasi-judicial*. The legislature, however, continues to bear ultimate responsibility for actions of agencies, to which it delegates power.

To ensure that powers given to agencies such as the board of nursing are not exceeded, the judicial branch of government sits as an overseer of administrative law. This "watchdog" function of the judiciary is used when it is alleged that an agency improperly exercised its power, failed to follow its own rules and regulations or administrative procedure, or infringed on the constitutional rights of individuals (Northrop and Kelly 1987).

Federal agencies that function under administrative law include the National Labor Relations Board (NLRB), Food and Drug Administration, and Department of Health and Human Services. The

NLRB is empowered to resolve labor disputes that arise under the National Labor Relations Act. Its role in collective bargaining is described more fully in Chapter 11.

Statutory Law

Statutory law is made by the US Congress and state legislatures. For the most part statutory law is restricted only by the US Constitution and state constitutions. Called *statutes,* these laws are grouped together in codes. Federal statutes become part of the United States Code (USC). State statutes become part of state codes. In Illinois, for example, statutes are recorded in the Illinois Revised Statutes, and have various names, such as Code of Civil Procedure and Criminal Code. These laws are broad-based and cover a wide range of subjects. For instance, Medicare and Medicaid are federal statutes that were amendments to the Social Security Act. Nurse practice acts and child abuse and neglect reporting acts are examples of state statutory laws.

State legislatures have a great deal of power to enact statutes to protect their citizens. Many of these statutes give state agencies the power to intervene in order to provide for the general welfare of individuals. This power to intervene is termed *police power.* Thus, until a full hearing can be held, the state, through its respective courts and administrative agencies can (1) take a minor into protective custody if the minor is being abused and/or neglected, (2) appoint a temporary guardian for an alleged disabled (incompetent) person, and (3) issue an injunction prohibiting a health professional from practicing medicine because that practice threatens the health and safety of the public.

The process of making and passing statutory law in a democracy is by nature a political one. Because legislators are elected and thus accountable to the people, the decisions they make about what laws to pass are based on input from voters. Constituents who make their concerns known, either by direct contact or lobbying, are the ones whose views are most likely represented in the laws legislators pass. Thus, it behooves nurses to voice their concerns directly to legislators or indirectly through the lobbying efforts of various organizations.

State legislatures cannot pass statutory laws that conflict with federal statutes. As with state and federal constitutional law, state statutes can add, but cannot take away protections provided by federal laws. Moreover, legislatures cannot pass statutes that infringe on individual constitutional rights. Thus, as with administrative law, the judicial branch of government sits as an overseer of statutory (legislator-made) law.

Local legislatures, such as city councils, can pass laws that affect their city or municipality. Usually called *ordinances*, these laws are subject to the same limitations as other statutory laws, including those rights guaranteed by the United States and state constitutions.

Common Law

Common law, in contrast to other types of law, is "court-made" rather than being made by administrative or legislative bodies (Christoffel 1982). Common law consists of precedents (earlier decisions), customs, and tradition. Two concepts permeate common law: *stare decisis* and *res judicata*.

Stare decisis means to stand by things decided. In common law the court attempts to look at past decisions to resolve present disputes. This practice provides some consistency in decisions handed down by the courts. Although past decisions may be useful, a case currently before the court may present slightly different facts than prior cases or may raise a new argument for overturning prior cases. Thus, each and every case that comes before a court may result in the formation of new common law.

Res judicata means a thing or matter settled by judgment. It provides that once a decision is handed down and no further appeals are possible, the parties cannot take the case to court again. This practice avoids duplication and unnecessary cost.

Functions of the Judicial System

The purpose of the judicial system is to administer justice without partiality. It carries out its purpose by resolving disputes, modifying behavior, allocating gains and losses, and making policy (Baum 1986).

As an *arbiter of disputes*, the court may interpret administrative rules or regulations, determine whether or not the civil rights of individuals have been violated, and resolve contract disputes between individuals.

As a *modifier of behavior*, the court may impose sanctions on behavior that is not condoned, such as indecent exposure. The court may reward behavior that is acceptable, such as reducing a jail sentence for "good behavior."

As an *allocator of gains and losses* in a contract dispute, the court may be asked to decide which party will bear the cost of breaking an agreement. For example, the court may be asked to determine if a hospital has broken a labor contract with its nurses and if so, how much compensation it should pay. How the court functions in this role is discussed later in this chapter under the trial process.

As a *policy maker* the court may recognize new causes for action or may determine that individuals have a clear personal interest in suing (standing to sue) for injuries.

Types of Law

Civil Law

Law is divided into two general types: civil and criminal. *Civil law* is concerned with harm against another individual. It seeks redress for wrongs and injuries suffered by individuals, usually in the form of monetary compensation. Two examples of civil offenses include breach of contract and tort.

A *contract* is a legally binding agreement between two or more parties, such as exists between employers and employees. Breaking such an agreement is called a *breach* of contract.

A *tort* is any civil wrong other than a breach of contract. It includes violations of statutes, administrative rules and regulations, and common laws. Examples of tort actions are malpractice, false imprisonment, and sexual harassment suits. In order to win a civil suit, proof must be established by a preponderance of the evidence.

Criminal Law

Criminal law is concerned with harm against society, that is, with actions that directly threaten the orderly existence of society.

It deals with violations of criminal statutes and their resultant punishment. Criminal acts, while aimed at individuals, are offenses against the state. Fenner explains, "to tolerate such actions would directly endanger the state's right to maintain an orderly social existence" (1980). Therefore, in criminal cases the state attorney, on behalf of the people, is the prosecutor.

When a guilty verdict is returned, the victim usually does not receive *redress* (compensation). Instead, the person who committed the crime is punished in some way, such as being sentenced to jail, fined, or placed on probation. Conviction of a criminal offense requires proof beyond a reasonable doubt.

As a rule, criminal offenses are categorized into three types: felonies, misdemeanors, and juvenile offenses (Baum 1986). *Felonies* are the most serious offenses and include a wide variety of crimes such as murder, driving under the influence of alcohol, and evading income taxes. Conviction of a felony often mandates a year or more of incarceration and may require payment of large fines to the government.

Misdemeanors are lesser criminal offenses such as traffic violations and unlawful assembly. Conviction of misdemeanors usually results in jail sentences of less than a year and relatively small fines.

Juvenile offenses are crimes committed by juveniles (minors) as defined by state statutes. These cases are handled in juvenile rather than adult courts. In some states juveniles who commit especially heinous crimes and are over a certain age can be treated as adults and tried in regular criminal courts.

Violations of both Civil and Criminal Law

A single incident may generate both criminal and civil legal actions. For example, if a nurse administered a lethal dose of meperidine to a 35-year-old husband and father, a criminal action could be filed against her. If convicted of homicide, the nurse might be sentenced to prison. A civil action could also be filed against the nurse by the man's family. If found guilty of malpractice, she might be liable to the man's family for thirty years of lost wages, court costs, and emotional suffering.

The Trial Process

The trial process can be confusing and frightening to nurses, just as it was to Mary in the vignette. That confusion and fright can be reduced by understanding the adversarial nature of trials and the difference between civil and criminal trials.

Civil Trials

Initiation of a Suit

A civil case is initiated when individuals believe they have been injured by someone or some group. They consult an attorney who advises them as to whether or not there is a viable *cause of action* (grounds for legal action). If so, the attorney drafts a *complaint,* which details the alleged wrongs. Persons who initiate a suit are called *plaintiffs* and those who are alleged to have caused an injury are called *defendants.* A complaint is composed of *counts* (separate statements), alleging facts upon which plaintiffs bring the *cause of action.* When and if a case goes to trial, plaintiffs must prove their allegations.

In addition to the complaint, a *summons* is prepared that accompanies the complaint. A summons tells the defendant when and where to file (make) an appearance to answer the complaint. Both the summons and complaint list the names of all parties, including attorneys for the plaintiff, addresses, telephone numbers, and other identifying information required by the court in which the suit will be filed. In the vignette Mary received a summons and complaint.

Filing the Complaint

When the summons and complaint are prepared they are taken to the courthouse for *filing.* The clerk in the courthouse stamps the complaint with the date and time it is filed and assigns a number to the case. That number, along with the names of plaintiffs and defendants, must appear on all other court documents associated with the case.

Service

Once filed and assigned a number, the complaint and summons are given to a legal service agent or the sheriff to serve on defendants. *Service* (giving a copy of the summons and complaint to defendants) is required in order for the court to have jurisdiction over them. Once served, defendants have a specified time within which to appear and answer the court. Defendants usually retain (hire) attorneys to represent them. It is customary for attorneys of defendants to contact attorneys of plaintiffs to let them know they have been retained. No action takes place on a case unless defense attorneys are notified.

Unless there is an objection by defense attorneys to the manner in which service occurred, or to the jurisdiction of the court over their clients, attorneys usually make an appearance on behalf of their clients.

Strategies to Avoid a Trial

Defense attorneys then determine if there is any way the suit can be disposed of at that time without going to trial. One strategy is to find a flaw in the complaint. State laws require that certain elements must be included in a complaint for a particular cause of action. If a complaint is drafted so that it does not meet these requirements, the attorneys can present a pretrial motion to dismiss the case for "failure to state a cause of action." If this and other strategies to dismiss the case are not available, then the defense attorneys prepare an *answer to the complaint* with the help of the defendant. The answer must specifically admit or deny each and every allegation in the complaint. The answer is then filed with the court. If and when the case goes to trial, defendants will be required to support their answers.

Counterclaims

Attorneys for defendants may decide that a counterclaim should be filed. A *counterclaim* is a separate cause of action against plaintiffs (Grigis 1975). It is filed in order to oppose claims of plaintiffs. The basis of counterclaims must be the "same transaction or occurrence" that formed the basis for the initial suit. For example, if the original claim is based on an incident in which a patient is burned by a hot-water bottle, the counterclaim must be based on the same incident.

In addition, either attorneys for defendants or for plaintiffs may determine that a third party, not named in the original suit, had a part in the injury that formed the basis of the suit. If so, a *third-party complaint* may be filed.

Discovery

Although allowable time-frames vary from state to state, a *period of discovery* usually begins after all defendants have been served. During this period, all parties attempt to discover as much information as they can about the cause of action. Discovery rules set down in civil practice acts of each state must be obeyed. These include giving proper notice to all parties, avoiding harassment and delay during discovery, and following proper procedures. Three common discovery methods are written interrogatories, notices to produce, and depositions.

WRITTEN INTERROGATORIES. *Written interrogatories* are written questions prepared by attorneys to obtain information from the other party. For example, in the malpractice case against Mary in the vignette, attorneys for the plaintiff would prepare questions for her to answer in writing, under oath. The questions might cover such topics as Mary's educational background and license, whether her license had ever been suspended or revoked, whether she had ever been involved in any previous suits alleging malpractice, and whether she knew of any witnesses in the emergency department (ED) who might have information about what happened. Once prepared, written interrogatories are filed with the court, with copies sent to all parties in the suit. The defendant and the attorneys review the questions. The defendant must answer them, sign the document, and *attest* (certify) to the truthfulness of the answers. Defense attorneys then file the response with the court and send copies to all parties. In like manner, attorneys for defendants file interrogatories on the plaintiffs.

NOTICES TO PRODUCE.   A *notice to produce* is a second discovery method. The notice is prepared by the attorneys and directed to other parties in the suit. The notice asks the parties to produce for inspection specific documents, papers, or other data. For example, attorneys representing the plaintiff in the malpractice action against Mary might ask for the nurses' and physicians' notes, policies and procedures of the hospital, a floor plan of the ED, and other relevant data. When such information is obtained it must be shared with all parties in the suit.

DEPOSITIONS.   A third discovery method is *deposition*. It is an oral statement, in question and answer form, given under oath, with all parties present (Grigis 1975). As such, it is an *adversarial proceeding* (the parties are opponents). Attorneys have the right to cross-examine the *deponent* (person giving the deposition) and the entire proceeding is transcribed by a court reporter. Testimony obtained during a deposition can be used at the trial to challenge the credibility of deponents, especially if their testimony changes radically. When a deposition is taken as an *evidence deposition* it can be introduced at the trial.

MOTIONS TO RESOLVE THE CASE.   During the period of discovery, any one of the attorneys may present motions to resolve the case. Defense attorneys may, for example, decide that during the discovery no evidence to support the case was found and may move for a *summary judgment* by the court because there is not a *material issue of fact* on which a jury must decide. Likewise, attorneys for the plaintiffs may move for a *voluntary dismissal,* if the plaintiffs decide not to go forward with the case at that time.

Pretrial Hearing

If a case is not resolved during the discovery period, then it is placed on the *pretrial call* (list to be reviewed by a pretrial judge). When the case is on the pretrial *docket* (list of cases) before it goes to trial, a pretrial judge attempts to help the parties resolve the dispute. If successful, the case is settled or otherwise resolved. If a resolution cannot be reached, the case is placed on *trial call.*

The Trial Procedure

When the case is sent to trial, it is assigned a trial judge. Again, there is an attempt to resolve the dispute without going through a full trial. If the dispute is not resolved, the trial begins.

JURY SELECTION.   If one or the other of the parties in a trial have filed a *jury demand,* the first step in the trial procedure is to select a jury. Depending on the state, either the trial judge or the respective attorneys conduct the *voir dire,* literally, "to see, to say." This is an examination of prospective jurors to determine their qualification for jury duty. Qualifications for jury duty depend on the type of case being heard. In malpractice cases against nurses, for example, attorneys for defendants may want nurses on the jury, but attorneys for plaintiffs might not. The attorneys can exercise a *preemptory challenge* and excuse a prospective juror from service on the jury without stating a reason. Each attorney has a certain number of challenges that can be used without explanation to the court. Once exhausted, however, further objections to jurors must be supported by stated reasons. Because of these challenges, jury selection can be a very long process. However, it is an important part of the judicial process and the right of individuals to a fair trial.

If neither party files a jury demand, then the trial proceeds as a *bench trial,* that is, with the judge acting in a fact-finding, law-deciding capacity. Jury trials are more common for malpractice cases.

OPENING STATEMENTS.   Once a jury is selected, the actual trial begins. It is initiated by opening statements of attorneys for both the plaintiffs and the defendants. In their opening statements attorneys give their positions concerning the case and what they will prove. They ask the jury to return a verdict in their favor against the other party.

TESTIMONY.   After the opening statements, attorneys for the plaintiff begin. In civil cases they must present and prove the case by a preponderance of evidence. Plaintiffs testify for themselves and may have witnesses testify to support their case. In malpractice actions expert witnesses will probably be called to testify. An *expert witness* is one who by training, education, experience, or all three, can testify as to whether of not a standard of care in a particular situation was upheld (Scully 1982). After the plaintiffs present their case, the defendants present theirs. Defendants must defend, or dispute, evidence presented by plaintiffs. They, too, may testify for themselves or have witnesses or expert witnesses testify to support their case.

THE VERDICT.   Once both sides have presented their respective cases, either or both sides may ask the judge for a *directed verdict in their favor.* That is, they may ask the judge to rule in their favor because the evidence presented was insufficient or insufficiently rebutted, with the result that proof by a preponderance of the evidence was not (or was) demonstrated. If the judge grants the request, the trial is over. If the judge denies it, the case goes to the jury. The judge instructs the jury as to its responsibilities and applicable law. The jury then "retires" to a private room to deliberate. When the jury reaches a decision it returns to the court room and states the verdict. In civil cases a unanimous decision by the jury may not be required.

Appealing a Verdict

If either party is unhappy with the verdict, that party can appeal the decision to an appellate court. The person who appeals a decision is called an *appellant;* the one who defends a lower court decision is called the *appellee.*

Criminal Trials

Initiation of a Suit

A criminal case begins when law enforcement officers present their investigative data to either state or federal prosecutors. These attorneys determine whether there is sufficient evidence to prosecute an individual for a particular crime. If they believe there is, a *complaint of information* or *indictment* is issued.

When the crime in question is a felony and a violation of federal law, a grand jury is convened. An assistant attorney general presents the evidence to the grand jury. The grand jury then decides whether or not there is *probable cause* to believe a crime was committed. When a crime is a violation of a state law, police and other officers work with the office of the state attorney. If the state attorney believes a crime has been committed, a complaint is filed. Some states use grand juries to decide probable cause just as in federal cases.

Arraignment

If alleged violators of criminal laws have been arrested prior to issuance of a complaint, they must be brought before a judge or magistrate to determine if they can be released on bail until their trial. If individuals are not arrested prior to the complaint, an *arrest warrant* is issued. After the individual is arrested an *arraignment* or *bail hearing* takes place.

Pleas

During an arraignment, alleged criminals must plead "guilty" or "not guilty" to the charges. Most often, at this stage, defendants plead "not guilty" (Northrop and Kelly 1987). If defendants plead "guilty," judges are required by both the US Constitution and state constitutions to determine if the plea has been made voluntarily (Northrop and Kelly 1987). This is important, because by pleading "guilty" defendants waive their right to all due process protections afforded by the US Constitution. Those rights include the right to a jury trial when an offense carries a sentence of imprisonment of more than six months, the right to confront witnesses against them, and the right to a speedy and public trial.

Discovery

When alleged offenders plead "not guilty" a period of discovery ensues. Because criminal trial verdicts can result in loss of life or liberty, criminal defendants are given certain protections that are not given to defendants in civil trials. For example, prosecutors are required to give defense attorneys evidence concerning the guilt or innocence of the defendants. Additional requirements may be necessary, depending on state law and whether the alleged crime violates federal law. After reviewing the evidence, defense attorneys may make motions seeking to exclude evidence based on constitutional protections.

During the discovery process, defense attorneys may attempt to arrange a *plea bargaining agreement* whereby the defendant may plead "guilty" in exchange for a more lenient sentence. Recent statistics indicate that more convictions result from guilty pleas associated with plea bargaining than from judicial decisions (Baum 1986).

Trial

If defendants do not plead "guilty" and no plea bargaining agreement is made, then the case goes to trial. The process of jury selection in criminal trials is the same as described for civil trials. Judges are always present, and like their colleagues on civil benches, they preside over the proceedings to ensure compliance with court procedures, to rule on motions, and to instruct the jury prior to its deliberation.

In criminal trials, government prosecutors must prove their case against defendants *beyond reasonable doubt.* Unlike in a civil trial, defendants do not have to rebut (disprove) the state's case. They can remain silent, or they may choose to waive their right to refrain from self-incrimination and can testify on their own behalf. They also may present witnesses to testify in their defense.

The Verdict

Once both sides have presented their respective cases, the judge instructs the jury as to its responsibility and applicable law. Then the jury retires to a private room to deliberate. When a unanimous decision is reached the jury returns to the court room and delivers its verdict. If the jury cannot agree, a *mistrial* is declared. If the jury finds a defendant "not guilty" the individual must be allowed to go free. The case is over. If found "guilty" the defendant is sentenced. Of course, defendants may appeal their conviction to a higher court.

Roles of Nurses in the Legal Process

Nurses may be involved in the legal process as plaintiffs, defendants, factual witnesses, or expert witnesses.

As *plaintiffs,* nurses may be the initiators of suits alleging harm from the actions of others. For example, nurses may believe that their professional competence has been injured by untrue oral or written statements of other health professionals. As plaintiffs in such suits they might seek compensation from defendants for damage to their reputations caused by slanderous (oral) or libelous (written) statements.

As *defendants,* nurses may be charged with committing civil wrongs such as professional negligence or crimes such as homocide. In either case, nurses who are defendants can make sure that their rights are protected by obtaining competent legal advice about their options.

As *factual witnesses* nurses give testimony about what they saw or remember about events or occurrences. It may be, for example, that a nurse was present when Mary administered a drug to which the patient reacted. The suit alleges that Mary breached the duty of care when she gave the drug, resulting in injury to the patient. The nurse who witnessed the incident is *subpoenaed* (summoned) to testify as to what she saw and heard relative to administration of the drug. Even before the trial, the witness probably would be subpoenaed to give a deposition of the incident.

Participating as an *expert witness* is perhaps one of the more challenging and rewarding roles in the legal process for nurses. This role demands a thorough knowledge of nursing practice, the nurse practice act of the state, and standards of care in the same field as the case at issue. The function of an expert witness in a malpractice case is to inform the jury what the standard of care would be in a particular situation. He or she would also state whether or not a defendant upheld that standard, functioning as an ordinary, reasonable, and prudent nurse in the same or similar circumstance in the same or similar community. Many professional malpractice cases are won or lost as a result of the testimony of expert witnesses.

Violations of Nurse Practice Acts

The purpose of nurse practice acts is to protect the public by setting and enforcing standards of nursing education and practice. As an extension of that purpose, regulatory boards make rules that can affect many issues, including entry into practice and titling, as described in Chapter 3. When institutions or individuals believe that a nurse has violated a provision of a nurse practice act, they can complain to the state regulatory agency. The agency then investigates the allegations. If an investigation supports the allegations, the agency files a complaint against the licensee.

Although nurse practice acts vary from state to state, they contain similar grounds for complaints. The complaints include: (1) diverting controlled substances from the facility for the nurse's own use, (2) obtaining a nursing license by fraudulent means, (3) being convicted of a felony in any state, and (4) practicing nursing in a grossly incompetent or negligent manner.

Because a state license cannot be taken away without due process, licensees have the right to a hearing about alleged violations. They have the right to be represented by an attorney and the right to present witnesses in their own behalf. The results of such hearings may be that: (1) no action is taken against the nurse, (2) a reprimand is given, (3) the license is suspended or revoked, and (4) the nurse is placed on probation. Because conviction of violations of a nurse practice act has such serious consequences, nurses facing alleged violations should obtain legal counsel at once.

Malpractice

Malpractice is professional negligence. It is an area of law that directly affects nursing practice. To address this concern, nurses first must understand the meaning of negligence.

Negligence

Negligence concerns injuries and damages to persons and property. It is an example of a tort, a civil cause of action. When individuals sustain injuries or suffer damages they seek redress, usually money, in *negligence actions.* If their allegations are proven, they are awarded compensation (Prosser 1971, p 143).

Four elements must be pleaded and proven for a cause of action alleging negligence to be successful:

1. There must be a *duty,* usually established by law or expert testimony, that dictates expected behavior in order to avoid unreasonable and foreseeable risk of harm to another.

2. There must be a *breach of that duty,* or a failure to uphold that duty.

3. The breach must be the *proximate (probable) cause* of injury to the victim.

4. *Actual damages* recognized by law must be suffered (Prosser 1971).

When negligence is alleged, the conduct of the person who is allegedly negligent is measured by *what an ordinary, reasonable, and prudent person would have done in the same or similar circumstances.* This provision ensures that an objective standard is used by the court to determine whether or not negligence was present.

Another important concept in any negligence situation is the principle that *each person is responsible for his or her own behavior.* Even when other persons or organizations are involved in a situation it is difficult for any one person to remain free of all responsibility and shift entire liability to others. Therefore, having additional parties named in a suit does not take away potential liability for negligence from each codefendant. Nurse managers share responsibility with staff for patient care to the degree expected by standards of care.

Respondeat superior is another principle important to an understanding of negligence. Literally, it means "let the master speak." This doctrine holds employers indirectly and vicariously liable for any negligence of their employees when employees were acting within the scope of employment and when negligent acts occurred during employment (Prosser 1971). This doctrine allows an injured party, or plaintiff, to sue only the employer, or to sue both the employer and the employee for alleged injuries.

Professional Negligence

Professional negligence deals with the negligence of professionals such as nurses, physicians, and attorneys. All of the elements and principles that apply to negligence also apply to professional negligence, with one exception. The principle of standard of care is different for professionals than nonprofessionals. When judging alleged negligent behavior, the conduct of nurses is measured by a standard of care that is *what an ordinary, reasonable, and prudent professional nurse would have done in the same or similar circumstances in the same or similar community* (Prosser 1971). The "same or similar community" part of the definition sounds as if it is the standard of care found in the local community. This is not the case. The "community" for health-care professionals is the national community, the entire United States. Thus, it is imperative that nurses know national standards of care for nursing practice. These standards are set forth by well-known experts and authors and by professional organizations such as the American Nurses' Association and National League for Nursing.

Most states compare alleged negligent behavior of nurses with that of professional nurses in the same or similar circumstances. A few states may use lay standards to evaluate more basic caregiving nursing activities. However, using lay standards is becoming more and more obsolete as judges recognize the need for experts to determine acceptable behavior.

By contrast, there have been attempts to apply physician standards of care to evaluate the conduct of nurses. In *Fein v. Kaiser Permanente Medical Group* (1985) a lower court attempted to apply physician standards to the conduct of a nurse practitioner. On appeal, although the California Supreme Court stated that physician standards were incorrectly applied to the nurse in the case, the court held that use of physician standards was not *reversible error* (always wrong). Thus, even though the decision was helpful in that particular case, it may not prevent future application of physician standards to nursing.

When health professionals, including nurses, represent themselves as specialists they are held to a standard of care that is *what the ordinary, reasonable, and prudent specialist in that particular area of expertise would do in the same or similar circumstances in the same or similar community*. Thus, when nurses represent themselves as nurse practitioners, for example, they must be certain to conform to nurse practitioner standards.

Good Samaritan Laws

Good Samaritan laws protect nurses and physicians from civil liability when they give emergency care. When nurses come to the aid of accident victims two kinds of law protect them: common (court-made law) and statutory (legislature-made law), often called *Good Samaritan acts*. All states now have Good Samaritan laws that cover nurses and physicians when they aid disaster and accident victims. Some states have *duty to rescue statutes*, requiring all citizens to come to the aid of anyone they know is in grave danger. In all cases, nurses must observe professional standards of care. The following are guidelines to help nurses reduce risk of malpractice action:

Do:

1. Move victims only to protect them from further injury.
2. Give cardiopulmonary resuscitation as needed.
3. Stop bleeding.
4. Keep victims warm.
5. Assess level of consciousness, pain, and the possibility of fractures.

Do not:

1. Move victims unnecessarily.
2. Force victims to walk.
3. Allow unskilled persons to attempt to treat victims.
4. Leave scene until skilled personnel assume care.
5. Give property of victims to anyone except police or family members.
6. Give any advice that, if wrong, could result in serious or permanent injury (*Nurses' Legal Handbook* 1985).

Selected Malpractice Cases

Wound Monitoring

In the case of *Daniel v. Gladewater Municipal Hospital* (1985), John Daniel, the plaintiff, incurred a leg injury and was treated at Gladewater Municipal Hospital. The injured leg developed osteomyelitis. In his complaint Daniel alleged that the condition was caused by negligent care of the nurses and the physician, Dr. Marashi. Specifically, Daniel alleged that the nurses were negligent because they failed to change his bandages and did not inform the physician of drainage from the wound. He alleged that the physician failed to properly monitor the wound and sued the physician and the hospital, as the nurses' employer.

At the trial, testimony showed that the plaintiff's bandage was changed only two times during his 39-day stay in the hospital. The first change occurred 13 days after surgery. Further testimony indicated that the surgical site drained heavily during this time and that the drainage was malodorous.

The plaintiff produced two expert witnesses: Dr. Jacobs, a physician, and Ms. Dole, a nurse. Dr. Jacobs testified that the physician who cared for Daniel did not uphold the standard of care of a reasonable, ordinary, and prudent physician in the same or similar circumstances in the same or similar community in relation to monitoring the wound and changing the dressings. Ms. Dole testified that the conduct of the staff nurses did not meet the standard of care of professional nurses because the nurses failed to change the dressings and to notify the physician of drainage from the operative site. Based on testimony by these expert witnesses, the jury returned a $100,000 verdict in favor of Daniel, against the physician and the hospital.

Patient Teaching

In another case, patient teaching became the focus of alleged negligence on the part of a nurse in an emergency room. In *Crawford v. Earl Long Memorial Hospital* (1983), the son of the plaintiff was involved in a fight during which the son was stabbed in the shoulder and hit on the head with a baseball bat. The injured man was rushed to one hospital, then transferred to Earl Long Hospital, where he was seen in the emergency room. The attending physician asked the nurse to call the mother and ask her to come and take her son home. The nurse did so. Later the nurse testified that when Mrs. Crawford arrived at the hospital she gave the mother specific instruction about how to care for her son at home. The nurse testified that she told the mother to awaken her son at regular intervals, question him to see if he was alert and knew who and where he was, and determine if his eye pupils were the same size. The mother seemed to understand the instructions and took her son home.

The mother testified that on arriving at home she went to bed and that her son stayed up a while longer. When Mrs. Crawford awoke the next morning, she went to check her son and found that he was dead.

Mrs. Crawford brought suit against the hospital as the employer of the nurse. She alleged that the emergency room nurse was negligent because she failed to give home care instructions. The nurse testified that she did give instructions to the mother, albeit orally. However, the nurse *did not* document the fact that she gave the instructions.

The court carefully evaluated the testimony of the nurse and concluded that the nurse was truthful when she testified that she had given the required instructions to the mother. By expert testimony, the court determined the standard of care in 1975, the year the injury occurred. Standard care was to give oral instructions to family members or other responsible persons for the care of individuals sent home with head injuries. The court gave great weight to the fact that the nurse insisted the mother come to the hospital to pick up her son, rather than send him home in a taxi as the mother requested. The nurse's insistence, they concluded, was evidence that she intended to give home care instructions directly to the mother. The court entered a verdict in favor of the hospital.

Although the verdict supported the nurse and hospital, the whole affair could have been avoided. The nurse should have given both written and oral instructions to the mother and noted her action in the record.

Drug Reaction Monitoring

In the case of *Torbert v. Befeler* (1985), four recovery room nurses and a cardiologist were sued for the death of a patient due to negligent care following surgery. Torbert, the plaintiff, was undergoing surgery for closure of a colostomy. He developed premature ventricular contractions (PVCs) of his heart shortly after the anesthesia was induced. Dr. Befeler, a cardiologist, was consulted. He ordered medication to suppress the abnormal heart contractions and then approved completion of the surgical procedure. In the recovery room the PVCs continued, and about three hours after surgery the patient had a cardiac arrest. Although revived, the man suffered brain damage and died several weeks later.

The family brought suit against the nurses and physician, alleging negligence on their part in not adequately monitoring the patient. Testimony at trial revealed that the head nurse in the recovery room interpreted existing protocols at the time of the incident to mean that one-to-one monitoring of the patient was to occur only until the patient stabilized. The team leader, also a nurse defendant, testified that she gave Demerol about 45 minutes before the arrest, but did not monitor the patient to detect an adverse reaction to the medication. It was determined that a reaction to the medication caused the arrest. Finally, the nurse assigned to monitor the man testified that she was not monitoring him at the time of his cardiac arrest. As a result, the patient was not attended by a nurse until at least ten minutes after the cardiac arrest.

The jury returned a verdict against the nurses and the cardiologist, apportioning fault at 45% for the head nurse, 45% for the team leader, 5% for the nurse who did not monitor the patient and 5% for the cardiologist.

It is clear that nurses are legally accountable for their actions whether they give patient care directly or supervise others. When they perform at a level below the standard of care for nurses and are found professionally negligent, liability can ensue.

Confidentiality

Nurses can be involved in other types of suits than those involving negligence. One area of concern involves patient rights and the duty of the nurses to protect those rights when providing care. For example, nurses must be sure that they protect a patient's *right of confidentiality*. This duty includes ensuring that information obtained during the course of providing care is not shared with anyone other than those involved in that care without the consent of the patient.

Confidentiality is particularly important when nurses work with patients receiving treatment for psychiatric disorders, including substance abuse. Federal and state laws provide additional protections of confidentiality for patient records and communications. The duty to adhere to those mandates is great.

Informed Consent and Refusal of Treatment

Another area of special concern to nurses is the patient's right to give *informed consent* and *informed refusal* of treatment. Nurses should not be involved in obtaining informed consent of patients. That is the physician's responsibility. However, nurses may discover that patients are not clear about impending surgery or treatment, or that the physician has not discussed the procedure with them at all. At a minimum, nurses must document their concerns in medical records and notify the physician and supervisor. Likewise, if patients tell nurses that they no longer want treatment or if they refuse a specific medication or treatment, nurses must document such refusal and notify the physician. Under no circumstance should nurses force treatment on patients. Both nurses and their employers could be charged with assault and battery as well as a breach of the rights of patients to informed consent or refusal.

Involuntary Commitment Protections

The rights of psychiatric client-patients are specifically protected. By statutes and case law, at both state and federal levels, psychiatric patients cannot be admitted involuntarily to mental hospitals without due process of law. The patient's behavior must meet the statutory definition of a need for commitment before involuntary commitment in that state can occur. What is more, restraints and seclusion can be used only when a clinical need re-

A Patient's Bill of Rights

1. The patient has the right to considerate and respectful care.
2. The patient has the right to obtain from his physician complete current information concerning his diagnosis, treatment, and prognosis in terms the patient can be reasonably expected to understand. When it is not medically advisable to give such information to the patient the information should be made available to an appropriate person in his behalf. He has the right to know by name the physician responsible for coordinating his care.
3. The patient has the right to receive from his physician information necessary to give informed consent prior to the start of any procedure and/or treatment. Except in emergencies, such information for informed consent should include but not necessarily be limited to the specific procedure and/or treatment, the medically significant risks involved, and the probable duration of incapacitation. Where medically significant alternatives for care or treatment exist, or when the patient requests information concerning medical alternatives, the patient has the right to such information. The patient also has the right to know the name of the person responsible for the procedures and/or treatment.
4. The patient has the right to refuse treatment to the extent permitted by law, and to be informed of the medical consequences of his action.
5. The patient has the right to every consideration of his privacy concerning his own medical care program. Case discussion, consultation, examination, and treatment are confidential and should be conducted discreetly. Those not directly involved in his care must have the permission of the patient to be present.
6. The patient has the right to expect that all communications and records pertaining to his care should be treated as confidential.
7. The patient has the right to expect that within its capacity a hospital must make reasonable response to the request of a patient for services. The hospital must provide evaluation, service, and/or referral as indicated by the urgency of the case. When medically permissible a patient may be transferred to another facility only after he has received complete information and explanation concerning the needs for and alternatives to such a transfer. The institution to which the patient is to be transferred must first have accepted the patient for transfer.
8. The patient has the right to obtain information as to any relationship of his hospital to other health care and educational institutions insofar as his care is concerned. The patient has the right to obtain information as to the existence of any professional relationships among individuals, by name, who are treating him.
9. The patient has the right to be advised if the hospital proposes to engage in or perform human experimentation affecting his care or treatment. The patient has the right to refuse to participate in such research projects.
10. The patient has the right to expect reasonable continuity of care. He has the right to know in advance what appointment times and physicians are available and where. The patient has the right to expect that the hospital will provide a mechanism whereby he is informed by his physician or a delegate of the physician of the patient's continuing health care requirements following discharge.

Table 7-3 (*continued*)

A Patient's Bill of Rights

11. The patient has the right to examine and receive an explanation of his bill regardless of source of payment.
12. The patient has the right to know what hospital rules and regulations apply to his conduct as a patient.

Reproduced by permission of the American Hospital Association. © 1975.

quires them, not to convenience the staff or to punish the patient. Nurses who work in psychiatric facilities need to know state and federal laws pertaining to patient rights.

Privacy and Nondiscrimination Protections

Patients have a right to privacy and nondiscriminatory treatment. While nurses cannot guarantee that they will never violate the rights of patients, a working knowledge of those rights may help them avoid violating them. To emphasize the rights of patients guaranteed by the US Constitution, the American Hospital Association approved *A Patient's Bill of Rights* in 1973 (see Table 7-3) and the National League for Nursing published the *NLN Patient's Bill of Rights* in 1976 (see Table 7-4).

Professional Liability Insurance

As Mary in the vignette found out, the likelihood of a nurse being sued is real. An experienced liability attorney once said to a group of nurses, "Let me follow you around on the job for a few hours and even though you're a good nurse, I may catch you in enough situations to get you sued for malpractice" (Nurses' Service Organization 1987). Lawsuits are costly events. Awards may reach thousands, even millions of dollars. Even when a verdict is favorable, the price of defending oneself can be enormous. Given these realities, nurses need to become informed consumers of liability insurance, considering the following:

NLN Patient's Bill of Rights

National League for Nursing believes nurses are responsible for upholding these rights of patients:

1. People have the right to health care that is accessible and that meets professional standards, regardless of the setting.
2. Patients have the right to courteous and individualized health care that is equitable, humane, and given without discrimination as to race, color, creed, sex, national origin, source of payment, or ethical or political beliefs.
3. Patients have the right to information about their diagnosis, prognosis, and treatment, including alternatives to care and risks involved, in terms they and their families can readily understand so that they can give their informed consent.
4. Patients have the legal right to informed participation in all decisions concerning their health care.
5. Patients have the right to information about the qualifications, names, and titles of personnel responsible for providing their health care.
6. Patients have the right to refuse observation by those not directly involved in their care.
7. Patients have the right to privacy during interview, examination, and treatment.
8. Patients have the right to privacy in communicating and visiting with persons of their choice.
9. Patients have the right to refuse treatments, medications, or participation in research and experimentation, without punitive action being taken against them.
10. Patients have the right to coordination and continuity of health care.
11. Patients have the right to appropriate instruction and education from health care personnel so that they can achieve an optimal level of wellness and an understanding of their basic health needs.
12. Patients have the right to confidentiality of all records (except as otherwise provided for by law or third-party payer contracts) and all communications, written or oral, between patients and health care providers.
13. Patients have the right of access to all health records pertaining to them, the right to challenge and to have their records corrected for accuracy, and the right to transfer all such records in the case of continuity of care.
14. Patients have the right to information on the charges for services, including the right to challenge these.
15. Above all, patients have the right to be fully informed as to all their rights in all health care settings.
    The National League for Nursing urges its membership, through action and example, to demonstrate that the profession of nursing is committed to the concepts of patient's rights.

Reprinted with permission of the National League for Nursing.

1. If nurses are the only named insured on a professional liability insurance policy they have more power to control decisions about cases than if they are insured only as employees on the insurance policies of their employers.

2. Even when nurses are insured by policies of employers, they may need to retain their own counsel at high hourly rates. If nurses have their own insurance, however, and are named in a suit, the insurance company usually assigns them their own attorney and the cost is covered by their personal policy.

3. If nurses purchase their own policy, it covers them wherever they work, providing the policy has no restrictions about place or scope of employment. By contrast, liability insurance policies of employers cover nurses only when they are working for those employers.

4. If alleged negligent acts are outside the scope of the job description of a particular employer, the insurance coverage of the employer does not apply. Accused nurses may be told that, although the employers' insurance company may defend the suit, monetary awards to plaintiffs would have to be paid by the nurses.

5. When purchasing insurance, nurses should be sure the amount of coverage gives adequate protection.

6. In professional liability insurance policies, inclusions and exclusions are significant. Many exclude coverage for criminal acts, intentional torts (assault, battery, false imprisonment), and disciplinary actions brought against nurses by boards of nursing or state agencies that license nurses.

7. Nurses need to understand the rights and responsibilities of the insured. For instance, nurses need to know if they would have the right to decide about the settlement of the case, or if the decision would rest with the insurance company alone.

8. Definitions of nursing contained in the policy should be examined to ensure that, in fact, professional responsibilities of nurses fall within that definition.

9. Nurses should know whether they are relying on an occurrence policy or a claims-made policy. An *occurrence policy* is one that covers any claim that arises during the time the policy

is in effect, even if the claim is filed in court after the policy is no longer in existence. A *claims-made policy,* on the other hand, covers only claims made during the time when the policy is in effect. Thus, only those cases filed in court while the policy is in effect are covered by the policy. Understandably, occurrence policies are more costly than claims-made.

Tail-coverage is offered by many insurance companies offering claims-made policies. Tail-coverage covers the period after the original policy ends so that coverage is possible if a suit is filed after the original policy is terminated. Of course, tail-coverage adds to the cost.

10. With more and more competing insurance companies to choose from and various group plans, staff nurses can shop for the best buy in insurance. Independent nurse practitioners, however, may find liability insurance expensive and difficult to obtain except through their professional organizations.

Possible Actions if Served

This chapter is intended to provide an overview of the legal issues for nurses and not to provide specific legal advice or professional services. If such services are needed, they should be obtained by the reader. In general, however, if a summons and complaint is served, nurses may want to consider taking the following actions:

Do (if personally insured):

1. Immediately telephone the company that provides your liability insurance. Usually a toll-free number is given on the cover-letter that accompanies the policy.

2. Fill out the informational forms that come from your insurer as completely as possible.

3. Follow any other instructions that the insurance carrier gives, such as telephoning a specific attorney in your area.

4. Contact the legal department of the institution where the incident occurred.

Do (if not personally insured):

1. Contact the legal department of the institution where the incident occurred, notifying them that you have been served.

2. If it seems that your interests are not being protected, you may decide to retain your own legal counsel.

Do not:

1. Talk to anyone about the incident except the insurance carrier and your attorneys, including personal and professional acquaintances and news media.

2. Sign any papers or give any written statements to plaintiffs or their attorneys without legal counsel.

Summary

The legal system in the United States is based on old English law. The organization of the government into an executive, legislative, and judicial branch reflects the doctrine of separation and balance of powers. The laws of the land include constitutional, administrative, statutory, or common law, depending on their source. Civil law is concerned with harm against individuals and includes torts and contracts. Criminal law is concerned with harm against society and includes felonies, misdemeanors, and juvenile offenses. The trial process of both civil and criminal cases follows a step-by-step sequence. Malpractice (professional negligence) is decided by measuring nursing action against what an ordinary and prudent professional nurse would do in the same or similar circumstances and community. To protect themselves against costly malpractice litigation, nurses may want to obtain their own professional liability insurance.

———————————— *C* ————————————

Learning Activities

1. Visit the state legislature and talk with a representative from your legislative district about some health-related bill going through the process of becoming a law.

2. Observe a trial, preferably one involving professional negligence.

3. Interview a nurse who has been an expert witness at a trial; determine what made that person an expert and what kinds of questions were asked at the trial.

4. Examine a patient's chart in a health-care agency; in your judgment, would the nurse's documentation be considered complete if that record were presented as evidence in a trial?

5. Review protocols established in a health-care agency for reporting unusual occurrence, accepting telephone prescriptions, administering controlled substances, obtaining permission for surgical procedures, and applying physical restraints.

6. Review a professional liability insurance policy; is it a claims-made or occurrence policy? What are its inclusions and exclusions?

7. Read the vignette at the beginning of this chapter. In a group discussion role-play explaining the trial process to Mary.

Annotated Reading List

Freidman L: *A History of American Law,* 2nd ed. Simon and Schuster, 1985.

This text traces the history of the United States legal system from its beginnings to the present. It provides perspective and gives the reader an understanding of the traditions found in the current legal profession.

Meubauer MP: Careful charting, your best defense. *RN* Nov 1990; 77–80.

The author asks, "How does your charting measure up against these examples?" She gives examples of sketchy charting that leaves little defense, then clearly states what to include and what to omit in what she calls "defensive" record keeping. The article is brief, but fact-filled and useful.

Nursing: A Social Policy Statement. ANA, 1980.

In this 32-page pamphlet the ANA Congress for Nursing Practice presents a description of the scope of nursing practice. By offering a definition of nursing and description of the characteristics of specialization in nursing practice, it provides a foundation for consideration of the legal implications of practice.

Roach W, et al: *Medical Records and the Law.* Aspen Systems, 1985.

In this valuable text, legal issues associated with medical records are explored in detail. Such topics as release of information from medical records, documentation of events, and related concerns of nurses are discussed. Its up-to-date descriptions offer valuable information for the practicing nurse.

References

Baum L: *American Courts: Process and Policy.* Houghton Mifflin, 1986.

Christoffel T: *Health and the Law: A Handbook for Health Professionals.* Free Press, 1982.

Crawford v. Earl Long Memorial Hospital, 431 So. 2d 40. (La. App.) 1983.

Creighton H: *Law Every Nurse Should Know,* 5th ed. Saunders, 1986.

Daniel v. Gladewater Municipal Hospital, 694 S.W. 2d 619 (Tx. App.) 1985.

Darling v. Charleston Community Hospital, 694 S.W. 2d 619 (Tx. App.) 1965.

Fein v. Kaiser Permanente Medical Group, 695 P 2d 655 (Ca.) 1985.

Fenner KM: *Ethics and Law in Nursing, Professional Perspectives.* Van Nostrand, 1980.

Grigis S: *Law Dictionary.* Barron's Educational Series, 1975.

Northrop C, Kelly M: *Legal Issues in Nursing.* Mosby, 1987.

Nurses' Legal Handbook. Springhouse, 1985.

Nurses' Service Organization: Advertisement. *RN* Sept 1987; 8.

Prosser W: *Handbook on the Law of Torts,* 4th ed. West Publishing, 1971.

Rhodes A, Miller R: *Nursing and the Law,* 4th ed. West Publishing, 1971.

Scully P: Are you expert enough to be an expert witness? *Nurs Life* July/Aug 1982.

Torbert v. Befeler, No. L-17463-81, Union City Superior Court, April 25, 1985, *Atlanta Law Reporter* Dec 1985.

Twenty-eighth United States Code 1331, 1332. 1982.

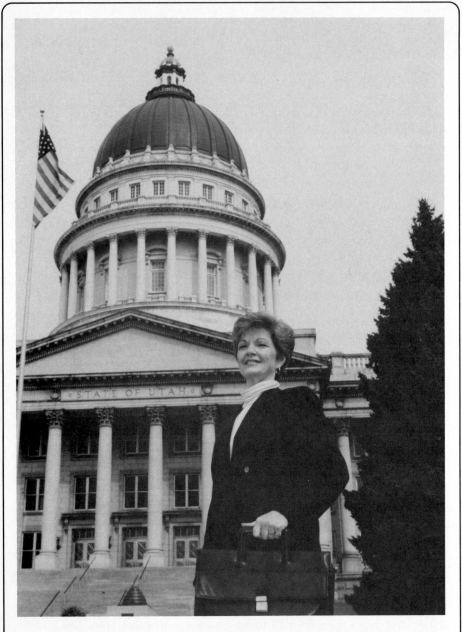

In 1988, Paula Julander became Utah's first RN legislator. By taking political action nurses bring about change, exert power, and influence the delivery of health care. (Courtesy Paula Julander)

CHAPTER 8

Change, Power, and Politics

LEARNING OBJECTIVES

1. Define change, change agent, and target system.

2. Describe the characteristics and types of change.

3. Compare rational, paradoxical, normative, and coercive models of planned change.

4. Identify criteria for choosing each model for planned change.

5. Define power and state its characteristics and types.

6. Discuss the various sources of power, giving examples of individuals who exert power based on each source.

7. Explain how nurses can use power with themselves, their peers, subordinates, superiors, and the public.

8. Define politics, political strategies, and political action.

9. Discuss the use of political strategies and describe specific instances when each might be employed.

10. State the "do's" and "don'ts" of writing to elected representatives.

11. Discuss political actions nurses can take relative to the government, professional organizations, workplace, and community.

12. Discuss the socialization of women relative to power and politics.   251

Julie was so upset she could not speak. She left the old man's room and stalked down the corridor. How could they discharge Tom to a hotel for transients on skid row! With no one to care for him, he would surely get worse. It was no wonder he had developed pneumonia and nearly died before they found him, living in a cold, dingy room without enough food. His last meager social security check had been stolen. To avoid eviction he used what money he had for rent. Social services had done all they could, they said, but with DRG constraints, the number of allotted days for his diagnosis was used up. Tom had to go. The hospital would be bankrupt if it kept everyone like Tom.

Julie felt angry, sad, and powerless. In our great and wealthy nation, how could this happen? Why was there no money to care for sick and hungry people? What could she do to change things? What could a single woman, a nurse, do to influence the delivery of health care?

The realities of contemporary health care do not always fit the humanistic ideals of nursing. Yet nurses traditionally have accepted the passive role they learned as women and have not taken a leadership role in creating change. As sex roles have begun to change, nurses have begun to realize that they can have a say in the delivery of health care. To do this they must understand the concepts of change, power, and politics. They must learn to use this knowledge in government, the community, their professional organizations, workplaces, and personal lives.

Change

The primary reason for nurses to learn about power and politics is to produce change. But what is *change?* Change is action, movement, alteration, and transformation. It is conversion from one state to another. Brooten et al (1978) defined change as "the process which leads to alteration in individual or institutional patterns of behavior." Bennis et al (1976) said that "planned change is a conscious, deliberate, collaborative effort to improve the operations of human systems through the use of valid knowledge, . . . a goal-directed process." *Change agents* plan and implement change in *target systems*.

Characteristics of Change

In open, living systems, change is inevitable. It may occur quite slowly and subtly or quickly and dramatically. Regardless of the speed, change in any part of a system affects the whole system. By continually adapting to change, systems have a tendency to maintain a uniform, steady state within and between their parts. Some systems are more stable than others. However, the more stable they are, the more they resist change. For example, a newly formed health agency may be more open to innovation than an old, established one.

Change, like power, is neither good nor bad in itself. It is the use of change that gives it value. Some changes are inherently unwise and some are actually destructive. Such change should be resisted. Of course, change for the sake of change is of no value and the disruption it creates actually may damage a system. Nonetheless, positive change produces growth, relieves boredom, increases productivity, heightens self-esteem, and invigorates participants.

Many factors influence the way people respond to change. Such things as past experiences, values, culture, and present needs affect the way people respond to change. Group norms, social climate, roles, accepted leadership style, and even approaches used to bring about change affect the way people respond. People resist change for a variety of reasons. It may violate an established norm, disrupt an established routine, or threaten a cherished tradition. It may be implemented too rapidly, before people in a system have had time to adapt. Sometimes change penalizes people in terms of time, money, or effort and sometimes it frightens them because its effects are unknown.

Types of Change

Change has been categorized in various ways by different scholars. In one of his early writings, Bennis (1968) identified eight types of change: indoctrination, interactional, socializing, coercive, technocratic, natural, emulative, and planned. Sampson (1971) suggested the types be reduced to three: developmental, spontaneous, and planned change. Duncan (1978) further reduced the number to two types: haphazard and planned change. Notice that planned change was identified by each scholar.

Models of Planned Change

There are several approaches (models) to planned change. The amount of resistance to change governs the choice of an approach. It is imperative that change agents charged with the responsibility of bringing about change make an accurate assessment of resistance before they choose a model. Listed from the least to the greatest amount of power needed to overcome resistance, models for change are: rational, paradoxical, normative, and coercive. Each model has an appropriate use.

Rational Model

The *rational model* for planned change is based on the belief that people would change if they knew a better way of accomplishing some goal. Therefore, there are no strategies for overcoming resistance to change in this model. The focus is on the change rather than the resistant system. One of the best known rational approaches is called *diffusion of innovation* (Rogers and Shoemaker 1971). The diffusion of innovation model has three steps:

1. Invention of the change
2. Diffusion (communication of information, with success depending on compatibility with existing values, complexity in using or understanding, trialability (use on a trial basis), and observability of positive results
3. Consequences: adoption or rejection

Application of the Rational Model

The rational model often takes the form of public information campaigns such as those initiated to reduce the incidence of street drug abuse and teen pregnancy ("Just say NO!") and to control the spread of AIDS by using condoms ("Safe sex"). Accurate data on the effectiveness of these approaches is not readily available.

Paradoxical Model

A paradox is a contradictory, illogical event. This model grew out of the study of human communication by Watzlawick et al (1974). These researchers are remembered for their description of "double bind" communication and for the paradoxical psychotherapy of "prescribing the symptom." They proposed that change occurs at two levels: a logical, first order and an illogical, second order.

First order change involves rearranging existing elements of a system in a logical fashion. Such change may prove frustrating when the harder the system tries, the more persistent the problem becomes.

Second order change requires a creative new approach to an old problem. It asks change agents to look at a problem creatively, from a different perspective called *reframing*. The process of creating second order change is as follows:

1. Define the problem in concrete terms.

2. List the solutions attempted so far.

3. Clearly define a realistic change.

4. Create an innovation to solve the problem and implement the innovation.

Application of the Paradoxical Model

The long-term care unit regularly exceeded its budgeted supply of clean linen. Hospital administration decided to mount a campaign to reduce expensive linen use. The supervisor of the long-term care unit (the change agent) set up meetings with staff nurses to publicize the high cost of clean linen, asked staff to reduce linen use, and finally, issued a quota of linen per patient per day. The nurses tried to comply, but it seemed as if the more they tried, the less they were able to reduce linen use. After a three-month trial period, linen use was just as high as before the campaign. First order change had not been effective.

The supervisor, working with the staff, decided to implement the paradoxical model. Together they:

1. Defined the problem:
   Patients require frequent bed baths and linen changes because they are incontinent, even though bowel and bladder training is ongoing.

2. Listed possible solutions:
   (a) Use paper diapers on patients; use paper towels to clean up after incontinence, changing bed linen but once a week
   (b) Install a washing machine and dryer on the unit and ask the staff to wash the linen if it becomes soiled
   (c) Give fewer baths and only minimum cleaning after incontinence
   (d) Get patients up into bath chairs and wash them thoroughly in the shower

3. Defined realistic change:
   A 10% drop in linen use.

4. Created an innovative solution:
   Remodel the bathroom into a shower room with a hand-held spray unit, purchase shower chairs with wheels, and give inservice education to staff on how to use the new facility and equipment.

The supervisor presented the idea to the hospital administrator, who convinced the board of trustees to authorize the construction project.

Three months after the new system was instituted, evaluation of the change showed a 15% reduction in linen costs, fewer decubitus ulcers, greater mobility of patients, and higher staff morale. Although the solution required the initial cost of remodeling the bathroom and purchasing shower chairs, the expense was recovered in savings, patient welfare, and staff morale.

The unique thing about second order change is *innovation*. New equipment, even a different building design, may be necessary. Second order change is not merely a rearrangement or improvement of old methods. It is a fundamentally different approach to the problem.

Normative (Natural) Models

Normative models of planned change are more holistic than rational ones. They take into account the nature of the change, the change agent, and the target system. They recognize the effects of feelings, needs, attitudes, and values on the people who are to change. Two well-known normative approaches are Lewin's phases of change model and Havelock and Lippitt's steps of the change model.

LEWIN'S MODEL.   Lewin identified three phases that occur in all change: unfreezing, changing, and refreezing (Lewin 1951). Lewin recommended that the process of planned change begin with a thorough analysis of the target system and its environment to identify forces for and against change. Those that push the system to-

Driving forces: Restraining forces:

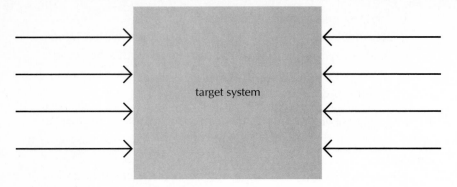

Figure 8-1   *Forces For and Against Change in a Target System*

ward change he called *driving forces;* those that pull the system away from change he called *restraining forces.* Such information is portrayed graphically in Figure 8-1.

Unfreezing.   Once the driving and restraining forces are known, Lewin recommends using three tactics to unfreeze, or destabilize, the system in order to get it moving in the direction of change. He described these tactics as: disconfirmation, inducing guilt and anxiety, and providing psychologic safety.

   Disconfirmation is confronting the target system with conflicting evidence so that people will feel uncomfortable or dissatisfied with its present condition and will want to change. Disconfirmation may consist of information or experiences that challenge the present condition.

   Inducing guilt and anxiety is done by demonstrating that important goals or values are not being met or upheld. This is done to upset the balance between driving and restraining forces and raise the level of tension within the system.

   Psychologic safety is offered so that people will feel comfortable enough to reduce their defensive behavior and attempt to change.

Changing.   Once the system is unfrozen and moving toward change, the change agent begins putting the planned change into effect. Tappen (1983) suggested the following activities for the change agent:

1. Introduce information needed to implement changed behavior.

2. Encourage new behavior when possible, and allow practice and experimentation with changed behavior.

3. Continue supportive climate to reduce defensive behavior and resistance.

4. Provide opportunities to ventilate feelings of frustration and anxiety regarding the change.

5. Provide feedback on progress and clarify goals to reinforce change and keep up momentum of change.

6. Encourage trust and keep communication open.

7. Continue to use disconfirmation, guilt, and anxiety to overcome resistance.

8. Be enthusiastic, keeping interest high and the change process moving forward.

Refreezing.   The purpose of refreezing is to stabilize the system and integrate the change so that it becomes a part of the regular functioning of the system. During this phase the change agent continues to guide the process, acts as an energizer so that the change will continue, and increasingly delegates responsibility to others in the system.

APPLICATION OF LEWIN'S MODEL.   Administrators of a state psychiatric hospital were smarting under media criticism. Patient violence had caused many serious injuries of staff nurses and other patients. They appointed a panel of experts to study the problem. The panel recommended that patients be assigned to nursing units on the basis of aggressive behavior, diagnosis, and age. Such an assignment method would replace the regional one that had been in effect for 20 years. In the regional method patients were assigned to units according to their geographic area. Administrators decided to make the change.

Unfreezing began by analysis of the system to identify driving

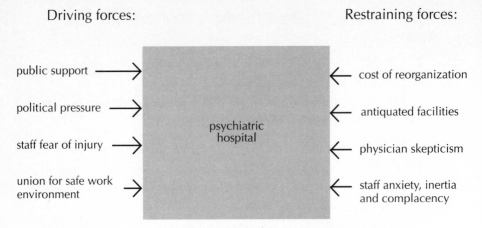

Figure 8-2   Forces For and Against Change in a Psychiatric Hospital

forces that would facilitate the change and restraining forces that would work against change, as shown in Figure 8-2. To unfreeze the system the change agent (administrators) used: disconfirmation by citing safety records of other psychiatric hospitals, guilt and anxiety by citing recent deaths and serious injury to patients and staff members, and psychological safety by encouraging staff participation.

The general plan for reassignment of patients was announced. It was to be implemented gradually. Staff members were asked to sort patients according to twelve categories, including age, aggressive behavior, and level of functioning.

The change was planned to occur over two years. Before, during, and after, staff and administrators exchanged information by written communications and group discussions. During these meetings staff had the opportunity to ventilate concerns. Administrators clarified goals and kept the momentum going. To reduce anxiety a detailed calendar for each move was published well in advance so that patients and staff members knew when and where they were going. Administrators visited the nursing units to encourage and keep the process moving forward.

Refreezing took several months. After the initial large-scale moves of patients and staff, administrators delegated more and more of the process to supervisors. An impartial priority system for transfer of personnel was instituted. The system gradually stabilized as it integrated the change into its regular functioning. Although resistance to change was substantial at first, gradually the staff saw the benefits of the change, adjusted to their new assignments, and accepted the change. The incidence of staff and patient injury dropped significantly.

HAVELOCK AND LIPPITT'S MODEL.   The change process described by Havelock and Lippitt (Havelock 1973) focuses on how the leader brings about change using a democratic style of leadership. In fact, the term *change agent* came from this model. It assumes a good working relationship between the leader and target system. The six steps in this model are: (1) build a relationship, (2) diagnose the problem, (3) assess resources, (4) set goals and select strategies, (5) implement the change, (6) stabilize, consolidate, and reinforce the change.

Build a Relationship.   The first task of the change agent/leader is to gain the respect of the target system. This is done by providing information about credentials and past relevant experiences of the change agent. It is essential that the leader develop a relationship of trust and respect within the system and demonstrate leadership ability.

Diagnose the Problem.   The next step in the change process is to identify a problem that the target system considers important and in need of changing. The leader acts as the energizer and promotes a climate of trust, encouraging and guiding movement toward the development of consensus on the problem.

Assess Resources.   The third step is to assess the resources available to the group or leader to bring about the identified change. Resources include: motivation and commitment, needed knowledge and skills, power for implementation, financial backing, time and energy, social norms, roles, and values that support the change.

Set Goals and Select Strategies.   After diagnosing the problem and assessing available resources, the group sets goals and specific objectives. Group members in the target system are actively involved just as they were in the second and third steps. The leader acts as guide, supporter, resource person, and energizer.

Implement Planned Change.   Implementation of planned change is greatly facilitated by beginning at a *leverage point*. A leverage point is a person or group that is most likely to be receptive to change. By instituting the change at the leverage point, resistance may be softened and change demonstrated.

Stabilize, Consolidate, and Reinforce.   In the final step, the change agent works to stabilize the system, consolidate, and reinforce the changes. The leader continues to give participants feedback and support the change.

APPLICATION OF HAVELOCK AND LIPPITT'S MODEL.   A new director of nurses was hired for a 35-bed hospital in a small town. She had excellent credentials and a reputation for effective leadership, but the staff was skeptical. Soon after arriving the director set up individual and group meetings with staff members to learn about their problems. Gradually, she gained their confidence by her openness, honesty, fairness, and evident knowledge.

So many problems were identified, a decision had to be made about where to begin. A poll of the nurses indicated that the most vexing problem was the performance evaluation "nonmethod" used by the hospital to determine salaries and promotion.

Assessment of resources from all available sources was the next step. The director gained the support of the hospital administrator. Sample copies of performance evaluation methods of other hospitals were collected. Information on evaluation was obtained from the National League for Nursing. Nursing staff offered their time and effort to work on the project and hospital volunteers agreed to provide secretarial assistance as needed.

With the director of nursing as leader, a coordinating committee was formed. At the first meeting the committee identified goals and strategies:

Goal: To develop performance evaluation criteria for each staff position and a fair, comprehensive process for promotions.

Strategy: The director and nursing staff would work together to develop a new evaluation process. When completed it would be presented up the chain of command for hospital board approval and then implemented by the director.

The leverage point was identified as the shift lead nurses, the ones who were most dissatisfied with the old method. They were asked to serve on the coordinating committee.

The project was a big one, involving much time and effort. The director of nurses gave ongoing support, encouragement, and co-ordination to the project. After it was completed and approved by the hospital trustees the director continued to support the plan during its implementation.

Coercive Model

The coercive model is an authoritarian approach to change. It assumes that there will be a great deal of resistance to a proposed change. It is used when more democratic, participatory approaches have failed or are expected to fail. This model recognizes human needs, values, feelings, and attitudes, but does not necessarily bow to them. Leaders may *use* human needs to bring about desired change. Those who use this approach enter a win-lose situation. Before they begin they should make a careful assessment of their power to be sure it can overcome all resistance.

The change agent/leader reassesses the target system, decides on the change to be made, plans the sequence of steps for its implementation, and decides strategies for overcoming resistance.

The coercive model is what groups of people, using the political process, employ to make change. By getting enough votes to pass a legislative act they gain the police power of the state to enforce a law that will mandate change. It is this kind of change in the health-care system of the United States that Julie longed for in the vignette.

Application of the Coercive Model

Several nurses complained to the director of nurses that many of their peers arrived late to work, took many coffee breaks, and long lunch periods. The concerned nurses said such behavior placed an unfair burden on the nurses who were punctual, that it was unethical, and violated their employment contract.

The director of nurses discussed the problem with the hospital administrator and checked the employment contract. Indeed, such behavior was a clear violation of the nurses' contract. The director decided to monitor the situation informally for a week to see if the complaints were legitimate. She found they were.

The director decided to use a coercive approach to change. She sent a notice to all units reminding nurses that they were expected to report to work on time and were allowed two ten-minute breaks and a thirty-minute lunch period. If consistent tardiness or excessive break-taking continued, a time-clock would be installed, pay would be docked for missed time, and attendance records would become an item in performance evaluations.

Change occurred immediately. The hospital had the legal and ethical power to overcome resistance and to enforce the change.

Power and Politics

Power and politics are discomforting concepts to nurses. Indeed, power and politics are foreign notions to members of the caring profession, although nurses use them every day, in every sphere of life. Understanding these concepts and learning strategies to use them is essential if nurses wish to manage their personal and professional lives and influence the delivery of health care.

Power

Power is defined as the ability to influence behavior. Hendricks (1982) said "it is a positive force for creative change and is a central issue in nursing's struggle to define itself." Stevens (1979) said that "power is the capacity to modify the conduct of others in a desired manner, while avoiding having one's own conduct modified in undesired ways by others." Ferguson (1985) said that "power is the ability to do or act . . . [to have] possession or control or command over others . . . is access . . . [to] the ability to deliver goods and services on your terms . . . to achieve the desired result."

Characteristics of Power

Power is a neutral concept, neither good nor bad. However, it can be used constructively or destructively and has the ability to effect change. McFarland (1982) said that "power and change are inevitably present in all organizations. . . . Understanding the two concepts is vital to effective nursing performance."

Power is a reciprocal process. When one person assumes control, the other gives it up. Power cannot be assumed without the permission or coercion of the one who surrenders it. By studying the reasons people willingly relinquish control of themselves to others, one can learn power-gaining and power-keeping strategies.

The possession of power is temporary, in constant flux, never permanently owned and held. It is forever subject to challenge by those who seek to gain or regain control.

Types of Power

Power has been typified as personal, shared, political, and professional. *Personal power* is defined as "the drive within a person to overcome both internal and external resistance to reaching one's goals . . . not a desire to exercise control over others, but to have control within oneself . . . having the energy and means to use what is needed to reach the "pot of gold." . . . [It is] a way of living, not a way of responding" (Hamilton and Kiefer 1986). Personal power develops as a result of life experiences, values, and how one views one's place in the world.

Shared power has been described as team power, or the empowering of others. In its application to leadership, Kelly (1987) said that "shared power placed an emphasis on interdependence in relationships and human interaction as a source of power . . . differing from the personal power seen in a male style of leadership which is direct, aggressive, and competitive." Research indicates that women tend to prefer shared power rather than to depend on personal power (Gorman and Clark 1986). Kelly (1987) suggests that this preference may occur because women are socialized to act as part of a group.

Political power is associated with governmental control of the people, using the prestige and coercive power of the state. In a broad sense, political power is a type of shared power. In a democracy the citizens have a say in laws that govern them. Often they feel powerless, however, because changing those laws and influencing the people who interpret them is so difficult and expensive. Julie in the vignette experienced this sense of powerlessness. By banding together with others of like mind, citizens gain political power.

Professional power is described as "the ability of nurses to reach goals with patients, function autonomously, and effect change within a work setting, such as knowing how to work within the system . . . to reach goals" (Hamilton and Kiefer 1986). Nurses exercise professional power in many ways, including demonstrating expert clinical skills and knowledge, participating in quality assurance activities, and working through official nursing organizations to advance the profession.

Sources of Power

The ability to exercise power by influencing the behavior of others is derived from a number of sources. Some are more available and more ethically acceptable to nurses than others. However, recognizing that there are such sources and what they consist of is the first step toward developing power strategies. Sources of power have been described in a number of articles, including those by French and Raven (1959), Hersey et al (1979), and Stevens (1979), as follows:

Informational power (expert knowledge) comes from a perception of an ability to access, withhold, or possess key information, exceptional talent, skill, or expertise. It is possessed by such persons as researchers, clinical specialists, and "old hands" (experienced nurses).

Legitimate power (positional) derives from a formal position or title in an organization that gives the holder authority to make decisions. It is possessed by such persons as directors of nurses, members of faculty, and deans of nursing schools.

Associative power (connection) arises from a perception of an important relationship with others who have power. Those with associative power include office nurses of famous physicians, alumni of great universities, and friends of elected officials.

Reward power comes from a perception of an ability to bestow rewards or favors on others, such as promotions, grades, money, and days off. This power is possessed by such persons as instructors, scheduling clerks, and performance evaluators.

Coercive power (legal, physical, financial) arises from a perception of an ability to punish, threaten, or withhold rewards. It is possessed by such persons as nursing instructors, officers of the law, and nursing supervisors.

Collective power arises from the sheer weight of numbers of people, as possessed by organized groups of voters or potential donors such as the American Medical Association and American Nurses' Association.

Referent power (charismatic, personal) arises from a personal sense of self and an ability to communicate personal attributes so that others admire, identify with, and are motivated to follow that person. It is possessed by "natural" leaders, respected teachers, and role models.

Uses of Power

We have said that power is a neutral concept of control, neither good nor bad in itself. It is the use of power that is constructive or destructive. Nurses use power in relation to the self, their peers, subordinates, and superiors.

WITH THE SELF.   To use power constructively with themselves nurses must take control of their lives and manage them to achieve personal and professional goals. (See Chapter 12, Career Management.) The first step in using personal power is to "know thyself," as Socrates advised. Nurses need to make an accurate assessment of their physical, emotional, and intellectual capacities, values, beliefs, talents, limitations, prejudices, aspirations, and needs. With such knowledge nurses move to the second step, setting down large general goals they want to achieve. From these general goals they list specific, attainable objectives to be accomplished in a certain time span.

The third step in using power is to achieve objectives. Here are some strategies to help you achieve your objectives:

1. Package yourself to fit your objectives. For example, if you want to be considered for promotion to an administrative position, dress with impeccable care to "look like" an executive. If you want to be a university professor, earn higher academic degrees. If you want to have friends, be friendly.

2. Be adaptable and flexible, temporarily altering your course, if necessary, in order to reach ultimate goals. For example, as a new graduate you may have to work a year on a medical-surgical unit before the hospital will permit you to work in a specialty such as maternity.

3. Demonstrate adult behaviors and practice assertive communication. For example, do not sulk and complain if your application to transfer to another unit seems to have been ignored. Go to the supervisor, state specific facts of the case, state how you feel, and ask for what you want. Such behavior is honest, direct, and mentally healthy (Hamilton and Kiefer 1986).

WITH PEERS. People can exert destructive as well as supportive power. *Destructive power* is exhibited by mean criticism and lack of support of others. Too often nurses are critical of one another, competitive, and downright cruel. If someone makes an error such nurses are the first to tell the supervisor, magnify the significance of the error, and disassociate themselves from the errant one. Such unfortunate lack of charity may stem from the autocratic style of leadership so often found in hospitals. The classic research of Lewin et al (1939) on styles of leadership revealed that in authoritarian-led groups, members are more competitive, hostile, and less creative than in democratic-led groups. However, nurses do not need to remain victims of such a system. Using personal power they can change their individual behavior towards others. Using shared power they can change the work environment to one that fosters collegiality.

Supportive power with peers is characterized by mutual respect for other nurses, kindness, collegiality, accountability for the performance of self and peers, and professionalism. (See the discussion of shared governance under "Participative Management" in Chapter 10.)

WITH SUBORDINATES.   Nurses use power constructively with those they supervise by accepting responsibility and not lording power over subordinates or using it capriciously. The constructive use of power includes assessing subordinates accurately, fitting assignments to capacities, delegating duties appropriately and fairly, giving compliments and reproofs sincerely without favoritism, and explaining rationales for decisions. When change is needed, the constructive use of power means selecting an appropriate model. Wynd (1985) said that "the effective use of power is associated with a high degree of responsibility, accountability, the ability to form alliances and procure resources, and the courage to take action, often in a competitive mode, in the face of obstacles and outside power."

WITH SUPERIORS.   Nurses exercise power with superiors by demonstrating professional competence, using assertive communication, and being flexible and willing to compromise. Even when nurses behave in these ways, problems sometimes arise. When they do, remember that a group is more powerful than an individual. Professional organizations can offer expert advice on the use of collective power with superiors to effect change.

WITH THE PUBLIC.   The media has not been kind to nursing. It has portrayed nurses as sex-craved females, incompetent servants with time to sit at a desk, flirt with male physicians, and gossip. Too often sensational stories of unethical and criminal acts by nurses get front-page coverage while noble and autonomous acts of nurses go unnoticed. Nurses can change their public image individually and collectively in many ways. They can (1) support health and human welfare legislation, publicizing their stand; (2) "toot their own horn" by submitting news stories of courage, achievement, and independence to the media; (3) communicate their objections about demeaning, sexist TV nurse roles and state the case for roles that portray nurses as independent professionals with high ethical standards and rewarding personal lives; (4) maintain high standards of professional competence; and (5) deliver sensitive nursing care to patients.

Politics

Political Strategies

While *politics* is the art or science of government, *political strategies* are activities people can take to gain governmental power in order to institute change. The following political strategies, coupled with energy and commitment, have been suggested by Talbott and Mason (1987) and others:

1. Develop a sense of self and the ability to communicate effectively.

2. Seek positions that give the authority to grant rewards and mete out punishment.

3. Become an expert in various fields of study, earn degrees, and gain special skills that command respect.

4. Form alliances or coalitions with powerful persons of like mind; guard against association with people with sullied reputations.

5. Control information, either by giving or withholding it.

6. Foster a public image of nurses that portrays them not as uniformed servants but as dedicated, autonomous professionals.

7. To gain collective power, join professional organizations such as the American Nurses' Association.

8. Be ready to move on issues; "strike while the iron is hot."

9. Compromise, if necessary; "half a loaf is better than none."

10. Display confidence; "nothing ventured, nothing gained."

11. Be prepared to give something in return; "quid pro quo."

12. Be patient; "Rome was not built in a day."

13. Watch for any change or weakening of position; "get your toe in the door."

14. Gather as many facts as possible; do your homework.

15. Become sensitive to hidden agendas; "read between the lines."

16. Refrain from commitments that limit maneuverability or influence.

17. When upset with others, try to understand their position; "walk a mile in the other person's mocassins."

18. Don't be discouraged by setbacks; "look at the big picture."

Political Action

Political action means getting involved in the process of change. Such involvement is most effective when nurses use what Connie Vance (1985) called the three "Cs" of political action:

Communication that is assertive, clear, and concise,

Collectivity, a source of power and the foundation for networking, coalition-building, and collaboration, and

Collegiality, a sense of community, camaraderie, and sisterhood that is the foundation for building esteem and trust and supporting and nurturing associates.

Nurses use these three interpersonal skills to take political action in the government, community, professional organizations, workplace, and personal lives.

GOVERNMENT

Become Informed.   The first step for nurses to become politically active is to become informed. They (1) listen to daily news and in-depth reports of radio and television stations; (2) read news magazines and news sections of professional journals; (3) seek out special reports of such nonpartisan groups as the League of Women Voters and Common Cause, or of partisan groups such as the Republican Party and Democratic Party; (4) talk to people with similar concerns; (5) learn the names and addresses of elected representatives by calling a public library, the local newspaper, or a chapter of the League of Women Voters; (6) obtain copies of proposed state laws by asking for them by number from elected representatives and state printing offices. Send for proposed federal laws from:

Senate bills: US Senate Documents Office
                Washington, DC 20510

House bills: Doorkeeper of the House of Representatives
                US Capitol
                Washington, DC 20515

Vote.   The most fundamental political action citizens can take is to vote. It is the responsibility and privilege of every citizen. Nurses may feel they are too poor to contribute money, too busy to work for candidates, or too involved in other interests to serve on boards or committees. However, nurses everywhere can become informed and vote.

Communicate with Representatives.   Elected officials represent the people of their district or state. They want, seek, pay attention to, and vote in accordance with the wishes of their constituents. Those who make their opinions known influence the outcome of issues. Address letters to:

US representatives: Honorable _____
                      House Office Building
                      Washington, DC 20515

US senators: Senator _____
               Senate Office Building
               Washington, DC 20510

When you write *do:*

1. Identify the issue or the bill by number.
2. Time letter or telegram to arrive before a vote.
3. Be brief and to the point. "Please vote 'no' on Bill # _____."
4. Give reasons; state how the bill affects people. "Because . . ."
5. Be constructive; offer an alternate approach if you can.
6. Give praise when it is due.

7. State your own views, in your own words, on your own stationery. (Form letters and petitions are less effective.)

When you write, *do not:*

1. Threaten, berate, or demean.
2. Send long, rambling essays.

Contribute Time, Money, and Effort.   Political action takes time, money and effort. Besides writing letters and sending telegrams, nurses can work in election campaigns of individual candidates and referendums, testify at public hearings, contribute money, and participate in demonstrations. Nurses can offer to serve on various voluntary boards and commissions. By so doing they can provide pertinent facts and give the viewpoint of nursing, increasing the visibility of nursing. Nurses can influence health policy and practice by being appointed to positions of authority. Of course, the ultimate political action occurs when nurses run for public office and become elected representatives.

COMMUNITY.   Nurses can become politically active in their communities in countless ways, from serving on school lunch committees to becoming mayors of cities. Because nurses are articulate, intelligent, highly motivated, and energetic individuals, they are natural leaders. Their interests are found in every area of life, in health clinics and prisons, with infants and aged care, in highway safety, air quality, self-help groups, and food distribution centers. Wherever there are people, nurses have concerns. By applying their knowledge of change, power, and politics nurses can help create a more healthful society.

PROFESSIONAL ORGANIZATIONS.   Professional nursing organizations are devoted to advancing the profession and influencing health care. They exercise collective power by presenting a united voice for nursing. Individual nurses can participate in the activities of these organizations in many ways, from simple membership to serving as officers and committee members at local, state, and national levels. Although they are not legally "political," professional organizations do influence the delivery of health care by serving in advisory capacities to governmental agencies and supporting many public and private initiatives.

Political action committees (PACs) are organizations devoted to advancing the interest of a particular group. Many are single-issue organizations. Because not-for-profit organizations such as the American Nurses' Association cannot engage in political action, these groups pursue their political efforts by means of PACs. Nurses can support the work of the ANA-PAC in a variety of ways. (See Chapter 4, Nursing Organizations.)

WORKPLACE.   Nursing is hard work. It requires enormous amounts of energy and concentration. Not much energy is left over for political action in the workplace. However, if nurses leave decisions about patient care and scarce resources to others, others will make the decisions. If nurses are to exert power they must become involved. By applying the interpersonal skills of political action (communication, collectivity, collegiality) and their knowledge of the sources of power, nurses can effect changes in their workplace in the following ways:

1. Volunteer to be members of standing committees that make policy recommendations, such as patient safety, employee welfare, and ad hoc committees.

2. Use both the formal and informational network of the agency. Many hospitals and health agencies have their own in-house newsletter or other official communications network. People who control information exercise power.

3. Use employee representatives if the agency has a collective bargaining organization.

4. Pursue activities that gain recognition and respect, such as research projects and excellence in nursing care.

5. Seek positions of authority. Nurses are excellent managers, well qualified for administrative jobs. By serving in such positions nurses gain the power to make decisions and gain access to other persons with power.

PERSONAL AND PROFESSIONAL LIVES.   Nurses can take charge of their personal and professional lives by applying the concepts of change, power, and politics to their own careers. Chapter 12, Career Management, focuses on this task.

RESTRICTIONS ON POLITICAL ACTIVITIES.   There are some restrictions on the political activities of employees of tax-supported agencies. The Hatch Act prohibits public employees from engaging in activities on the behalf of a political party or in support of legislation that could be construed as support from a government agency. The act does not interfere with employee rights as private citizens to support parties, candidates, or ballot measures. However, employees must be careful only to speak and act as private citizens, not as representatives of an agency. Because many states have their own versions of the Hatch Act nurses employed by government agencies need to learn what restrictions apply to them.

Women, Power, and Politics

In our culture, power and politics are associated with masculinity. Until recently, women have been socialized to be noncompetitive, meek, compliant, passive, subservient, and to shun power. They have been taught that authority and power are the birthright of men and obedience the lot of women. In most world cultures men are the rulers and spiritual leaders. Only when family inheritance outweighs sexual bias, and efforts to produce a male heir fail, are women given the reins of government. Small changes are being made, but women have a long way to go before they acquire a significant proportion of the positions of power.

Because nursing is a woman's profession (97% are women) it is no wonder that nurses have difficulty assuming power or using power in the political arena. Like Julie in the vignette, they have felt angry and sad, but also powerless to change the system. Many nurses still think of power as antifeminine, inappropriate, and antiprofessional and view powerful nurses with suspicion and fear. This negative view of power may explain why nursing continues to be a subservient occupation and why so few men choose nursing as a career. As nurses of both sexes learn more about power they will be able to take charge of their personal and professional lives and make changes without fear.

Summary

A working knowledge of the concepts of change, power, and politics can help nurses make a difference in government, the community, their professional organizations, workplaces, and personal lives. Change is a process for altering a system. It can be haphazard or planned. To institute planned change, change agents use rational, paradoxical, normative, and coercive models. Power is the ability to influence behavior. Neither good nor bad, power may be personal, shared, political, or professional. Its sources are informational, legitimate, associative, reward, coercive, collective, and referent power. Power can be used with self, peers, subordinates, superiors, and public. Politics has to do with government; political strategies are useful tactics for change. Political action means applying these tactics in various arenas. As a profession of women, nurses must change their view of power and take charge of their personal and professional lives.

Learning Activities

1. Identify a change in some health-care system that would improve employee morale or patient care services. Select a model for planned change and state the rationale for the selection. Outline the steps of the plan, including a timeline.

2. Explain the steps of Lewin's model and Havelock and Lippitt's model for planned change to a group of nurses; give your own example.

3. Give a five-minute talk entitled, "Women, power, and politics."

4. Write a brief character sketch of someone who possesses each of the following sources of power: informational, legitimate, asso-

ciative, reward, coercive, and referent power. State why collective power is an extension of reward and coercive power.

5. Assign one or more political strategies to each of a group of students. Ask each one to state when that strategy might be useful, how it could be used, if it would violate her or his ethical standards, and how she or he would feel using it.

6. In a small group discuss how power can be used constructively and destructively in relation to the self, peers, subordinates, and superiors.

7. Write to the US House or Senate printing office for specific health-related bills.

8. Write a draft letter to a member of Congress about an issue of concern. Critique the letters in a small group discussion.

9. Take a specific political action in the workplace or community. Write a description of that action.

Annotated Reading List

Mason DJ, Talbott SW (editors): *Political Action Handbook for Nurses: Changing the Workplace, Government, Organization, and Community.* Addison-Wesley, 1985.

Awarded the *AJN* Book of the Year Award, this comprehensive book contains writings of 83 nursing leaders. The work is divided into seven units. Many case studies and vignettes illustrate the political process in action. A readable, practical, and comprehensive text, it is appropriate for all nurses, from student to well-informed, involved political activist.

McCloskey JC, Grace HK: (editors): Governance. Chapter 6 in: *Current Issues in Nursing,* 2nd ed. Blackwell, 1985.

This book-length chapter focuses on the inherent power of nursing, specifically asking the question, "Does nursing have the power to change the health-care system?" Well-known nursing leaders give their answers in seven articles that follow, essentially affirming that nursing does have the power but also must have the will to make changes.

References

Bennis WG: New patterns of leadership for adaptive organizations. In: *The Temporary Society,* Bennis WG, Slater PE (editors). Harper and Row, 1968.

Bennis WG, Benne KD, Chin R, Corey KE: *The Planning of Change,* 3rd ed. Holt, Rinehart, and Winston, 1976.

Brooten DA, Hayman L, Naylor M: *Leadership for Change: A Guide for the Frustrated Nurse.* Lippincott, 1978.

Duncan WJ: *Essentials of Management,* 2nd ed. Dryden Press, 1978.

Ferguson VD: Power in nursing. Chapter 9 in: *Political Action Handbook for Nurses,* Mason DJ, Talbott SW (editors). Addison-Wesley, 1985.

French JRP, Raven B: The bases of social power. In: *Studies in Social Power,* Cartwright D (editor). University of Michigan, 1959.

Gorman S, Clark N: Power and effective nursing practice. *Nurs Outlook* May/June 1986; 129–134.

Hamilton JM, Kiefer ME: *Survival Skills for the New Nurse.* Lippincott, 1986.

Havelock RG: *The Change Agent's Guide to Innovation in Education.* Educational Technology Publications, 1973.

Hendricks D: The power problem. *Nurs Management* Oct 1982.

Hersey P, Blanchard K, Nayemeyer W: Situational leadership perception and impact of power. *Group Org Studies* 1979; 4:148–28.

Kelly LY: *The Nursing Experience: Trends, Challenges, and Transitions.* Macmillan, 1987.

Lewin K: *Field Theory in Social Science: Selected Theoretical Papers.* Harper and Row, 1951.

Lewin K, Lippitt R, White RK: Patterns of aggressive behavior in experimentally created "social climates." *J Soc Psych* 1939; 10:271–299.

McFarland D: *Managerial Innovation in the Metropolitan Hospital.* Praeger, 1982.

Rogers EM, Shoemaker FF: *Communication of Innovation,* 2nd ed. Free Press, 1971.

Sampson E: *Social Psychology and Contemporary Society.* Wiley, 1971.

Stevens BJ: Power and politics for the nurse executive. *Nurs Health Care* Nov 1979; 1:208–210.

Talbott SW, Mason DJ: Politics and power. Chapter 6 in: *Fundamentals of Nursing,* Kozier B, Erb G, 3rd ed. Addison-Wesley, 1987.

Tappen RM: *Nursing Leadership: Concepts and Practice.* Davis, 1983.

Vance C: Political influence: Building effective interpersonal skills. Chapter 14 in: *Political Action Handbook for Nurses,* Mason DJ, Talbott SW (editors). Addison-Wesley, 1985.

Watzlawick P, Weakland J, Fisch R: *Change: Principles of Problem Formation and Problem Resolution.* Norton, 1974.

Wynd C: Packing a punch: Female nurses and the effective use of power. *Nurs Success Today* Sept 1985; 2:15–20.

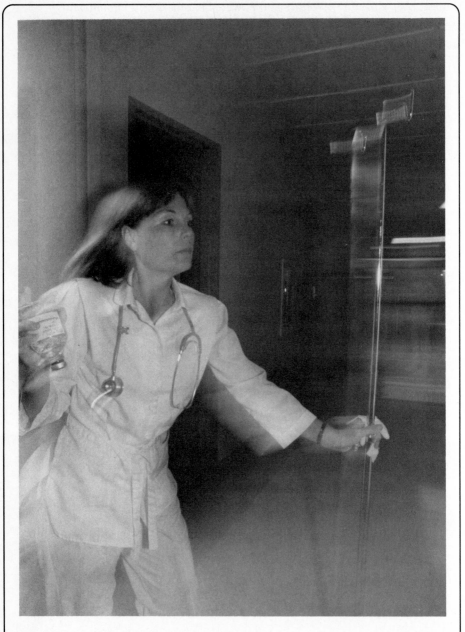

Stressed and overwhelmed by demands that exceed resources, a nurse races down the hall to add more intravenous fluid before a bottle runs dry. (Photograph by Chuck O'Rear, Westlight)

CHAPTER 9

~

Managing Stress Effectively

LEARNING OBJECTIVES

1. Compare definitions of stress according to the stimulus, response, and transactional models.

2. Identify physiologic and psychologic manifestations of stress.

3. Discuss the definition and purpose of self-awareness.

4. Explain the causes and dynamics of stress.

5. Discuss stress management and describe emotion-focused and problem-focused coping.

6. Describe various strategies for coping.

7. Discuss networking as a social support resource.

8. Explain the dynamics of burnout.

9. Discuss how the biologic clock affects nurses' work performance.

10. Describe strategies to cope successfully with shift work.

As Emily *returned from dinner to her medical-surgical unit the chronically exhausted charge nurse sighed, "I've given you another patient, a transfer from ICU, multiple fractures, Tom something, a drunk who flipped his car, room 312." This was her first job as an RN and Emily felt overwhelmed by her other six patients. How could she manage another? Other nurses did it. Emily felt she should, too. She nodded numbly.*

Emily went to pour the 6:00 PM medications. Something was wrong with the heating system; it was freezing cold. The LPN interrupted her to report that Ms. Gaw's IV had infiltrated and Mr. Fall's temperature was 102° F. Just then an orderly wheeled the new patient onto the ward, with a retinue of family members trailing behind. Orthopedic scaffolding framed the patient's bed. Emily hurried down the hall to meet the procession. The family let her know how upset they were about the transfer. She assured them she would take good care of Tom. But as Emily helped position the bed, fear swept through her. Never had she seen so many pins, ropes, and pulleys! Emily sped back to the nurses' station with the chart. She would do the paper work later. Right now she had to check the IV, Mr. Fall's temperature, supervise Mr. Stein giving himself insulin, and administer the other medications. Just then a physician stopped her and asked for assistance with a dressing. Emily looked around for help. Everyone was busy. She felt alone, anxious, frustrated. Her head throbbed.

How could Emily manage stress more effectively? How could she prevent the burnout she saw in her toilworn charge nurse?

Stress

Stress, like the weather, is something everyone talks about, but nobody does much about. School teachers, nurses, policemen, and business executives talk of stress in the workplace. Journalists call our era "a generation of stress." Since the publications of Hans Selye in 1956 and 1976, the term has become a public watchword. Perhaps the concept of stress as a tension that threatens equilibrium caught on because it gave a name to a universal human experience. Stress affects the whole person, physically, emotionally, socially, intellectually, and spiritually. It is of great concern to nurses because it is a significant factor in the health-illness continuum, having been linked to diseases such as hypertension and gastric ulcers.

Many studies have been conducted in an attempt to understand the concept of stress. Lyon and Werner (1987) found that between 1975 and 1984, there were 82 stress-related studies. Three models dominated the studies. One viewed stress as a stimulus, another saw it as a response, and a third regarded stress as a transaction between people and their environment.

Stress as Stimulus

The stimulus model defines stress as a stimulus that causes disruption in a person's life. The event or set of circumstances causing a disrupted response is called a *life-change* or *life-event*. The model proposes that too much life-change increases one's vulnerability to illness (Williams and Holmes, 1978). It focuses on major life-change events using a tool known as the Social Readjustment Rating Scale (SRRS) (see Table 9-1).

The stimulus model is based on the following assumptions: (a) life-change events are similar for each person in that they require the same amount of adaptation, (b) a person's view of an event as positive or negative is not relevant, and (c) illness occurs

Social Readjustment Rating Scale

Rank	Life Event	Life-change Unit (LCU) Value
1	Death of a spouse	100
2	Divorce	73
3	Marital separation	65
4	Detention in jail	63
5	Death of a close family member	63
6	Major personal injury or illness	53
7	Marriage	50
8	Termination of employment	47
9	Marital reconciliation	45
10	Retirement from work	45
11	Major change in health of family	44
12	Pregnancy	40
13	Sexual difficulties	39
14	Addition of a new family member	39
15	Major business adjustment	39
16	Major change in financial state	38
17	Death of a close friend	37
18	Changing to a different line of work	36
19	Major change in arguments with spouse	35
20	Mortgage or loan over $10,000	31
21	Mortgage foreclosure	30
22	Major change in work responsibilities	29
23	Son or daughter leaving home	29
24	In-law troubles	29
25	Outstanding personal achievement	26
26	Spouse starting or ending work	26
27	Start or end formal schooling	26
28	Major change in living conditions	25
29	Major revision of personal habits	24
30	Trouble with employer	23
31	Major change in working conditions	20
32	Changing to a new school	20

Table 9-1 (continued)

Social Readjustment Rating Scale		
33	Change in residence	20
34	Major change in recreation	20
35	Major change in church activities	19
36	Mortgage or loan of less than $1,000	17
37	Major change in sleeping habits	16
38	Major change in family get-togethers	15
39	Major change in eating habits	15
40	Vacation	13
41	Christmas	12
42	Minor violations of the law	11

Found in Williams CC, Holmes TH: Life change, human adaptation, and onset of illness. In: *Clinical Practice in Psychosocial Nursing: Assessment and Intervention,* Longo DC, Williams RA, p 72. Appleton-Century-Crofts, 1978.

when a common point or score is reached. The model portrays a person as a passive recipient of stress. Stress is viewed as a non-changing, additive phenomenon that can be measured by selected life events with assigned scores. A stress score is obtained by adding weighted responses or by counting events that have occurred (Williams and Holmes, 1978). The score disregards a person's perception of an event, relationship between events, or the physical and mental disruption that such events produce.

While the scale may be helpful as a tool to identify people who are "at risk," therapists find that it is not very useful as a way to understand and manage stress. On the basis of a total stress score the model suggests that individuals should avoid additional life-change events, even though such avoidance may not be possible or practical. In some cases a major life-change actually may be desirable, such as moving away from an abusive spouse. The model does not account for the people who remain well even though they have high scores. It seems reasonable to conclude that viewing stress simply as the sum of stimuli oversimplifies a far more complex phenomenon.

Stress as Response

The response model defines stress as a nonspecific response of the body to demands placed on it (Selye 1956, 1976). The stress response is represented by the *General Adaptation Syndrome* (GAS) (Figure 9-1). The GAS has three stages: (1) alarm reaction, the body's first response when exposed to a stressor; (2) adaptation or resistance to demands, called stressors; and (3) exhaustion, the result of prolonged exposure to stressors. Every stressful response is characterized by the same three stages. The response model is based on the following assumptions: (a) all stressors elicit the same response, (b) stress is not cognitively mediated, and (c) there is a finite amount of adaptive energy (Lyon and Werner 1987). Selye acknowledged the role of perception in stressful experiences but did not modify his theory to include such things as the cause of the stress, context of the event, or meaning to the person. He maintained that stress is a nonspecific response of the body to stressors, manifested by the General Adaptation Syndrome.

The response model, like the stimulus model, does not allow for individual difference in perception or response. Therapists who use this model advise individuals who are "at-risk" to take a vacation or relocate to reduce their stress. Such action does not address life-change events. Wherever they go, stress follows.

Stress as Transaction

The transactional model views stress as a concept that is neither in the environment nor in the person, but a product of their interplay (Lazarus and Folkman 1984, p 354). The person and environment are seen as constantly intertwined, each affecting the other and affected by the other (Lazarus 1966). Stress includes cognitive, affective, and adaptational factors that arise out of person-environment transactions. Unlike stimulus and response models the transactional model allows for individual differences in perception, response, and outcome. It acknowledges that some environmental demands produce stress in most people. The transactional model emphasizes that people differ in sensitivity and vulnerability, as well as interpretation and reaction to demands. For ex-

Principal Neuroendocrine Pathways that Mediate
the Response to Stress

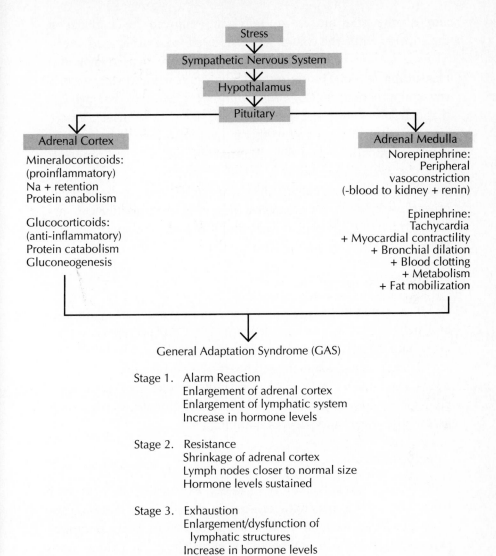

Stage 1. Alarm Reaction
Enlargement of adrenal cortex
Enlargement of lymphatic system
Increase in hormone levels

Stage 2. Resistance
Shrinkage of adrenal cortex
Lymph nodes closer to normal size
Hormone levels sustained

Stage 3. Exhaustion
Enlargement/dysfunction of
lymphatic structures
Increase in hormone levels
Depletion of adaptive hormones

The stress syndrome evolves in three stages. Stage 1 and 2 are
repeated continuously throughout a lifetime cycle. If resistance
cannot be sustained, exhaustion (stage 3) occurs, with its altered
psychophysiologic functioning.

***Figure 9-1** Physiologic Responses to Stress: General Adaptation Syndrome
(GAS)*

From Smith MJ, Selye H: Reducing the negative effects of stress. *AM J Nurs* Nov 1979; 79
(10): 1953–1964.

ample, other staff nurses on Emily's unit enjoyed the challenge of their work, while the charge nurse suffered from prolonged stress.

Assumptions of the transactional model are that stress is not measurable as a single concept and that cognitive appraisal modifies stressful experiences. *Cognitive appraisal* is an evaluative process that determines why and to what extent particular transactions are stressful. Stress, according to this model, is an interactive process between individuals and their internal and external environment.

The transactional model is useful for nurses, both as a way to assist others and to manage their own stress. Interventions focus on exploring how people perceive or appraise a stressful event, assessing their coping mechanisms, and if need be, helping them develop more effective coping strategies.

Manifestations of Stress

Stress is manifested by physiologic and psychologic symptoms and behaviors. These vary, depending on the perception of an event and effectiveness of coping strategies. Typical physiologic manifestations include increased heart rate, respirations, sweating, headaches, insomnia, and digestive disturbances. Typical psychologic manifestations of stress include emotional responses such as anxiety, anger, and procrastination.

Self-awareness

Self-awareness is the ability to assess realistically one's external behaviors and internal characteristics, especially those that indicate stress-produced tension. These include behaviors such as finger-tapping, teeth-grinding, and fist-clenching. They also include traits such as impatience, procrastination, detachment, and feelings of inadequacy. The development of self-awareness involves noticing bodily sensations, inner thoughts, and feelings. Such self-awareness opens the door to understanding and constructive change.

Causes of Stress

Stress occurs when demands exceed resources and a person feels threatened. Such demands may come from the environment, from other people, and as internalized values and beliefs. *Environ-*

mental demands include such things as sounds, odors, air movement, temperature, light, and aesthetics. *People demands* come
from the people with whom we associate. *Internalized value and
belief demands* are those such as Emily's belief that nurses like herself "should be able to care for several patients."

In the vignette, Emily experienced demands from the cold environment, the many people she was trying to please, and her internal beliefs about what nurses "should" do. When she could not
meet all these demands, Emily felt anxious and frustrated. As her
stress level rose she experienced the physical symptom of a throbbing headache.

Dynamics of Stress

From a transactional viewpoint, stress is neither an environmental stimulus, a personal characteristic, nor a response. It is a
relationship, a balance between demands and capacity to respond
to demands without unreasonable cost. People interpret situations
with respect to the effect they have on their well-being. Then they
consciously or unconsciously decide if they are able to deal with
demands and what they should do about them. The two-step interpretation process looks like this: (1) an evaluation of the significance of an event to oneself: "Does it matter to me? Am I in
trouble?" and (2) a judgment concerning options, coping responses, and constraint: "Can I handle this? If so, what can I do
about it?" Stress interpretation includes the potential for future
harm or loss. This constitutes a threat. The most frightening life
events are those where the self or significant others (extensions of
the self) may be harmed or lost. When such a threat is anticipated,
something must be done to manage the situation and reduce the
danger. Therefore, what might and can be done becomes critical.
The person must decide what coping strategies are available and
what the consequences will be for each one.

In any situation where a person asks, "Does it matter to me?
Am I in trouble?" the potential for stress exists. If the answer comes
back, "No! There is no possible gain or loss," implications for the
person's well-being are minimal and so is the stress. If the situation
holds a potential for gain, implications for the person may be positive. However, if the answer comes back, "Yes it matters; I am in

trouble," then the situation is interpreted as threatening and negative because it may cause harm or loss. Stress then occurs. For instance, Emily interpreted her work situation as extremely important. This was her first job and she desperately wanted to succeed. She feared being judged incompetent. Other nurses managed similar assignments and she felt she had to prove she could, too.

The second part of stress interpretation regards the person's resources. When the situation is judged to be threatening a person asks: "Can I handle this? If so, what can I do about it?" If the person has a history of prior success and a large repertoire of coping strategies, the answer may be, "Yes, I can handle this. I have in the past and I know what to do." However, if the answer is, "No, I don't think I can cope; I don't know what to do," the situation produces even greater stress. Emily recognized that she was in trouble and she didn't know what to do about it. As a consequence, her stress increased even more and she developed a throbbing headache.

Stress Management

Coping

Stress management is a process of balancing demands and resources, regulating feelings, and if need be, changing something in the situation. The person who is managing stress and the emotions it generates is said to be *coping*. *Coping mechanisms* usually imply managing the physiologic, automatic responses portrayed in Figure 9-1. *Coping strategies* imply managing deliberate, conscious responses.

The choice of coping strategies addresses the question, "Can I handle this and what can I do?" Although many characteristics of the person and environment are involved, the ways people cope depend on resources available to them and their ability to use them. The greater a person's store of coping strategies (resources), the greater the ability to handle demands. Therefore, coping is a crucial variable in a person's efforts to adapt and feel good about the self.

Coping has two functions: (1) to manage the somatic and subjective components of stress-related emotions, called emotion-focused; and (2) to change the situation for the better, called problem-focused (Lazarus and Folkman 1984). *Emotion-focused coping* addresses the emotional response to a stressful situation. *Problem-focused coping* addresses the situation itself. When emotion-focused coping is used, the troubling situation remains the same, but the emotional response may change. When problem-focused coping is used to change the situation, the threat is dissolved and emotional responses are avoided.

Emotion-focused Coping

Emotions are powerful forces originally developed in humans to help them survive. Plutchik (1980) defined an emotion as a complex sequence of events involving cognitive appraisal, feelings, impulses to action, and overt behaviors. He identified eight primary emotions: fear, sadness, anger, disgust, surprise, anticipation, joy, and acceptance. Although fear is a common emotion of stress, other emotions such as anger, joy, sadness, and anticipation also may produce stress. Emotion-focused coping addresses the events that produce an emotion, namely, cognitive appraisal (thinking), feeling, and behaviors.

(1) *Cognitive appraisal* involves using the mind to assess an emotion produced by a stressful situation. For example, Emily experienced stress as a result of demands made on her. Had she used the emotion-focused strategy of cognitive appraisal, she would have assessed and identified her feelings of fear and anger: *fear* of censure by herself and others and *anger* at the charge nurse, patients, and physician for blocking progress towards completing her work.

(2) *Feeling* is the intense subjective experience of an emotion. Emotion-focused strategies involve acknowledging and allowing oneself to experience emotions generated by demanding situations. For example, Emily felt the uncomfortable distress of frustration (anger). Had she acknowledged the anger, she would have been able to gain better control and reduce its intensity.

(3) *Behaviors* are actions associated with the emotions. Emotion-focused strategies involve taking various actions to avoid, reduce intensity of, or gain control of feelings. For example, had Emily counted to ten or taken a one-minute deep-breathing break when she identified her anger, she might have reduced

her sense of frustration. Other useful behaviors of emotion-focused coping are physical exercise, self-hypnosis, and biofeedback training.

Problem-focused Coping

Problem-focused coping is directed towards defining a problem, generating alternative solutions, weighing the alternatives in terms of their costs and benefits, choosing among them, and acting. Problem-focused coping embraces a wider array of strategies than problem-solving alone. It involves an objective, analytic process focusing on the environment, people, and inner values and beliefs.

(1) *Defining the problem* involves becoming aware of the manifestations of stress and identifying their cause. When Emily noticed her anxious feelings she needed to stop and define the problem. She was angry about her assignment and fearful that she could not meet the demands made on her.

(2) *Generating alternate solutions* means thinking of various ways to solve the stressful situation. This is accomplished by decreasing demands, increasing resources for meeting demands, or changing the way one views demands. Emily might have assertively told the charge nurse she could not take the added assignment. She might have asked for help from a co-worker. She might have informed the physician she was unable to assist him just then. She could have given herself permission to accomplish only essential tasks or to do so at a more relaxed pace.

(3) *Weighing alternatives in terms of costs and benefits* means identifying the pros and cons of each solution. Emily needed to weigh the risks of each solution. Would it be more costly to admit that she could not manage another patient, or to take the patient and not manage the care properly? Would the physician make an issue of her refusal to assist, or would he or she accept it? Would she be judged more incompetent for asking for help than for not asking for help? Could she feel good about herself even if she didn't get her work done on time?

(4) *Choosing* from among alternative solutions involves making a decision. Emily might have decided the best solution was to accept the additional patient but ask for assistance, to refuse the phy-

sician's request for help at that time, and to give herself permission to complete only necessary tasks.

(5) *Acting* means doing what one has decided is the best choice. To act, Emily would carry out her decisions.

Effective Coping

Coping effectiveness in a specific encounter is based on both emotion-focused and problem-focused coping. People who manage to change a situation, but at great emotional cost, cannot be said to be coping effectively. Neither can people who regulate emotions successfully but do not deal with the source of problems. Effective coping involves both regulation of emotions and management of situations.

Strategies for Coping

Coping strategies are purposeful, thoughtful responses people can use to manage stress. They require that nurses balance demands and resources, change stress-producing factors in the situation, and regulate feelings.

Balance Demands and Resources

Strategies to balance demands and resources are important tools for a busy nurse. Lyon (1984) described several such strategies:

1. *Cognitive rehearsal* uses imagery to visualize successful coping, and self-talk to talk oneself through stressful events.

2. *Delaying tactics* uses time to gain perspective by putting off tasks that produce overload or waiting until more information is available and more alternatives are identified.

3. *Setting limits* controls such things as interruptions during work or leisure, number of tasks one agrees to do, and the time one spends on activities.

4. *Planning activities ahead of time* limits experiences to those that are truly desired.

5. *Controlling the timing of activities* keeps them at an optimum pace.

6. *Developing personal assets* such as money, problem-solving skills, and one's spiritual life maximizes resources.

7. *Developing environmental assets* such as support systems, a comfortable home, and sources of information maximizes coping resources.

In the vignette, Emily could have used many of these coping strategies to balance demands and resources. By planning ahead, prioritizing tasks, and setting some limit on the number of tasks she attempted to accomplish, Emily would have reduced her stress. In addition, she could work to develop a collegial relationship with other staff nurses, helping them when they needed help and asking for help when she needed it.

Change Situational Factors

Strategies to change the threatening aspects of a situation help reduce stress. To accomplish such change Lyon (1984) suggested a number of strategies:

1. *Reappraising the situation* changes the interpretation of an event, such as decreasing the importance of the event, modifying expectations of oneself and others, and finding something good or humorous in the situation.

2. *Expressing emotions* helps ventilate feelings and resolve problematic conditions.

3. *Talking through concerns with others* helps objectify problems and identify alternative perceptions and actions.

4. *Modifying one's values from absolute to relative* reduces threat and is more realistic.

5. *Seeking feedback from others* and using it to assist in self-evaluation removes some threat of unexpected censure.

6. *Focusing self-talk statements on accomplishments and abilities* is encouraging, while focusing on failures is negative and discouraging.

Emily could have used many of these coping strategies to reduce the threat she experienced. She might have modified her expectations of herself and adopted relative, instead of absolute values. She could have ventilated her feelings of frustration to a co-worker and asked for help in finding alternate solutions. She might have focused self-talk on her accomplishment in completing her assignment, rather than on how long it took.

Manage Frustration and Anger

Anger is the experience of a blocked goal or unmet need. It ranges in intensity from mild irritation, to frustration, to rage. In spite of conventional wisdom, research shows that anger is magnified by venting, not lessened (Travis 1983). What, then, can people do to manage anger?

They can: (1) acknowledge the experience of anger and frustration, (2) identify the goal that is being blocked, (3) identify who or what is doing the blocking or denying, (4) list assumptions about one's right to attain the goal, (5) decide how important the goal really is, (6) use assertive rather than passive-aggressive communication, and (7) decide to fight for the goal, abandon the goal as not worth the effort, or compromise and let go of the frustration and anger. Exercises to manage frustration and anger are found in Tables 9-2 and 9-3.

Manage Guilt and Blame

Guilt is an experience of sadness, self-anger, and fear of consequences from doing, thinking, or feeling something that is inconsistent with internalized ideals or values. *Blame* is the experience of feeling anger toward others because they failed to behave according to internalized ideals or values.

Coping strategies for guilt and blame are: (1) acknowledge feeling angry toward oneself or others, (2) apologize or make restitution to those who have been damaged by guilt-producing behavior, (3) recognize that ideal actions are not always possible in nonideal situations, (4) view shame-producing events as learning experiences, (5) recognize that intensity of feelings diminishes with time, and (6) forgive oneself or others and go on; the past cannot be changed. Exercises to manage guilt and blame are found in Table 9-4.

⬛ Table 9-2

Exercise to Manage Frustration

Answer These Questions:

1. What is my goal?
2. What is the time-frame for accomplishing my goal?
3. What ingredients does it take to accomplish my goal?
4. Is the goal realistic for me?
5. Am I able to provide the ingredients to ensure accomplishment of my goal?
6. Am I able to manipulate my environment so that I can facilitate accomplishing my goal?
7. Am I capable of developing over time necessary ingredients to accomplish my goal?
8. Is the time-frame for goal accomplishment realistic?
9. If not, have I broken the goal down into accomplishable steps?
10. As I move toward accomplishing my goal do I need to experience early gratification?
11. What blocks prevent me from accomplishing my goal?
12. Is the block an internal one, such as lack of skill or knowledge, fear of success, or unwillingness to spend the necessary time, effort, and energy?
13. Is the block an external one, such as institutional policies, or funds, or other persons?
14. Have I imagined that there is a block without concrete evidence that it actually exists?
15. If the block is real, have I tried to overcome the block?
16. Do I need to consider modifying my goal?
17. Would failure to accomplish my goal have negative consequences on what I think of myself?
18. Have I had similar experiences of frustration in the past?
19. Was I able to deal with those experiences successfully?
20. Can I use similar strategies in the current situation?
21. Am I expending a lot of energy responding to this situation?
22. Do I experience frustration as an opportunity to problem-solve in a creative way?
23. In what ways can I facilitate successful management of my frustration?

Adapted from Lyon BL: *Stress Management, an Essential Ingredient for Good Health.* 1984. (Available from author: Indiana University, 610 Barnhill Drive, Indianapolis, IN 42620.)

⧉ *Table 9-3*

Exercise to Manage Anger

Answer Each Question "Yes" or "No":

1. Is my expectation a self-expectation?
2. Is my expectation an expectation of another?
3. Is my expectation realistic?
4. Have I verbalized my anger?
5. Have I attempted to change my expectations?

Strategies:

A. If you answered "Yes" to questions 1 and 4, then you need to work on changing unrealistic aspects of your self-expectation.
B. If you answered "Yes" to questions 2 and 4, then you need to work on changing unrealistic aspects of your expectations of others.
C. If you answered "Yes" to question 2 then you need to work on changing unrealistic expectations.
D. If you answered "Yes" to questions 2 and 3, then you need to learn to verbalize your anger appropriately.
E. If you answered "Yes" to 2, 3, 4, and 5, you are well on your way to managing anger.

Adapted from Lyon BL: *Stress Management, an Essential Ingredient for Good Health.* 1984. (Available from author: Indiana University, 610 Barnhill Drive, Indianapolis, IN 42620.)

Nuture Self-esteem

People with low self-esteem are especially vulnerable to the stress-related emotions of fear, anger, and guilt. Therefore, strategies that build self-esteem help prevent damaging levels of stress. Some of these include: (1) engaging in positive self-talk, (2) setting realistic personal goals and expectations, (3) viewing "failure" as a learning experience, and (4) focusing on the positive aspects of difficult situations.

Accept the Given

People who base their expectations and actions on the ideal rather than the real set themselves up for failure and frustration.

⁵⁵ *Table 9-4*

Exercise to Manage Guilt

Answer Each Question "Yes" or "No":

1. Is your self-expectation realistic?
2. Is your self-expectation part of your value system?
3. Was someone hurt as a consequence of your actions?
4. Can you correct the situation?
5. Are you punishing yourself for your actions?
6. Can you learn something from the situation?
7. Have you attempted to correct the situation?

Strategies:

A. If you answered "Yes" to questions 2, 5, and 6, re-examine your expectations in relation to your values and the situation.

B. If you answered "Yes" to questions 1, 2, 4, 5, and 6, attempt to correct the situation.

C. If you answered "Yes" to questions 1, 4, 5, 6, and 7, refer to the anger management guide.

D. If you answered "Yes" to questions 2, 3, 5, 6, and 7, identify what you can learn from the experience, avoid repeating such actions in the future, accept the reality of the situation, forgive yourself, and go on.

Adapted from Lyon BL: *Stress Management, an Essential Ingredient for Good Health.* 1984. (Available from author: Indiana University, 610 Barnhill Drive, Indianapolis, IN 42620.)

Coping strategies to avoid such unrealistic expectations include: (1) learning what is and is not possible in the real work-a-day world; (2) accurately assessing one's values, beliefs, limitations, abilities, competencies, priorities, experience, and energy levels; (3) accurately assessing the work environment and people who work there; and (4) making the best use of what is, not what would be ideal.

Learn to Relax

Learning to relax is an effective coping strategy for regulating stress-related emotions. Relaxation exercises help reduce tension, relax muscles, promote peripheral blood flow, and normalize heart and breathing patterns (Davis et al 1982). One of the many exercises one can use to relax and cope with stressful feelings is found in Table 9-5.

Develop a Social Support Network

A network is a group of individuals with whom one communicates for information, support, and guidance (Hamilton and Kiefer 1986). Networking is the process of communication between members of a network to share information and resources.

A network provides: (1) esteem support, (2) instrumental support, (3) informational support, and (4) social companionship (Cohen and Syme 1985). *Esteem support* supplies a sense of belonging, acceptance, and encouragement, helping to liberate creativity and foster productivity. *Instrumental support* gives financial aid, material resources, and services, offering concrete assistance when it is needed most. *Informational support* provides facts, and guidance in decision-making. *Social companionship* offers pleasurable activities and recreation. Thus, a social support network provides many resources to balance demands and reduce stress.

One of the great advantages of a network is that it is made up of people with various talents, contacts, experiences, and skills. Networks are different for every person and change over time. Social support networks consist of individuals with whom one works, organizations to which one belongs, schools in which one enrolls, neighbors where one lives, services or shops from which one buys, and members of one's family.

Networking is not all take and no give. A network makes demands on its members as well as providing them with resources. It is dynamic and reciprocal in nature and members expect assistance and support in return for what they give. A network functions because the members identify with and feel positively toward one another. If one member becomes overdependent or is in conflict or competition with other members, mutuality is destroyed and the network ceases to exist. A social support network in which one gives as much as one takes is a valuable coping resource. Had

Autogenic Relaxation Exercise

Choose a quiet area and assume a comfortable position. Repeat each statement several times slowly as you passively concentrate on a particular part of your body.

My feet feel warm.
My feet feel heavy.
My feet are warm and heavy.
  I feel very much at ease.
  I feel comfortable and relaxed.
My right leg feels warm.
My right leg feels heavy.
My right leg feels warm and heavy.
My left leg feels warm.
My left leg feels heavy.
My left leg feels warm and heavy.
Both my legs feel warm and heavy.
  I feel very much at ease.
  I feel comfortable and relaxed.
My right arm feels warm.
My right arm feels heavy.
My right arm feels warm and heavy.
My left arm feels warm.
My left arm feels heavy.
My left arm feels warm and heavy.
Both my arms feel warm and heavy.
My hands feel warm.
My hands feel heavy.
My hands feel warm and heavy.
  I feel very much at ease.
  I feel comfortable and relaxed.
My abdomen feels warm.
My abdomen feels heavy.
My abdomen feels warm and heavy.
My chest feels warm.
My chest feels heavy.
My chest feels warm and heavy.
  I feel very much at ease.
  I feel comfortable and relaxed.
My shoulders feel warm.
My shoulders feel heavy.
My shoulders feel warm and heavy.
My head and neck feel warm.
My head and neck feel heavy.
My head and neck feel warm and heavy.
  I feel very much at ease.
  I feel comfortable and relaxed.

Adapted from Lyon BL: *Stress Management, an Essential Ingredient for Good Health.* 1984. (Available from author: Indiana University, 610 Barnhill Drive, Indianapolis, IN 42620.)

Emily had a social support network, she might not have felt so alone and fearful.

Communicate Assertively

Assertive communication is the honest, forthright exchange of information. It enables individuals "to act in their own best interest, to stand up for themselves without undue anxiety, to express honest feeling comfortably, and to exercise personal rights without denying the rights of others" (Alberti and Emmons 1972). Assertive communication is the opposite of passive-aggressive communication, in which anger is clothed in sarcasm or vented by libelous gossip. Assertive communication involves an objective, nonemotional, nonjudgmental exchange of information, based on respect of self and others.

To communicate assertively, one (1) states what one believes to be true, using "I" rather than "you" statements; (2) states how one feels about the situation, owning up to emotions; and (3) states what one wants relative to the situation. For example, when the charge nurse gave her an additional patient, Emily might have said, (1) "I am already caring for six patients and I do not believe I can manage another one adequately," (2) "I'm feeling pretty frightened and overwhelmed already," and (3) "I do not want to take on the care of a seventh patient."

Assertive communication is not a one-way dialogue. It includes a willingness to listen to another point of view. When people listen to another perspective, they gain new information. This data opens the door to compromise. As a result, emotions as well as desires may change. For example, in response to Emily's assertive communication the charge nurse might have said, "I can see your point. I'll see if the special procedure nurse can give us a hand for a while."

Assertive communication is especially useful as a coping strategy to reduce stress. It helps objectify nebulous emotions by stating clearly what the problem is and what emotion is being experienced. Assertive communication provides a tool to either change a situation or alter negative feelings about the situation. It affirms respect for oneself and others.

Burnout

Burnout is a condition in which people in the helping professions lose concern and feelings for those they are trying to help, treating them in detached, dehumanized ways. It is an attempt to cope with the stresses of intense interpersonal work by distancing oneself from the source of painful experiences (Wilson and Kniesl 1988).

Symptoms of burnout can be heard in the words the charge nurse in the vignette used to describe the new patient, and in jokes nurses make about serious problems, such as "You'd think by now she'd figure out what makes babies!" Burnout can be seen in the way nurses withdraw from patients, hiding in the nurses' station. It may be evidenced in the rigid application of rules, keeping nurses from thinking about individual patients. Burnout changes caring persons into mechanical bureaucrats. People who suffer from burnout experience emotional and physical fatigue, lack of enthusiasm, and feelings of helplessness and hopelessness. They may have insomnia, gastrointestinal disturbances, headaches, and difficulty in concentration. However, burnout is not physical exhaustion, nor is it mental fatigue from prolonged concentration. It is the result of an unsuccessful attempt to manage stress.

Causes and Dynamics

Burnout is believed to be caused by two interrelated factors: idealism, untempered by reality, and inappropriate identification.

Caregivers such as nurses and social workers place a high value on unselfish altruism, relief of suffering, and empathetic understanding of human beings. These caregivers translate their values into idealized performance expectations for themselves, believing that they "should be able to help." They are encouraged to establish relationships with patients, using the self as a therapeutic tool. They learn that one of the most important aspects of a therapeutic relationship is to give empathetic understanding to patients.

Empathy means to experience the emotions of another. It has four phases: (1) *identification,* allowing oneself to become absorbed in another person's experience; (2) *incorporation,* taking in the experiences of another; (3) *reverberation,* interplaying the internalized emotions of another with one's own emotions; and (4) *detachment,* withdrawing from subjective involvement, resuming one's own identity, and offering useful responses to the other person. When caregivers do not detach themselves from the people they seek to help, they experience burnout (Wilson and Kniesl 1988).

Strategies to Reduce Burnout

To reduce burnout:

1. Avoid prolonged direct patient contact through shorter work shifts or rotating work responsibilities.

2. Use a social support network to express, share, and analyze feelings of frustration and to gain constructive feedback and new perspectives.

3. Become informed about burnout, its symptoms, causes, and management, and share that information with others.

4. Focus on positive, nonproblem aspects of patients' lives and work toward reduction of staff-patient ratios through collective bargaining.

5. Work toward provision of sanctioned breaks (mental health days) to replace nonsanctioned, guilt-producing escapes.

6. Explore motives for pursuing a career as a caregiver, especially in regard to a need to be needed or to control others.

7. Appraise the real work situation as compared to an ideal one and adjust self-expectations to the real one.

Emily's charge nurse exhibited many symptoms of burnout, including chronic fatigue and distancing from patients. She sorely needed a break from the pressures of work. She needed to learn strategies to reduce burnout.

Surviving Shift Work

Most clinical experience of student nurses takes place during the day. Often, however, when new nurses graduate they must work during the evening or night. This change in work-sleep cycle greatly increases the stress new graduates experience. Sleep research studies suggest ways to reduce such stress and cope successfully with shift work.

Sleep and Health

By nature, humans are diurnal creatures, that is, they are awake and active during light hours of the day and asleep and quiet during dark hours of the night. Americans normally sleep about one-third of every 24-hour cycle, or about six to nine hours a day. Very few people can sleep less than five hours per day without feeling sleepy and suffering serious mood and performance deficits. In fact, death rates are higher in people who sleep less than seven hours and more than ten hours per day (Coleman 1986). Adequate sleep, therefore, is essential to health and a feeling of well-being.

Sleep and Performance

Not only is the number of hours of sleep important, but the time of sleep is critical to performance. When workers are sleepy they make serious mistakes. The accident at Three Mile Island, the Union Carbide explosion in Bhopal, and the nuclear disaster at Chernobyl all occured late in the evening and during the night shift. Since nurses must work at peak performance at all hours of the day and night, they should sleep when their bodies say it is time to sleep.

Biologic Clocks

The timing of bodily functions is set by the biologic clock, an innate physiologic system in humans that measures the passage of time. Each physiologic function has its own unique pattern that cycles over a 24-hour period. The body temperature cycle is of particular interest to shift-workers because the mental alertness cycle closely follows its curve. During the daylight hours body temperature is high. During the night it drops by 2 to 3 degrees. As long as people stay on regular day schedules their clock operates efficiently and they barely notice its effects. However, when the biologic clock is asked to adjust to a new schedule, either as a result of work shifts or jet travel, the system becomes seriously stressed. Fig-

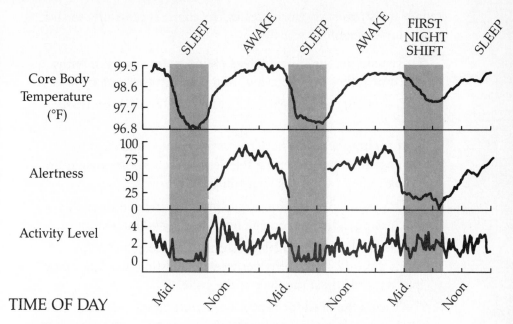

Figure 9-2   *Sleep and Alertness Cycle of a Worker Starting a New Night-Shift Rotation*

From Coleman RM: *Wide Awake at 3:00 A.M. By Choice or by Chance.* Stanford Alumni Association, 1986.

ure 9-2 shows the sleep and alertness cycle of a worker starting a new night-shift rotation after being off for two days.

Resetting the Clock

Shift-workers and jet travelers need not despair. Within certain limits the biologic clock is capable of free-running and resetting. Since the internal clock, left on its own, gravitates to a 25-hour day, it is much easier for people to stay up later than to go to bed earlier. In general, the 25-hour clock can be reset about two hours each day, allowing humans to live comfortably on a 23- to 27-hour day. Thus, when adjusting to a new sleep cycle, it is much easier to move in a clockwise direction than a counter-clockwise one. Therefore, *if one must adjust to a new schedule, the most natural biologic direction is to move from day to evening to night work.* The least natural is to move from night, to evening, to day work.

Since hospitals do not shut down at the end of the day, nurses who work during the evening and night need to adjust their lives to reduce the stress such work creates. To adjust successfully to shift work nurses should:

1. Remain on one shift, such as evenings, for several months at a time rather than rotating from one shift to another.

2. Follow the same sleep-wake cycle on days off as on work days.

3. If rotating schedules are necessary, rotate from days to evenings to nights, resetting the sleep-wake cycle by two hours (going to bed two hours later) during days off.

4. During sleep, duplicate night-time sleeping conditions as much as possible by reducing light, noise, and interruptions.

5. If offered, consider 12-hour shifts, since hospitals often count three 12-hour shifts per week as full-time work, leaving four days to adjust the sleep-wake cycle.

6. Discuss the need for restful sleep with family members and work out a mutually acceptable plan.

7. Make friends with other people working evenings or nights to reduce feelings of loneliness and isolation.

8. Participate in professional activities and hospital committees to avoid feeling powerless and paranoid.

9. Count the benefits of working evenings and nights, such as working in a less harried environment, more chances to meet patient needs, opportunities for school or hobbies during the day, and more pay per hour.

Had Emily tried some of these strategies she might not have been so stressed during her busy evening. Many nurses not only survive shift work, they adjust so successfully to it that they choose to work evenings or nights long after they are neophyte nurses. When promotion or life events require a change to day work, they look back on their time of working evenings or nights as a time of pleasure.

Summary

Much research has focused on stress. It is defined as a stimulus causing life disruption and portraying people as passive recipients.

The Social Readjustment Rating Scale gives point values to life-change events. Selye defines stress as a nonspecific response of the body to demands placed on it and advises people to reduce stress before they reach the exhaustion stage. Lazarus defines stress as cognitive, affective, and adaptational factors arising from people-environment transactions. He emphasizes differences in sensitivity and interpretation of demands and suggests people develop coping strategies to manage stress, including balancing demands and resources, regulating feelings, and changing situations. Coping strategies include anger and guilt management, self-nurturance, acceptance, relaxation, networking, and assertive communication. Burnout is an unsatisfactory attempt to manage stress by using detachment. It is caused by exaggerated idealism and identification. Both burnout and stress from sleep disturbances are preventable and curable.

Learning Activities

1. Using the Social Readjustment Rating Scale, add up your score for the past 12 months. Are you at risk for major life disruption (a score over 100 points)? If so, do you feel severely stressed? Can you make any changes in your life to reduce the score?

2. Focus on yourself. Are you exhibiting any of the psychologic and physiologic manifestations of stress described in the chapter?

3. List the demands that you are experiencing right now and the resources you have to meet those demands. Consider emotion-focused and problem-focused coping strategies that apply to your situation.

4. Practice using the exercises described in this chapter to reduce frustration, anger, guilt, and tension. Develop a social support network among your friends.

5. Practice assertive communication by telling a friend something you see as a problem between you. Ask that person to do the same for you.

6. Identify a person you would diagnose as suffering "burnout." What characteristic behaviors does he or she manifest?

7. Keep a record of your sleep-wake cycle for one week. If you work evenings or nights, take your temperature every three hours during your waking hours. Compare your alertness level with your temperature reading.

Annotated Reading List

Coleman RM: *Wide Awake at 3:00 A.M. By Choice or by Chance.* Stanford Alumni Association, 1986.

This delightfully written little book presents the essence of research studies of biologic clocks, sleep, dreams, and sleep dysfunctions. It applies the information to such practical problems as shift-work and jet travel and gives instructions to improve sleep for chronic insomnia. A glossary of terms used in sleep research and therapy adds to the usefulness of the book.

Davis M, Eschelman RT, Mckay M: Time management. In: *The Relaxation and Stress Reduction Workbook,* pp 151–161. Harbinger, 1982.

This is a practical, easy-to-follow chapter dealing with the management of time. It relates time to decision-making, describing symptoms of poor time management, gives a process for readers to analyze the way they spend their time, and offers three steps for managing time more effectively. It also describes methods to overcome procrastination and set priorities.

Plutchik R: A language for the emotions. *Psychology Today* Feb 1980; 68–70.

This relatively brief article describes many years of research devoted to identification of the basic emotions and their original function in evolution: survival. The author defines an emotion as a "complex sequence of events having elements of cognitive appraisal, feeling, impulses to action, and overt behavior—all of which are designed to deal with a stimulus." The eight basic emotions are identified as fear, anger, sadness, disgust, joy, acceptance, anticipation, and surprise. They vary in intensity and combine to form related emotions.

References

Alberti R, Emmons M: *Your Perfect Right*. Impact, 1972.

Cohen S, Syme SL: Issues in the study and application of social support. In: *Social Support and Health*. Cohen S, Syme SL (editors), pp 3–22. Academic Press, 1985.

Coleman RM: *Wide Awake at 3:00 A.M. By Choice or by Chance*. Stanford Alumni Association, 1986.

Davis M, Eshelman ER, McKay M: *The Relaxation and Stress Reduction Workbook*. Harbinger, 1982.

Hamilton JM, Kiefer ME: *Survival Skills for the New Nurse*. Lippincott, 1986.

Lazarus RS: *Psychological Stress and the Coping Process*. McGraw-Hill, 1966.

Lazarus RS, Folkman S: *Stress, Appraisal, and Coping*. Springer, 1984.

Lyon BL: *Stress Management, An Essential Ingredient for Good Health*. 1984. (Available from author: School of Nursing, 610 Barnhill Drive, Indianapolis, IN 42620.)

Lyon BL, Werner JS: Stress. In: *Annual Review of Nursing Research*, Fitzpatrick JJ, Tauton RL (editors), Vol 5, pp 3–22. Springer, 1987.

Plutchik R: *Emotion: A Psychoevolutionary Synthesis*. Harper and Row, 1980.

Selye H: *The Stress of Life*. McGraw-Hill, 1956.

Selye H: *The Stress of Life*, 2nd ed. McGraw-Hill, 1976.

Travis C: *Anger: The Misunderstood Emotion*. Simon & Schuster, 1983.

Williams CC, Holmes TH: Life change, human adaptation, and onset of illness. In: *Clinical Practice in Psychosocial Nursing: Assessment and Intervention*, Longo DC, Williams RA, p 72. Appleton-Century-Crofts, 1978.

Wilson HC, Kniesl CR: *Psychiatric Nursing*, 3rd ed. Addison-Wesley, 1988.

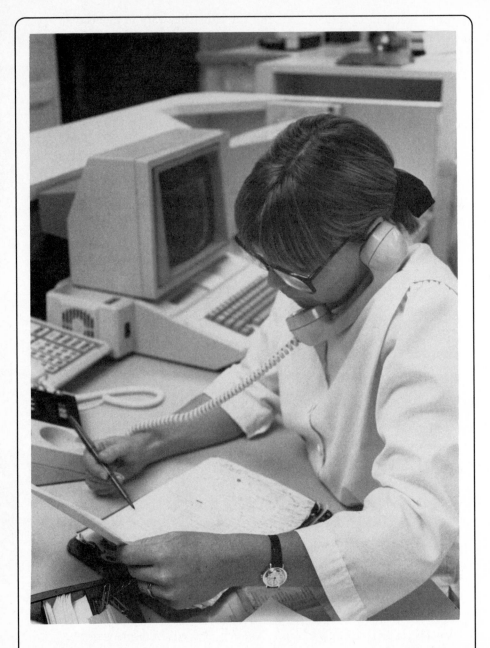

Using interpersonal skills to direct patient care, a nurse manager communicates with a physician about a patient's condition. (Photograph by Chuck O'Rear, Westlight)

CHAPTER 10

Management-leadership

LEARNING OBJECTIVES

1. Describe characteristics of an open system and explain how the management process fits into such a system.

2. Compare management with leadership.

3. Discuss participative management and shared governance as they apply to nursing practice.

4. Discuss the decision-making process, creativity, and computer technology as they are used by nurse managers.

5. Describe the four phases of the budgetary process.

6. Identify measures to manage time effectively.

7. Compare bureaucratic structures with adaptive structures.

8. Describe the staffing process, from analysis of the work to be done to the scheduling of people to do it.

9. Discuss the leadership skills of communication, instruction, motivation, conflict resolution, and morale-building.

10. State the components of controlling and explain why accountability is its key.

11. Compare the purposes and programs of risk management and quality assurance.

12. Describe the purposes and process of performance evaluations that use assertive communication.

311

Steve *closed the door to the tiny office he shared with the other head nurse on the surgical floor. He had just returned from morning report. The preliminary budget was due for next year; he needed to prepare for the weekly departmental meeting, to schedule an inservice on the latest IV pump, and to write an evaluation of the new RN. How could he do it all? There was never enough time! Whatever made him take this thankless job?*

The phone intruded noisily. It was the nursing office. They needed to "borrow" one of his RNs; he was to send Bonnie to the medical unit right away. Steve protested. They were sorry but the acuity level on his unit indicated that staffing would still be adequate. He would just have to make do. As Steve hurried toward the nursing station he felt the hot flush of anger spreading from his neck to his cheeks. He was sick of acuity numbers and patient-staff ratios! The staff was already overworked and he needed to add more. They would blame him for allowing Bonnie to be reassigned. Steve decided to take two of her patients himself, leaving only one more for each of the other staff nurses. He had to be careful. Liz and Pearl compared workloads like children counting jelly beans. They found something to argue or complain about every day.

Steve made a quick assessment of his patients. Their care was relatively easy compared to being a nurse manager. What did he know about writing budgets, resolving conflicts, evaluating performance? Steve felt vulnerable and inept. He wondered if he would ever feel comfortable as a manager.

Management-Leadership Concepts

Although Steve did not realize it, he had been using the management process for patient care since he first became a nurse. However, to become a more effective and confident nurse manager, Steve needs to understand some basic management concepts and how to apply them to practice.

Organizational Systems

A general systems view of the world was developed by von Bertalanffy and others as a way to study various structures in the universe, including social structures (Emery 1969). For people who are interested in management, systems thinking is especially useful. A *system* is defined as an organized whole unit that produces an effect or a product whose interdependent component parts interact with the environment. Systems are classified according to their relationship to the environment (open or closed), their position in relation to other systems (supra, focal, or subsystems), and the nature of their component parts (animal, vegetable, mineral).

Closed systems are those in which there is no input or output of energy, therefore, no change in component parts, no renewal, and no life. A closed system represents the end result of a process where the components reach an inactive steady state.

Open systems are those in which there is an exchange of energy, materials, and information with the environment. Open systems are characterized by (1) uniqueness formed when separate parts come together; (2) internal organization, creating boundaries between the system and environment; (3) input of energy into the system; (4) throughput as the imported energy is processed, changed, and reorganized by the system; (5) output of energy in the form of goods or services into the environment; (6) feedback, by which a part of the output returns to the system, creating change (positive) or maintaining a steady state (negative); (7) interrelatedness of component parts so that a change in any part affects the whole; (8) dynamic equilibrium (as in homeostasis); (9) continual renewal; and (10) a cyclical pattern of events with a continual input-throughput-output-feedback sequence.

Management

Management is a process of integrating various parts of an organization into a working whole in order to accomplish specific objectives. The primary purpose of management is to take action to get a job done. To achieve this purpose organizations often use a hierarchy of managers to direct the work of others, including top, middle, and first-level managers.

Top managers are responsible for the overall operation of an organization. They establish goals, policies, and strategies, make business arrangements with outside firms, and represent the agency to the community. They report to the topmost manager, board of directors, or electorate, and have titles like vice-president, chief executive officer, and administrator.

Middle managers are responsible to coordinate several units within an organization. They convert broad policy and strategy into specific objectives and programs. They report to top managers, serve as links between first-level and top managers, and have titles like supervisor and coordinator.

First-level managers are directly responsible to deliver services and implement specific objectives and programs. They report to middle managers, serve as links between staff and middle management, and have titles like charge or head nurse.

The *management process* takes the goals of an organization and transforms them into concrete objectives, using people and resources. It does this within ethical, physical, cultural, and legal constraints in accord with agency philosophy and policy. The process is divided into four functions or operations: planning, organizing, directing, and controlling. Each function asks questions and calls for specific actions:

Planning:

Questions: What should be done to accomplish goals and objectives? When? Where? By whom? How? At what cost?

Actions: Identify goals and objectives in accord with organizational purpose and philosophy; select work that will accomplish objectives; establish policies and procedures; formulate an operating budget of time and materials; solve problems; modify the plan in response to evaluation (control) results.

Organizing (Staffing):

Questions: Who should do what work? In what place? In how much time? With how much autonomy?

Actions: Create organizational structure; write job descriptions; select, orient, socialize, and develop staff; make assignments and schedules; adjust organization in response to control results.

Directing (Activating):

Questions: What is the best way to motivate staff to perform at their highest level?

Actions: Communicate with staff; involve staff in solving problems; challenge staff to meet standards; develop potential; praise and reprimand fairly; resolve conflicts between members.

Controlling (Evaluating):

Questions: Are institutional goals and objectives being met? How well are tasks being performed? What can be done to improve performance?

Actions: Compare results with plans; identify ideal behaviors, evaluate process, product, and workers; work with labor representatives; take corrective action as needed.

Figure 10-1 illustrates the management process as an open system, with input, throughput, output, and a feedback loop. Notice that first-level managers are involved primarily in the throughput aspect of a system.

Participative Management

In recent years participative management has gained widespread popularity. Called by such names as shared power, democratic management, group decision-making, the method has three elements: group decision-making, decentralization, and management by objectives (Bower 1990). *Group decision-making* is the process of a formal or informal group, making decisions about specific tasks. *Decentralization* is the empowerment of subordi-

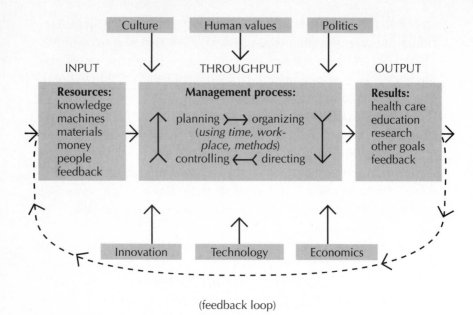

(feedback loop)

Figure 10-1 *The Management Process Within a System*

nates by superiors to make decisions at any level in the organization (Scanian and Keys 1979). *Management by objectives* (MBO)
is a system for accomplishing work that sets goals (written as objectives), works to carry them out, and evaluates how well they
have been met (Tappen 1983).

Shared governance is a type of participative management in
which managers and staff members make decisions and set rules
together, changing management from an oligarchy to a democracy. While executive authority remains with top managers, professional staff functions in a legislative role and has a say in the
development of practice policies. Shared governance is a model for
professional practice. It requires that nurses assume responsibility
for the quality of patient care in the whole institution, and that
nurses "confront, evaluate, and censor those who do not meet
standards. Shared governance permits nurses to become truly accountable for practice" (Bower 1990).

Leadership

Leadership is an interpersonal relationship in which a leader
employs specific strategies to influence individuals and groups

toward goals (Dossett et al 1988). It is a composite of personal abilities and characteristics, the environment, and relationships (Hutelmyer 1986).

Early studies identified a democratic style of leadership as more effective than authoritarian or laissez faire styles (White and Lippitt 1960). However, recent studies indicate that leadership effectiveness varies with followers and situations and that motivation plays a significant role (Hollander 1978). Thus, *authoritarian* leadership is useful for emergency situations, *democratic* leadership is useful for complex, nonemergency conditions, and *laissez faire* leadership is useful for circumstances that require innovation and self-motivation.

It is important to remember that without followers, there are no leaders. Leaders must produce commitment, trust, and loyalty in their followers. While no single list of personal traits or behaviors describes leaders, they are generally experienced, able to communicate, and possess qualities and competencies admired by their followers. Often they hold strong positions and take risks. *Formal leaders* have legitimate power by election or appointment. *Informal leaders* have no official authority, yet the group gives it to them. President Abraham Lincoln was a formal leader of the United States. The Reverend Martin Luther King, Jr. was an informal leader of the civil rights movement.

Leadership differs from management in that leadership is an ability and management is a process. In Table 10-1, managers and leaders are compared. Managers, regardless of level, are more effective when they exhibit leadership qualities, thereby earning the respect and loyalty of those they manage. Leaders are more effective when they use the management process to achieve goals.

Decision-making and Problem-solving

Nurse managers must make decisions and solve problems. These two processes are similar and often related. *Decision-making* is a process of selecting from among alternatives that may or may not involve a problem (Strader 1988), such as deciding between alternative assignment options. *Problem-solving* is a process of changing a condition that is a departure from a desirable state of affairs (Strader 1988), such as Steve's need to reassign Bonnie's patients to

52 *Table 10-1*

Comparison of Leaders and Managers	
Leaders	*Managers*
May or may not be officially sanctioned	Are officially sanctioned to fulfill a function
Have authority from followers to make decisions that affect the followers	Have authority from their superiors to plan, organize, direct, and control
Influence followers to achieve goals and accept decisions of leaders	Direct managed ones to carry out predetermined policies, rules, and regulations
Take risks, explore new ideas	Maintain orderly structure
Seek to fulfill personal goals and aspirations	Seek to fulfill goals of the organization
May or may not be skillful managers	May or may not be successful leaders

Reproduced with permission from Douglass LM: *The Effective Nurse*, 3rd ed., p 5. Mosby, 1988.

other staff members. The decision-making/problem-solving process is as follows:

1. Define the decision to be made or the problem to be solved; the more precise the definition, the more exact the result.

2. Gather information about the issue to be decided or the problem to be solved.

3. Analyze the information, categorizing it according to reliability, importance, time sequence, cause, and effect.

4. Develop criteria for selecting alternative decisions or solutions.

5. Develop alternative decisions or solutions.

6. Identify advantages and disadvantages of each alternative, considering the consequences (cost, benefit, effects).

7. Make a decision or solve the problem; consult, confer, and communicate the decision or solution.

8. Implement the decision or solve the problem.

9. Evaluate the decision or solution; compare the results.

Steve needed to make a decision about patient care assignments. Even though he may not have defined the process, Steve gathered data about patients needing care, abilities and personalities of staff, and his own need for approval. With this information he made a decision to assign himself two patients. By the end of the day Steve may evaluate his decision unfavorably and might choose a different alternative if the problem arises again.

Creativity

Creativity is the ability to generate new ideas, processes, and artistic expressions. It is a highly desirable ability, especially in nurses faced with complex problems that need solutions. Creative thinking seldom follows a step-by-step sequence. It is characterized by delays, inactivity, and unpredicted leaps. Creative people tend to be individualistic, have rich fantasy lives, exhibit less conformity to social norms, and use complex thought processes to combine various frames of reference. They find humor—a juxtaposition of logic—in many situations. Happily, the ability to think creatively can be learned (Adams 1974). It behooves nurse managers to encourage creative problem-solving in their staff.

Computer Technology

Computers crunch numbers and facilitate the flow of information. They store, sort, and retrieve data with incredible speed. Hospitals were quick to install these tools in business departments, but slow to put them in nursing stations. The nationwide shortage of nurses changed all that. Today computers in nursing stations are commonplace and nurses are expected to be computer literate.

Excellent computer programs are now available to assist nurses in managing patient care. One such program is *Patient Care Expert*

System (PACE), developed at the School of Nursing, Creighton University, Omaha, Nebraska. Formerly called COMMES, PACE provides individualized patient care, teaching, and discharge plans, and meets standards of the Joint Commission on Accreditation of Healthcare Organizations (JCAHCO). It gives nurses "an entire library of patient problems and nursing information, eliminates the need for time-consuming research, and increases time for actual patient care" (Kuster 1990).

Management Operations

Planning

The management process begins with planning, deciding in advance what to do. All other management functions, including organizing, directing, and controlling, depend on planning. To plan effectively, nurse managers identify the purpose and philosophy of an agency, clarify goals and objectives, review policies and procedures, prepare budgets, and assess resources.

Purpose

The first task of planning is to clarify the reason an organization exists. For most health care institutions, the primary purpose is to provide quality health care for patients. Other purposes may be to teach, to carry on research, to make money for investors, and to make converts to a belief system. Specialty areas within healthcare agencies have their own functions, but they all subscribe to the purpose of the institution. For example, the purpose of a hospital educational department may be to orient new staff members and provide up-to-date inservice education in order to provide quality health care for patients.

Philosophy

A philosophy is a statement of beliefs and values underlying the operation of an institution. Because a philosophy serves as an ethical guide for policy decisions, it needs to be written in clear terms, widely published, and reviewed periodically.

Goals and Objectives

Goals and objectives are central to the management process. They state what an institution seeks to do in order to achieve its purpose. *Planning* defines goals, *organizing* provides a way to accomplish them, *directing* uses personnel to attain them, and *controlling* evaluates how well they were achieved.

Goals are general statements of intent that may be short-term or long-term. They should be reviewed periodically to be sure they are still accurate. *Objectives* are specific aspects of goals. The more precise an objective, the more likely its attainment. For example, the goal is to provide quality care. An objective of this goal may be to make accurate assessments.

Policies, Procedures, and Methods

Policies, procedures, and methods are ways to attain goals and objectives. *Policies* serve as guides to define the scope of activities and explain how goals will be achieved. They serve as a basis for future decisions and actions. Policies may originate inside an institution at any level or they may come from law-making bodies and accrediting boards outside an organization.

Procedures are directions for taking specific action. They are more precise than policies and usually affect a department rather than an entire agency. For example, the procedure for administration of oral medication describes actions nurses take to administer oral medications. *Methods* are techniques for performing skills that affect efficiency, but rarely safety.

Budgets

A budget is a plan for allocating resources, monitoring expenditures, and controlling costs. Budgeting is part of the planning and controlling functions of management. Although budgets are made on an annual basis they may be subdivided into monthly, quarterly, or semiannual periods. A *fiscal year* (financial year) is any 12-month budget cycle. When the cycle begins in January the fiscal year coincides with the calendar year. Long-term budgets prepared by top managers may be for three or more years. Operating budgets prepared by nurse managers like Steve are for one year and follow the fiscal year of the agency. The four-phase budget process is continuous and cyclical, as follows:

PHASE I.   Top management determine requirements for the next fiscal year, anticipating activity levels of departments, such as number of patient care days, major surgeries to be performed, and meals to be served. This forecast is based on statistical data about past occupancy levels, proposed changes within the facility, and outside factors such as regulatory changes and population trends. The forecast is given to middle and first-level managers who translate it into needed personnel, supplies, and facilities, creating a preliminary budget. These budgets go to top managers for review, modification, and approval. Steve was expected to prepare just such a budget.

PHASE II.   When a preliminary budget is approved, first-level and middle managers develop formal budgets for each quarter of the upcoming fiscal year. These plans consider:

Salaries and wages. Managers determine staffing levels for each job classification, such as LPN, RN-I, and RN-II. They take into account anticipated changes in wages and staffing patterns and then total projected wage and salary costs for each quarter.

Other personnel costs. Managers calculate the cost of items such as disability insurance, fringe benefits, and overtime premiums, making sure that these projections include changes in policy or government regulation.

Supplies. Managers calculate projected supply costs based on services that are to be performed and expected costs of new products coming on the market.

Capital expenses. Capital expenses include new construction, physical plant changes, and acquisition of major equipment such as linear accelerators. Capital expenses usually are not included in the operating budget. Instead, they are financed by special expansion campaigns.

Other expenses. Managers include all other expenses in proposed budgets on the basis of forecasted levels of activity. In *zero-based budgeting,* no program is taken for granted. Each must be justified with every request for funds.

Statistics. In the preliminary budget, managers include expense projections and such statistics as are needed to support budget requests, such as average daily census, direct cost per patient day, and hours of work.

Revenue. The estimated income of a health-care agency is based on levels of anticipated revenue, changes in billing methods, new or expanded revenue-producing services, and third-party (insurance) reimbursement. While top managers make these estimates, middle and first-level managers must be alert to social and political change. Agencies cannot operate if income falls below expenses. When all preliminary departmental budget plans have been submitted and approved the accounting department consolidates them into a total hospital budget. The top manager presents the budget to the board of directors for final approval.

PHASE III.   The third phase of the budget process occurs as part of the controlling function. Managers are held accountable for keeping expenses within projected amounts. If a significant difference between budgeted and actual costs occurs, an exception is declared and corrective action is begun at once, a process called *management by exception.*

PHASE IV.   As the fiscal year proceeds, managers evaluate and revise the budget for ensuing quarters. With experience, time, and a stable economy, managers are able to forecast expenses and revenues with increasing accuracy, beginning Phase I again with less anxiety than Steve experienced.

Managing Time

Perhaps no one appreciates the phrase *tempus fugit* better than nurse managers. Steve found he never had enough time to accomplish what was expected of him. To do so he must:

Set priorities. When there are several things to be done, ask, "What is the relative importance of each one?" Then ask, "What is their relative urgency?" Doing the most important and urgent things first prevents frustration and supports composure.

Clarify objectives. When there is pressure to perform, ask, "What am I expected to do? What action is necessary to achieve the objective? How much time is required for each action? Can these actions occur concurrently or must they be sequential? Can they be delegated to someone else?"

Delegate tasks. Delegation is sharing responsibility and authority with subordinates and holding them accountable for performance (Baker and Heaton 1988). It is not the same as direction. *Direction* is telling others what to do; *delegation* is giving tasks to others and expecting them to do them. Before managers delegate tasks, they determine the amount and limits of authority, define expected behaviors, and hold delegates accountable. When managers fail to delegate they have less time for other tasks and deprive the staff of personal and professional growth. By taking a patient care assignment Steve shirked his management tasks, and his staff went unchallenged.

Reduce paper work. Even with the advent of computerized records, telephones, and word processors, nurse managers must fill out forms, write memoranda, compose letters, and read and write reports. Therefore, they need to (1) create a system of file folders or envelopes into which incoming papers are sorted by urgency and importance, (2) throw things away that no longer have value, (3) use word processors more, handwrite less, (4) delegate paper work and teach staff to handle it when possible, (5) purge files at least once a year, (6) combine or eliminate routine forms, (7) handle papers but once, (8) clear the desk for action: deal with, file, or discard papers.

Eliminate time-wasters. (1) Refrain from doing things that do not need to be done; (2) reduce telephone time by planning calls, minimize small talk, use a timer, ask for preferred call times, remember that people are more talkative in the afternoon than the morning; (3) reduce drop-in visitor interruptions by setting limits, encourage appointments, close the door or face away from it, go to talkative people so you can leave when your business is done; (4) become time-conscious, schedule activities.

Organizing

The second management function is organizing. Having planned, managers organize work so that workers can carry out the plan effectively and efficiently. Organizing involves installing a structure to accomplish the objectives of the institution. To function effectively, managers like Steve need to know about the purpose and process of organizing, organizational structures, staffing, assignment systems, and scheduling.

Purpose and Process

Organizing involves creating an orderly mechanism with channels of communication and authority relationships so that workers can cooperate to do a job. Its ultimate purpose is to increase productivity. To create such a mechanism managers (1) define goals and objectives, (2) establish policies and plans, (3) identify activities, (4) organize them into an efficient system using resources, and (5) delegate responsibility.

Organizational Structures

An organizational structure furnishes the framework in which the management process takes place. It provides an effective system for accomplishing the mission of the institution. Organizational charts graphically portray relationships within the institution so that managers like Steve can know at a glance the chain of command. *Line authority* is the responsibility assigned a position directly over another. *Staff authority* is the responsibility assigned the lowest position, the staff member. There are two general types of organizational structures: bureaucratic (hierarchical, centralized) and adaptive (participatory, decentralized).

BUREAUCRATIC STRUCTURES.   Bureaucratic structures have a clearly defined chain of command from a few at the top to many at the bottom (see Figure 10-2). Communication often moves in one direction from above, with employees viewed as work units. Loyalty and obedience are expected. Monetary reward, rather than autonomy, is the chief motivator. Most large health-care institutions are organized as bureaucratic structures.

ADAPTIVE STRUCTURES.   Adaptive structures are more flexible than bureaucratic ones because their underlying assumptions are based

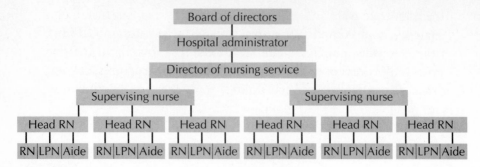

Figure 10-2   *Typical Bureaucratic Hierarchical Structure*

on humanistic principles. Adaptive structures affirm that job satisfaction and creativity are important, that motivation is more
powerful when it is derived from peer pressure and task-related
factors, and that leadership is more desirable than management
control.

McGregor described what he called *Theory X and Y.* Theory X
proposes that workers are basically lazy, desire security above all
else, and avoid work unless coerced; therefore, they need a rigid
hierarchy to manage and control them. Theory Y proposes that if
conditions are favorable and if workers enjoy their work, they will
be motivated to do a good job (McGregor 1960). Maslow cor-
roborated Theory Y by proposing that humans have basic needs
that they seek to fulfill, including survival, security, belongingness,
self-esteem, and self-actualization (1970). Several adaptive organizational models have been designed to improve worker satisfaction
and productivity, including free form, collegial management, project management, matrix, and task force.

Free form stresses flexibility with centralized control, decentralized operations, profit centers, and risk-taking managers. Self-
regulation, consensus, independent judgment, and open communication are maximized. Organizational charts, position titles, job
descriptions, and manuals are minimized.

Collegial management restricts single-person authority by maintaining a balance of power among top managers through collective
responsibility. Common in Europe, this design requires compromise and consensus. Policy decisions are made by a board of directors with each director representing functional areas within the
organization.

Project management (PM) assigns authority to a manager to accomplish some specified project within an existing bureaucratic structure. Such a design expedites projects, but since it uses workers already assigned to work within the central organization, PM places those workers under two bosses, with potential confusion and conflict. Thus, lines of authority need to be clarified.

Matrix combines project management and the central organization, but with clear lines of authority. The plan provides for both hierarchical and lateral coordination across departments and requires workers to report to more than one manager. Matrix structures work best in institutions where most employees are of equal status, as in colleges.

Task forces are used for special projects. They have clear missions, leaders, and completion dates. Personnel are relieved of usual duties and are given temporary assignments. While this plan avoids the problem of divided authority, it takes key people from established operations and disrupts normal work patterns.

Staffing

FROM JOB ANALYSIS TO PEOPLE SELECTION.   An organizational structure is but an impersonal framework until it is staffed with people. Staffing is the process of analyzing the work to be done, designing and describing jobs, recruiting, selecting, orienting, and developing people to fill jobs, and assigning and scheduling people to do the work.

Job analysis determines three sets of data: (1) principal responsibilities to be assumed, (2) specific tasks to be performed, and (3) knowledges, skills, aptitudes, and personal characteristics needed by the people who perform the tasks.

Job design divides tasks into clusters that become positions or jobs. It assigns monetary value, gives titles, and specifies the relationship of the job to others within the organization.

Job descriptions come from job analysis and design. They specify major duties, relationships, personal characteristics, and salary range for each position (see Table 10-2).

Recruitment involves attracting qualified applicants to a job. Its purpose is to provide a pool of applicants from which qualified workers can be selected (Decker and Hailstone 1988). Although

⎋ *Table 10-2*

Sample Job Description

Title: Staff Registered Nurse I   *Department:* Nursing Service
Reports to: Head nurse   *Wage scale:* $14.50 to $16.00/hr
Supervises: LPNs, nursing assistants   *Date applications close:* Open

Purpose of position: To provide direct patient care including assessment, planning, implementation, and evaluation.

Primary responsibility: Admits and provides ongoing assessment of patients using physical and psychosocial assessment skills, diagnostic data, and medical evaluations. Evaluates effectiveness of care as related to short- and long-term goals. Develops a plan for patient care including anticipation of discharge needs. Implements nursing actions and medical prescriptions to meet complex needs of patients and significant others. Documents care and patient responses in appropriate forms in records. Serves as a role model. Demonstrates leadership abilities and skills in communication, consumer relations, problem solving, and decision making. Participates in continuing education and research activities. Performs other job-related duties as assigned. Required to work rotating shifts.

Education and credentials: Graduate of a state-approved school of nursing. Current RN license in State of California or temporary work permit pending results of RN licensure examination. Current CPR certificate for nurses.

Special working conditions: Lifts weights over 25 pounds; often bends, squats, stoops, pulls, pushes; walks and stands for long periods. May be exposed to infectious diseases, toxic drugs, radiant and electric energy.

Experience: None

Application information: Rachel Hemway, RN, Nurse Recruiter
Regional Medical Center, Oakville, CA 94560

REGIONAL MEDICAL CENTER IS AN EQUAL OPPORTUNITY
AFFIRMATIVE ACTION EMPLOYER

---

hospital recruiters are assigned this task, first-level managers like Steve may be asked to conduct preliminary tours and describe the job to prospective applicants.

Screening is the process of choosing the best candidate for a given position. Staff nurse selection committees usually include the nurse recruiter, middle manager, and first-level managers where the recruit will work. Committee members gather data from written information and interviews, develop criteria, analyze the data, consider alternate applicants, and make a selection.

Application forms, resumes, tests, and letters of reference indicate whether an applicant meets minimum job requirements, furnish background data useful for planning the interview, and provide information about education and work experience.

Interviews gather information about personal traits, give information about the job, determine if applicants meet minimum standards, and garner goodwill for the agency. They are scheduled at convenient times and places.

To prepare for an interview managers review applications and resumes ahead of time, looking for discrepancies between job description and applicant. They formulate precise questions and use an interview guide to gather the same data from each applicant.

To conduct an interview, committee members (1) arrive on time; (2) welcome applicants and use proper names; (3) establish rapport by sharing something in common to help interviewees relax; (4) state the purpose and structure of the interview and that interviewers will take brief notes; (5) use an interview guide, following the order and content exactly; (6) probe to obtain details about negative or unclear information; (7) stay within the law (see Table 10-3); (8) listen attentively, noting verbal and nonverbal behavior; (9) if applicant looks promising, offer realistic information about the position; (10) ask applicant for comments and questions, answering truthfully; (11) if asked, state the salary range and refer the applicant to the personnel office for specifics; (12) explain the next step in the selection process; and (13) bid the applicant a friendly goodbye (Decker 1983).

Selection is the task of choosing the best candidate to fill a job. When the selection committee has interviewed all applicants, it considers the job description, evidence of qualifications, strengths, and weaknesses of applicants. It then makes a selection. Usually the nurse manager contacts the successful applicant by phone and the personnel department mails an official employment offer. When the terms of employment are agreed on, the nurse manager or personnel department write to unsuccessful applicants stating that the

Equal Opportunity and Affirmative Action Laws

Title VI and Title VII of the Civil Rights Act of 1964, as amended by the Equal Employment Act of 1972	Prohibits discrimination because of race, color, religion, sex, or national origin in any term, condition, or privilege of employment.
Title IX of the Education Amendments of 1972	Prohibits discrimination on the basis of sex in any educational program or activity receiving federal financial assistance.
Equal Pay Act, as amended by Education Amendments of 1972	Requires the same pay for men and women doing substantially equal work, requiring equal skill, effort, and responsibility under similar working conditions in the same establishment.
Age discrimination in Employment Act of 1967	Prohibits age discrimination against individuals between 40 and 70 years of age.
Executive Order 11246 as amended by Executive Order 11375	Prohibits all government contracting agencies from discriminating against any employee or applicant for employment; requires that contractors take affirmative action to ensure that applicants are employed, and that employees are treated during employment without regard to race, sex, color, religion, or national origin.
Section 503 and 504 of the Rehabilitation Act of 1973	Prohibits discrimination because of handicap in employment and in programs and activities receiving federal funds; requires contractors to take affirmative action to employ and advance in employment, qualified handicapped individuals.
Section 402 of the Vietnam Era Veterans Readjustment Assistance Act of 1974	Requires contractors to take affirmative action to employ and advance in employment qualified disabled veterans, particularly those of the Vietnam era.

position was filled and thanking them for their interest in the position.

ORIENTATION AND SOCIALIZATION. Having made a selection from available candidates, agencies help nurses succeed with orientation and socialization programs.

Orientation is the process of introducing new employees to the institution and to a specific job. In most hospitals this process is coordinated by the education department. Often this department prepares an orientation folder containing information about the agency, the department where the nurse will work, and a job description. Institutional orientation and departmental orientation include a tour, information about the institution, and fire safety. Work unit orientation includes a tour, introduction to co-workers, and discussion of work expectations.

Socialization is the process of acquiring the values and accepted modes of behaviors of a group. To facilitate this process, agencies provide various programs, including preceptorships, buddy systems, internships, and mentorships.

Preceptorships are formal arrangements between a preceptor and a novice, often arranged by hospitals for new employees. The goal is to assist new nurses to acquire the knowledge and skill needed to function effectively in a certain role. A preceptor acts as orientor, teacher, resource person, counselor, role model, and evaluator for a period of time, offering on-the-job training tailored to the needs of the learner. Preceptors gain recognition and sharpened clinical and teaching skills. Institutions gain well-socialized and oriented staff members.

Buddy systems are modified preceptorships in which a novice is paired for a few hours or days with an experienced nurse. Since no special preparation or contractual agreement precedes the assignment, the buddy usually is not accountable for specific teaching or evaluation. While new nurses gain some support, the quality of buddy systems varies considerably.

Internships are formal arrangements between agencies and interns to provide bona fide work experience. Interns receive formal credit for their work and may or may not receive money. Learning objectives and performance evaluations usually are a part of internship programs. The agency benefits because it gains the service of a near-professional at very little cost.

Mentorships are nurturing relationships between professionals that are not confined to a place or limited by time. Mentors serve as role models, friends, and sounding boards. They give their time, energy, and support, assisting goal-directed protégés to develop more fully. Mentorships are informal arrangements based on mutual respect and goodwill that develop over time. They may or may not be initiated by agencies, and may grow out of preceptor-preceptee relationships.

STAFF DEVELOPMENT.   Large health-care institutions usually have education departments that are responsible for staff development. They provide inservice education and continuing education programs.

Inservice education is offered by employers to help employees work more effectively. Inservice education begins with orientation and continues throughout employment. This includes general programs for the entire staff, such as fire safety, and specific programs for select staff, such as the nurses. Various educational techniques and tools are used, including lectures, computer simulations, demonstrations, discussions, and audiovisual tapes. Videotapes are especially useful because busy staff nurses can view them at their convenience. For instance, if Steve obtains a video on how to operate the new infusion pump he will not need to schedule a class, because the staff can view it during slack times.

Continuing education (CE) is much broader than inservice education. It builds on prior skills and knowledge and expands learning beyond current job functions. While inservice education is offered to improve the work performance of employees, CE is undertaken by individual nurses to achieve career goals. In states with mandatory CE regulations, hospital education departments often design inservice courses to meet state requirements (See Chapter 2, Education for Nursing and Chapter 12, Career Management.)

Patient education is a vital part of nursing practice. Its purpose is to give patients and their families the skills and knowledge they need to assume responsibility for their own health. Some hospital education departments provide health education for the community, offering classes on topics such as stopping smoking, nutrition, and stress reduction.

ASSIGNMENT SYSTEMS.   Nurse managers are expected to deliver the best patient care at the lowest cost, use available staff most effectively, and provide job satisfaction for caregivers. To meet this challenge managers must find an assignment system that matches local constraints with patient and caregiver needs. The system must be cost effective and realistic in regard to available staff and must give nurses maximum recognition and autonomy. Some common assignment systems are case, functional, team, and primary care. Each has advantages and disadvantages.

Case nursing is the oldest assignment system. By this method nurses give total patient care to one or more individuals during a work shift, reporting to a head nurse. The method is common with students, private duty, and special care unit nurses. Head nurses make assignments, supervise all activities on the unit, and report to their supervisors. Advantages of case nursing are that staff nurses gain a holistic view of patients, and managers are able to match patient needs with caregiver abilities. Disadvantages are that continuity of care from day to day is not assured and highly skilled nurses must perform unskilled, time-consuming tasks.

Functional nursing is an assignment system that was adapted from industry during the nurse shortage of World War II. It divides nursing into tasks, with different people doing different tasks according to their skill and knowledge. Nursing assistants give personal care, LPNs do treatments and give medications, RNs monitor IVs, do complex treatments, give medications, and assess critical patients. Responsibility and authority is delegated from the top. Staff members report to charge nurses who make assignments and supervise. Advantages of functional nursing are that it is efficient and economical. Disadvantages are that nurses do not gain a holistic view of patients, nor do they exercise autonomous accountability for care.

Team nursing is an assignment system that seeks to achieve patient care goals through group action. It was developed at a time of widespread interest in group dynamics (Lambertson 1953). In this system staff members are divided into teams. Each team consists of

RNs, LPNs, and nurse assistants. Team leaders make assignments according to caregiver abilities and perform the tasks team members are not qualified to do, such as starting intravenous infusions. At a daily patient care conference, team members review care plans. They care for the same patients each day and report to team leaders who report to the head nurse who manages the unit. Advantages of team nursing are that it gives nurses a more holistic view of patients and maximizes caregiver abilities. Disadvantages are that team leader workloads may be excessive and the system is less cost effective than other ones.

Primary care is an assignment system in which professional nurses assume total responsibility and authority for the care of several patients 24 hours per day from the time of admission to discharge (Marram et al 1974). On subsequent shifts, associate nurses, LPNs and RNs, follow the nursing care plan developed by the primary nurse and report to the head nurse who manages the unit. Advantages of primary care are that nurses gain a holistic view of patients, greater autonomy, and accountability. Patients have a nurse advocate and the system is cost effective. Disadvantages are that highly skilled nurses perform unskilled, time-consuming tasks, often carry excessive workloads, and burn out quickly.

STAFFING FORMULAS, PATTERNS, AND WORK SHIFTS.   *Staffing formulas* are ways to calculate the number of people to hire based on the average occupancy level of nursing units. These formulas take into consideration vacations, holidays, sick leave, and staff development time. For example, if a nurse works five days a week in a nursing position where coverage is needed for seven days, it takes $7 \div 5 = 1.4$ nurses to have one nurse on duty for each of the seven days. Schedulers use more complicated formulas to calculate sick leave and vacation coverage.

Staffing patterns are plans that show the number and mix of RNs, LPNs, and nurse assistants needed during a time period. When managers create these plans they consider institutional goals, policies, availability and qualifications of nurses, laws, assignment systems, and other factors such as beds per unit. They determine who is qualified to do what tasks, in how much time, and for patients of what acuity.

Task level analysis tells what qualifications caregivers need to perform tasks. *Time and motion studies* tell how much time it takes to do tasks. *Patients classification systems* (PCSs) tell the acuity of patients by grouping them according to how many hours of care they require per day. *Factor type* PCSs use lists of tasks, each with number values (eg, incontinent care = 3), with patients grouped into four or five categories according to the time it takes to do the tasks. *Prototype* PCSs use selective tasks that are critical indicators of required care, with patients grouped into four or five categories according to critical indicators. Both types of PCSs yield data about patient acuity and nursing care needs, translating it into hours.

To calculate the number of nurses needed, managers add the direct care time required by all patients on the unit to the indirect time needed for recording, reporting, and break time. They divide that number by the hours of a shift. For example, a group of 16 patients need a total of 30 hours of direct care plus two hours of indirect care during an eight-hour shift, or $32 \div 8 = 4$ nurses. The number and mix of required staff is then compared to the number and mix of those scheduled to work, minus absences.

The key to efficient use of resources is to match the required and available staff (Edwardson 1988). If more nurses are needed than scheduled, managers call a float pool of registry nurses or unscheduled employees. If more nurses are scheduled than needed, managers ask them not to work that day or to float to other units with greater need. In the vignette, Bonnie was asked to float to another unit because patient acuity on the unit did not justify her presence.

Work shifts, historically, were 12 to 24 hours, six days per week. In the mid-1940s nurses began to work five eight-hour shifts per week. Typically, shifts were 0700 to 1530, 1500 to 2330, and 2300 to 0730, with a half-hour lunch break and a half-hour overlap. To staff the hospital on weekends, evenings, and nights, some institutions mandated that all nurses rotate to evenings, nights, and weekends. Other hospitals employed permanent day, evening, night, and weekend workers.

With the advent of intensive care units, primary care, acute shortages, and increased autonomy, new work-shift patterns emerged. Today, a mosaic of shift lengths are used. Regular part-time positions and job-sharing are common. No longer bound to tradition, managers and staffs decide what will work best, considering quality of care, costs, and availability of nurses.

SCHEDULING.   The final step of the staffing process is scheduling people to fill specified work-force needs. In agencies that operate one shift a day, weekdays only, scheduling is not an issue. In health-care institutions operating 24 hours a day, 365 days a year, scheduling is a major concern. As a function of management, scheduling is either centralized or decentralized.

Centralized scheduling is done by an administrative clerk for personnel in all nursing units. The scheduler becomes an expert in impartially applying agency policy and observing budgeted nurse-patient ratios. While the process is fair and efficient, it is impersonal and nursing input is minimal.

Decentralized scheduling is done by managers on nursing units, taking into account patient needs and staff abilities. The task is time-consuming, and because managers must make hard decisions that do not please everyone, it is also thankless.

Directing

The third management function is directing. It is the connecting link between organizing for work and getting a job done (Douglass 1988). Directing informs workers what is expected of them and enables them to do it efficiently and effectively. When directing motivates staff members to achieve goals it is called *activating*. Directing requires technical activities and interpersonal skills.

Technical Activities

The technical activities of directing are aimed at achieving institutional goals. *Patient-focused activities* of nurse managers like Steve are to (1) initiate and update written nursing care plans; (2) maintain a healthy, safe, and comfortable environment; (3) accurately and concisely report and record essential information about patients to other responsible health professionals (see Table

⚡ Table 10-4

Guidelines for Giving a Shift Report of Patient Conditions

1. Assemble pertinent data such as intake-output and vital signs.
2. Speak clearly and slowly enough to be understood.
3. Introduce yourself, stating name, title, and room numbers of patients about whom you will report.
4. Report on each patient, as follows:
   a. State room number, patient's name, physician's name, medical diagnosis, and surgery or major treatment with date.
   b. Give pertinent assessment data, nursing diagnosis, and interventions. (For example, fluid volume: deficit; intravenous fluids: type, rate, amount; skin integrity: impairment; dressing changes: type, frequency; urinary elimination: deficit; indwelling catheter: describe urine, amount.)
   c. When patients are scheduled for surgery or other major treatment, state procedure, time scheduled, patient's status, and nursing interventions yet to be done, such as giving pre-op medications on call.
   d. Do NOT gossip, state subjective opinions as facts, or discuss personal problems. You are a professional speaking to professionals.
5. Offer information about expected admissions, discharges, scheduled inservice, and other matters of importance.
6. Conclude report by stating your name and an amiable wish.

10-4); and (4) provide information, assistance, and education to patients and their families.

Staff-focused activities of first-level managers are to (1) give formal and informal direction relative to nursing care; (2) oversee and advise staff regarding work assignments; (3) obtain supplies, equipment, and support services to facilitate quality nursing care; and (4) foster personal and professional growth of staff members.

Institution-focused activities of first-level managers are to (1) coordinate unit operations with other departments, (2) give information and assistance to other departments and physicians, (3) participate in meetings and projects, and (4) represent staff members to middle and upper level management.

Interpersonal Skills

Of all the management functions, directing is most dependent on the interpersonal skills of communication, teaching, motivation, conflict resolution, and morale building.

COMMUNICATION.   *Communication* is a process of exchanging ideas and feelings. It occurs when meaning is conveyed from one person to another, verbally and nonverbally. Communication is the key to all of the other interpersonal skills.

Assertiveness is behavior people use to stand up for themselves without violating the rights of others (Sullivan 1988). For centuries, passivity has been the hallmark of nurses. It is time that nurses, especially nurse managers, assert themselves, affirming their rights (see Table 10-5).

Assertive communication affirms one's observations, feelings, and needs without attacking or negating others. Passive communication discounts personal needs and yields without question to the needs of others. Passive-aggressive communication senses personal need, but yields to others, veiling hostility in sweetness or humor. Assertive communication acknowledges needs and feelings. When people communicate assertively they (1) report what they observe, (2) listen to the other point of view, (3) describe what they feel, and (4) state what they want.

Communication channels are networks through which information flows. They may be formal, official channels or they may be informal, unofficial channels, called *grapevines*. A grapevine transmits information much faster than an official channel because it fosters a feeling of camaraderie and delivers a message to clusters of people instead of one at a time (Marriner-Tomey 1988). Savvy managers use both official channels and grapevines to communicate with staff members.

Communication channels carry information down from above, up from below, and horizontally between equals. *Downward communication* tells subordinates what to do. Regardless of its quality,

Table 10-5

Ten Basic Rights for Nurses in the Health Professions

1. You have the right to be treated with respect.
2. You have the right to a reasonable work load.
3. You have the right to an equitable wage.
4. You have the right to determine your own priorities.
5. You have the right to ask for what you want.
6. You have the right to refuse without making excuses or feeling guilty.
7. You have the right to make mistakes and be responsible for them.
8. You have the right to give and receive information as a professional.
9. You have the right to act in the best interest of the patient.
10. You have the right to be human.

Adapted with permission from Chenevert M: *Pro-nurse Handbook*, p 109. Mosby, 1985.

it contributes to more dissatisfaction than upward communication (Marriner-Tomey 1988). *Upward communication* tells superiors what subordinates are thinking. Though often ignored, it is valuable. When encouraged, upward communication increases morale because it acknowledges the value of subordinates to the organization. *Horizontal communication* connects people at the same level. It includes sharing information, solving problems, and coordinating activities.

The American Management Association identified guidelines managers can use to improve communication (Koontz et al 1986):

1. Clarify ideas before communicating.

2. Examine the true purpose of the communication.

3. Consider the setting of the communication.

4. When planning communication, consult with others.

5. Be mindful of the nonverbal messages you send.

6. Communicate something helpful to the receiver.

7. Follow up on communication.

8. Be sure your actions support your communication.

ΒΩ *Table 10-6*

Principles of Teaching-Learning

Factors that Facilitate Learning:

Acceptance, freedom from fear and condemnation
Active involvement
Comfortable physical and emotional environment
Feedback that is both positive and negative
Logical presentation of information, simple to complex
Motivation, the desire to learn
Physical and emotional readiness
Practice, repetition, and immediate use
Relevance, value, meaning to the learner
Success, mastery

Factors that Hinder Learning:

Anxiety above moderate level
Cultural barriers of language, values, meanings, taboos
Physiologic discomfort, disease, and disability
Psychosocial discomfort, disease, and disability

TEACHING.   Teaching is an important aspect of directing. It is a deliberate action taken to help learners grasp new concepts, develop skills, and acquire attitudes. Because its purpose is to change behavior, teaching is most effective when it focuses on specific objectives. Yet it must respect the integrity and independent judgment of learners. Teaching is the responsibility of all nurses, especially nurse managers. Table 10-6 lists some important teaching-learning principles.

MOTIVATION.   Motivation is an energizing force for action, a powerful tool used by leaders to get things done. Nurse managers employ motivation to increase productivity, job satisfaction, and loyalty. Understanding that all behavior is caused and in an ultimate sense is motivated by self-interest, managers look for what motivates staff and how to motivate them.

Some theorists view motivation from a content view of *what* motivates. Others look at it from a process view of *how to* motivate. A content theorist, Freud proposed that instinct predisposes people to behave in certain ways and a "pleasure principle" causes them to seek pleasure over pain. Maslow proposed that a hierarchy of needs motivates people, including physiologic, safety-security, belongingness, esteem, and self-actualization (Maslow 1970). Skinner proposed that positive and negative reinforcers produce stimulus response bonds that modify behavior (Skinner 1953). Vroom added the notion of expectancy as a potent reinforcer (1964). These theories can be used to motivate nursing staff members, as suggested in Table 10-7.

CONFLICT RESOLUTION.   *Conflict* exists when two or more mutually exclusive goals, ideas, actions, roles, values, beliefs, feelings, or attitudes occur within or between individuals or groups. During childhood most people learn that all conflict is bad. In fact, conflict is neither good nor bad. It is the result of an inherent struggle for independence and survival. Conflict is destructive when it produces intolerable stress, aggressive action, or suppressed hostility. It is constructive when it educates, increases group cohesion, and generates personal growth, ideas, respect, and understanding. Conflict and its outcomes often proceed along a predictable path, with preexisting conditions, perceived threat, and manifest behavior. It is then suppressed or resolved and in the aftermath new attitudes and feelings evolve between the parties (Filley 1975).

Preexisting conditions include: (1) differences in beliefs, as between those nurses who support collective bargaining and those who do not; (2) structural issues, as between bureaucratic levels of authority; (3) scarce resources, as when intense competition develops between departments for available funds; (4) incompatible goals, as between the business office and social service; (5) role confusion, as when Steve identified with staff more than he did with management; (6) interdependence issues, as when operating room nurses depend on floor nurses to prepare patients for surgery; and (7) distancing, as occurs when day staff complain about night staff nurses.

When preexisting conditions develop into *perceived and felt*

Motivating Factors in the Work Setting

Physiologic Needs:

1. Work environment is comfortable and aesthetically pleasing.
2. Scheduling provides time for sleep and recreation.
3. Breaks are adequate for nourishment and stress reduction.
4. Employee health is enhanced by medical care, leave time, and infection control.
5. Salary is adequate to provide food, shelter, and health care.

Security and Safety Needs:

1. Hiring and firing policies are fair, with opportunity to learn by mistakes without harassment.
2. Patient assignments provide for continuity of care and are appropriate to ability of staff members.
3. Scheduling provides for regular, dependable work hours.
4. Emergency procedures are practiced with back-up and support.
5. Measures are taken to reduce physical, radiation, and biologic injury.

Belongingness Needs:

1. Conflict resolution is facilitated.
2. Attention is given to group dynamics to improve interpersonal comfort between staff members.
3. Team work systems, cooperation, and social contacts between staff members are encouraged.
4. Trust, honesty, assertive communication, and a degree of self-disclosure are modeled by nurse managers.

Self- and Other Esteem Needs:

1. Feedback on performance is objective and frequent.
2. Exceptional work is rewarded formally with merit raises and promotions and informally with timely recognition.
3. Assignments are individualized to suit abilities and interests of staff.

Self-actualizing Needs:

1. Staff members are included and consulted in planning.
2. Innovation is encouraged and acknowledged.
3. Opportunities for professional development are offered.
4. Management encourages testing of new projects and programs.
5. Staff members are included in decisions about assignments.
6. Staff members are encouraged to pursue professional activities.

threat, conflict may follow. There may be open aggression or passive-aggressive exchanges that escalate to intolerable levels. On Steve's unit the Liz-Pearl conflict created an unhealthy atmosphere. In a typical conflict, the battle rages until one opponent defeats the other. Unless destroyed or converted to the other viewpoint, the vanquished individual yields, but remains a threat. Suppressed hostility, mistrust, and fear continue until open battle flares again.

Strategies to manage conflict have been identified as withdrawal, smoothing, avoidance, forcing, naming a winner or loser, negotiation, compromise, and collaboration (Gustafson et al 1988).

Outcomes of conflict are lose-lose, win-lose, and win-win. In a lose-lose outcome, neither side wins and nobody is pleased. In a win-lose outcome, one side wins but bitterness may remain. In a win-win outcome, the needs of both parties are met. Table 10-8 outlines a collaborative strategy for conflict resolution that is useful with both individuals and groups.

MORALE-BUILDING.   Morale-building is a leadership skill found in the best nurse managers. It is the ability to foster enthusiasm, hope, faith, joy, and confidence. Morale is the esprit de corps, the "we" feeling that develops when people share common goals and experiences. When morale is high, people are able to accomplish extraordinary feats of courage and mastery.

To build staff morale nurse managers (1) set attainable goals and are realistic about what their staff can accomplish; (2) address conflicts, not waiting to deal with them until hostility and frustration destroy group unity; (3) consider staff abilities and preferences when making assignments (Douglass and Bevis 1979); (4) acknowledge individual accomplishment, complimenting staff personally; (5) invite and listen to suggestions of staff members, serving as a channel for upward communication to middle and top management; (6) encourage staff to participate in agency committees where they can have a voice; (7) model assertive communication and give prompt, genuine feedback; (8) maintain high standards and apply rules with absolute fairness, knowing that nothing demoralizes a staff more than unequal treatment; (9) institute clear lines of authority (Douglass and Bevis 1979) so that staff nurses know who is responsible for what and to whom; (10) defend and

Table 10-8

Conflict Intervention Using a Collaboration Strategy

1. The parties commit themselves to negotiate in good faith until an agreement is reached.
2. The parties agree to the following ground rules:
   a. No one walks out of the meeting before it ends.
   b. Everyone uses "I," not accusatory "you" statements.
   c. Everyone takes mutual responsibility for the outcome.
   d. Opponents A and B sit facing one another.
   e. Opponents have equal time.
   f. Moderator encourages, restates, maintains control, enforces rules.
3. A states A's perception of the problem to B.
4. B listens until B *experiences* A's point of view.
5. B states the problem back to A until A is satisfied that the statement truly represents A's feelings.
6. Reverse the process: B now states B's perception of the problem.
7. A listens until A understands and *experiences* B's point of view.
8. A and B then define the problem in terms of the needs of both parties, as follows: "A needs _____, and B needs _____." If the parties get stuck, go back to the beginning and repeat steps 3 through 7.
9. With the problem now clearly defined, A and B now generate possible solutions.
10. A and B discuss various solutions, assessing the potential of each.
11. Together A and B decide on a mutually acceptable solution, stated as follows: *Who* is to do *what, when?*
12. Session or sessions end with an agreement for a follow-up session to assess progress.
13. The solution is implemented.
14. At follow-up session moderator asks if the needs of both parties are being met. If not, parties go back to step 1 and begin again.

---

serve as an advocate for staff to others; (11) encourage staff development, showing sincerity by adjusting schedules, writing letters, applying for educational funds and undertaking research projects; (12) foster supportive behavior to reduce competition among staff members; and (13) model genuineness, nonpossessive warmth, and appropriate empathy, encouraging staff to extend to each other the same nonjudgmental caring they give to patients.

Controlling

Controlling is the fourth management function. It is the action taken to ensure that actual outcomes are consistent with those planned and anticipated (Schmude 1985). Controlling entails setting standards and criteria, measuring performance, and making corrections. Its watchword is accountability. Nurse managers are accountable in various degrees for the fiscal budget, risk management, quality assurance, and performance evaluations of staff members.

Fiscal Budget

Phase I and Phase II of the budget process are part of the planning function of management. Phases III and IV fall within the controlling function. Phase III takes place as an ongoing process throughout the fiscal year as managers strive to keep expenses and revenues within projected limits. If they notice a significant difference between budgeted and actual costs, managers take corrective action. During Phase IV they evaluate and revise the budget for ensuing quarters. With time and experience, managers like Steve learn to forecast revenues and expenses and to stay within budgeted amounts.

Risk Management

Risk management programs exist to prevent loss and control liability. They identify, analyze, and evaluate risks and create a plan to reduce the frequency and severity of accidents and injuries (England and Sullivan 1988). These programs set standards and criteria, measure performance, and take corrective action to reduce incidents that lead to liability suits. Some hospitals hire risk managers to coordinate activities. However, a large share of responsibility falls on nurse managers and staff because they are present or nearby when most incidents occur.

Reportable incidents are any unexpected or unplanned events that affect or potentially affect a patient or family member. The most common reportable incidents are: (1) medication errors, including intravenous fluids, (2) complications from diagnostic or treatment procedures, (3) falls, (4) dissatisfaction with care by patients or their families, and (5) refusal to sign a consent or to submit to treatment (England and Sullivan 1988).

Incident reports are made on two official documents: patient records and incident reporting forms. Nurses who are present write objective descriptions of events in patient records. On separate reporting forms, they describe incidents in greater detail than in patient records. These reports are vital to protect the institution and nurses from litigation. Managers use reports to analyze the frequency, severity, and cause, and to plan intervention to prevent future incidents. Incident reports tell what happened, to whom, when, where, under what conditions, who discovered the event, action taken to prevent further injury, who was notified and when, who is reporting the event, and how the event might have been prevented. When reports are omitted, inadequate, or faulty, hospitals are more likely to be sued and more likely to lose (Dixon 1980).

Many incidents go unreported because nurses fear discipline, feel pressured for time, and lack the knowledge of how to document events. Nurse managers can increase the accuracy and percentage of reported incidents by teaching staff how to follow an action plan for unusual events (see Table 10-9).

Quality Assurance

Quality assurance (QA) is the term used to describe the evaluation of products and services of an institution. QA sets standards and criteria, measures performance, and corrects deficits. Mandatory standards are set down by state boards of health. Voluntary standards are made by organizations such as the American Nurses' Association in its *Standards of Nursing Practice*. Standards set down by the Joint Commission on Accreditation of Healthcare Organizations (JCAHCO) are voluntary, but if hospitals are not JCAHCO-accredited, they are not reimbursed by third party payers such as insurance companies and Medicare.

Quality assurance programs aim to maintain quality health-care services. In 1982, JCAHCO began requiring that all accredited

Table 10-9

An Action Plan for Unusual Events

1. *Discover and report all unusual events.* Anyone can do this.
2. *Notify proper authorities.* Nurse informs physician immediately; if it is a major incident, nurse informs nurse manager or risk manager by phone and completes a reporting form within 24 hours.
3. *Investigate.* Physician, nurse manager, and risk manager investigate the incident immediately.
4. *Consult.* Nurse manager and risk manager consult with the physician and hospital risk management committee.
5. *Take action.* Nurse manager or risk manager explores the incident with the patient and family, as follows:
   a. Listen. Do not respond until patient and family have finished.
   b. Avoid reacting defensively. Convey sincere concern.
   c. Ask patient and family what solution they expect.
   d. If fitting, explain actions you can and cannot take.
   e. Agree on steps to be taken within a timeframe.
6. *Record information* in patient record and on reporting form; note conversations with patient and family; include agreements.

Adapted from England DA, Sullivan EJ: Quality assurance and risk management. In: *Effective Management in Nursing,* Sullivan EJ, Decker PJ, 2nd ed. Addison-Wesley, 1988.

hospitals have ongoing QA programs to maintain standards of care. Although some hospitals hire a QA manager, the responsibility often falls on nurses. Nurse managers must understand and apply JCAHCO Nursing Service Standards to patient care, incorporate them in management activities, and familiarize the staff with their interpretation (Fitzgerald 1986).

Quality assurance monitoring uses many procedures. *Nursing audits* are official evaluations of nursing care. Concurrent audits are made while patients are receiving care. Retrospective audits are conducted after patients are discharged. Auditors assess evidence that nursing care meets (or met) expected outcomes of care plans. If it does not, auditors recommend changes.

Peer reviews are made by practicing nurses who determine standards that indicate quality care. Their expertise is useful in evaluating the care of complicated cases where a synthesis of knowledge and experience is needed (Benner 1984).

Utilization reviews are mandated by Title XVIII of the Social Security Act for "maintenance of high quality patient care and assurance of appropriate and efficient utilization of facility services" (*Standards* 1976). These reviews evaluate medical care and length of patient stays. To receive Medicare reimbursement, facilities must have utilization review plans. While these plans do not focus on nursing, they impact patient care, such as length of stays.

Patient satisfaction rating scales are used to determine the level of patient approval. Patients may be asked to fill out a questionnaire before or after discharge. Though not scientific, these surveys help assess the usefulness of nursing interventions such as patient teaching.

Performance Evaluations

The words "performance evaluation" produce strong emotions in almost all nurses. Staff nurses may view evaluations as threats, while managers like Steve view them as time-consuming chores. Yet performance evaluations can be useful tools for professional growth. They give a formal appraisal of how well a nurse is meeting prescribed standards. Ideally, performance evaluations motivate, determine competence, recognize accomplishments, and suggest staff development needs. As with other control functions, performance evaluations set standards and criteria, measure behavior, and correct deficiencies.

Performance standards are given to nurses when they are hired, initiating the evaluation process. These standards should mirror job descriptions. Their clarity and specificity makes the evaluation process objective, consistent, and job-related. It reduces intimidation, and removes the element of surprise. Employee-employer contracts often describe the process, including an appeal mechanism for disputes. When hired, new nurses usually receive an evaluation schedule calling for an appraisal at the end of the orientation period, in six months, and on an annual basis thereafter unless problems arise.

To facilitate the process, managers keep an ongoing written

record of the performance of staff members. An annotated file works well. In it, they write brief notes, with dates, times, and both desirable and undesirable behaviors. If patients are endangered, managers do not wait for scheduled appraisals, but take immediate action. Written evidence objectifies the evaluation process and gives managers like Steve more power to effect change.

As the time draws near for a scheduled evaluation, nurse managers review their annotated file and fill out an approved form. They make appointments for evaluation conferences when minimal interruptions can be expected.

Nurse managers frame the conference as a feedback session for professional growth and career development. They are sensitive to human needs and focus on objective behavior, not personal attributes. They avoid accusatory "you" statements that create defensiveness and concentrate on objective evidence. The list of expected behaviors structures the discussion. Deficiencies are addressed as problems to be solved. Together, evaluator and evaluatee forge a plan of corrective action with specific criteria. For example, Liz and Pearl will begin conflict resolution sessions immediately and within four weeks each will exhibit specific cooperative behaviors. At the close of the conference, managers summarize decisions and confirm the time for the next appraisal.

When staff nurses have a plan to correct deficiencies, managers see that the plan is followed. When it is achieved, they acknowledge changes. If unacceptable behavior does not stop, managers follow the termination-for-cause policy of the agency. For example, four weeks after his session with Liz and Pearl, Steve will meet with each nurse to evaluate her progress.

Some behavior calls for immediate dismissal, such as theft and abuse of patients or drugs. To protect themselves from liability, managers must have first-hand knowledge, not hearsay. Therefore, they should write detailed notes about incidents and keep superiors apprised of problems.

Substance abuse or mental illness may cause a change in the disposition or appearance of a nurse. Managers confront such nurses with their observations and refer them for counseling with firmness and compassion. Managers report the matter to their supervisor. The institution reports the nurse to the state licensing board if the behavior calls for license suspension. Many states have diversion programs to identify and rehabilitate nurses (see the section on rehabilitation programs in Chapter 3).

Summary

Living organizations have all the characteristics of open systems, including interrelatedness and input-throughput-output feedback. The management process takes place inside systems. Leadership is a set of abilities. Decision-making is the process of selecting from alternatives. Creativity is an ability to generate new ideas. Computer technology assists nurses to manage patient care. The management process has four operations: planning, organizing, directing, and controlling. *Planning* includes identifying the purpose and philosophy of the agency, clarifying goals and objectives, reviewing policies, preparing budgets, and assessing resources. *Organizing* includes structures, staffing, assignment systems, and scheduling. *Directing* requires technical activities and interpersonal skills. *Controlling* entails setting standards, measuring performance, and making corrections. Nurse managers participate in all these functions.

Learning Activities

1. Spend a day with a first-level nurse manager. Classify each activity according to its management function (planning, organizing, directing, and controlling).

2. Design an orientation program for an acute care hospital for recent graduates entering the labor force for the first time.

3. Role-play assertive communication with a physician who is furious because a patient was fed breakfast when a fasting blood sample was ordered.

4. Using the conflict resolution strategy provided in Table 10-8, and resolve a real conflict between associates.

5. Compare a staff nurse job description in a local hospital and the same hospital's performance evaluation form. Do they match? If not, how would you change them?

Annotated Reading List

Baker LD, Heaton JB: Managing time. In: *Effective Management in Nursing,* Sullivan EJ, Decker PJ, 2nd ed. Addison-Wesley, 1988.

A little jewel of writing, this chapter addresses a chronic problem for nurse managers: using time wisely. It discusses a number of ways to manage time more efficiently. Full of useful suggestions, the chapter definitely is worth the time it takes to read it.

Gustafson DF, Sullivan EJ, Evans DO: Dealing with conflict. In: *Effective Management in Nursing,* Sullivan EJ, Decker PJ, 2nd ed. Addison-Wesley, 1988.

Conflict is an ever-present issue in the complex world of health care. In the chapter, the authors discuss the phenomenon, its importance, definition, process, and various resolution techniques. They discuss both individual and group conflict and describe strategies for dealing with conflict focusing on three outcomes: win-lose, lose-lose, and win-win.

Marriner-Tomey A: *Guide to Nursing Management,* 3rd ed. Mosby, 1987.

A comprehensive text on management, this book sorts every management topic into five management functions: planning, organizing, staffing, directing, and controlling. The writing is clear, understandable, and succinct. It is illustrated with graphic displays and charts. An extensive bibliography is provided for each chapter.

References

Adams JL: *Conceptual Blockbusting.* The Portable Stanford, Stanford Alumni Association; 1974.

Baker LD, Heaton JB: Managing time. In: *Effective Management in Nursing,* Sullivan EJ, Decker PJ, 2nd ed. Addison-Wesley, 1988.

Benner P: *From Novice to Expert.* Addison-Wesley, 1984.

Bower FL: Shared governance: A professional model for nursing practice. *California Nursing* Nov/Dec 1990; 29–32.

Chenevert M: *Pro-nurse Handbook.* Mosby, 1985.

Decker PJ: *Selective Interviewing Procedures for Health Care Managers.* Decker, 1983.

Decker PJ, Hailstone S: Recruiting and selecting staff. In: *Effective Management in Nursing,* Sullivan EJ, Decker PJ, 2nd ed. Addison-Wesley, 1988.

Dixon NE: *Quality, Trending, and Management for the '80s: A Hospital-wide Quality Assurance Program.* American Hospital Association, 1980.

Dossett DL, Jenkins RL, Decker PJ, Sullivan EJ: Leadership skills. In: *Effective Management in Nursing,* Sullivan EJ and Decker PJ, 2nd ed. Addison-Wesley, 1988.

Douglass LM: *The Effective Nurse Leader Manager,* 3rd ed. Mosby, 1988.

Douglass LM, Bevis EO: *Nursing Management and Leadership in Action,* 3rd ed. Mosby, 1979.

Edwardson SR: Productivity. In: *Effective Management in Nursing,* Sullivan EJ, Decker PJ, 2nd ed. Addison-Wesley, 1988.

Emery FE (editor): *Systems Thinking.* Penguin, 1969.

England DA, Sullivan EJ: Quality assurance and risk management. In: *Effective Management in Nursing,* Sullivan EJ, Decker PJ, 2nd ed. Addison-Wesley, 1988.

Filley AC: *Interpersonal Conflict Resolution.* Scott, Foresman, 1975.

Fitzgerald WD: Performance evaluation. In: *Handbook for First-Line Nurse Managers,* Schweiger JL (editor). Wiley, 1986.

Gustafson DP, Sullivan EJ, Evans DO: Dealing with conflict. In: *Effective Management in Nursing,* Sullivan EJ, Decker PJ, 2nd ed. Addison-Wesley, 1988.

Hollander EP: *Leadership Dynamics: A Practical Guide to Effective Relationships.* Free Press, 1978.

Hutelmyer CM: Leadership. Chapter 3 in: *Handbook for First-Line Nurse Managers,* Schweiger JL (editor). Wiley, 1986.

Koontz H, O'Donnell C, Weihrich H: *Management,* 4th ed. McGraw-Hill, 1986.

Kuster J: New software could revolutionize nursing industry. *Focus* Aug 1990.

Lambertson E: *Nursing Team: Organizational and Functional.* Columbia University Press, 1953.

Marram G, Schleger MW, Bevis EO: *Primary Nursing, A Model for Individualized Care.* Mosby, 1974.

Marriner-Tomey A: *Guide to Nursing Management,* 3rd ed. Mosby, 1988.

Maslow A: *Motivation and Personality,* 2nd ed. Harper & Row, 1970.

McGregor D: *The Human Side of Enterprise.* McGraw-Hill, 1960.

Scanian B, Keys JB: *Management and Organizational Behavior.* Wiley, 1979.

Schmude J: Nursing services. In: *Continuous Monitoring and Data-Based Quality Assessment,* Vol 3. Greeley Associates, 1985.

Skinner BF: *Science and Human Behavior.* Free Press, 1953.

Standards for Certification and Participation in Medicare and Medicaid Programs. Fed Reg, Vol 39, No 12, Part III, 1974. In: *General Administration in the Nursing Home,* Rogers WW, 2nd ed. Cahners, 1976.

Strader MK: Problem solving and decision making. In: *Effective Management in Nursing,* Sullivan EJ, Decker PJ, 2nd ed. Addison-Wesley, 1988.

Sullivan EJ: Communication skills. In: *Effective Management in Nursing,* Sullivan EJ, Decker PJ, 2nd ed. Addison-Wesley, 1988.

Tappen, RM: *Leadership: Concepts and Practice.* Davis, 1983.

Vroom VH: *Work and Motivation.* Wiley, 1964.

White RK, Lippitt R.: *Autocracy and Democracy: An Experimental Inquiry.* Harper & Row, 1960.

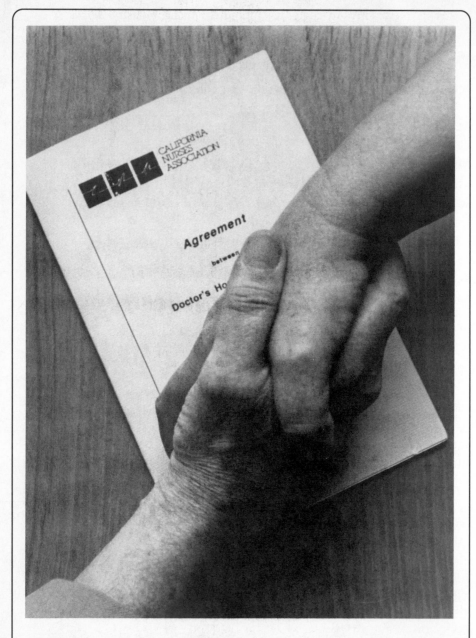

A representative of the nurses and a representative of the hospital shake hands over a collective bargaining agreement.

CHAPTER 11

Collective Bargaining

LEARNING OBJECTIVES

1. List the four essential elements of a legally enforceable contract.

2. Compare the following contracts: formal with simple, written with oral, and expressed with implied.

3. Discuss the elements of a sound employment contract.

4. Trace the history of labor laws in the United States since 1935, naming some of the most significant legislation as it impacts nurses.

5. Describe some important functions of the National Labor Relations Board.

6. Describe unfair labor practices that are prohibited for labor unions and employers.

7. Explain the steps nurses must take to organize a union.

8. Describe the collective bargaining process for negotiating a contract with an employer.

9. Explain the purpose for grievance procedures and describe a typical procedure.

10. Define and discuss arbitration, the arbitration process, and the Federal Mediation and Conciliation Service.

11. Describe grievances other than contract violations that may occur, who may file them, and to whom grievants may apply.

12. Discuss actions employers can take to prevent discontent and unionization among nursing personnel.

355

A **nurse** *from surgery opened the door to the nurses' lounge, thrust a note into Sue's hand, warned her to be careful, and disappeared. Sue looked at the note. It was the address of a hush-hush meeting with an organizer from the State Nurses' Association. Sue shrank from the conflict within her and looked about the windowless room as if for escape. The only decoration was a poster of a cat, desperately clinging to a tree limb. "That's how I feel!" Sue thought. "I've tried so hard to maintain my standards, but the more I try, the worse things get. Almost every day somebody else leaves for a better job. Maybe that's what I should do. But I'd rather stay here. I must be pretty desperate to consider joining a* union!"

Even the word union stuck in Sue's throat. She had grown up hearing that unions were evil and dangerous. Her father hated them. He believed unions were led by communists and controlled by the underworld, that they forced people to strike, cost members more than they gained, only created problems, got in the way of good employer-employee relationships, and served only low-class sloths. No "professional" would join a union. Certainly not a nurse! Not Sue!

Yet Sue knew she wasn't lazy. She knew the hospital paid low wages, gave few benefits, staffed at unsafe levels, granted promotions on the basis of "connections," and treated the staff like nameless pegs on a utility wall. As Sue thought about the situation, her anger rose. No wonder people joined unions! But could she? Sue really didn't know how unions worked and what they did to bring about change.

Nurses everywhere are concerned about economic status and working conditions, and they want to be heard and recognized. Adequate wages means economic security. Optimum working conditions mean job satisfaction and the opportunity to provide quality patient care. In recent years, an increasing number of nurses have felt the need to join an employee union to achieve these ends. Together they have joined forces to bargain with their employers for improved economic and working conditions. Many have realized their objectives (*Practices* 1984). Nonetheless, the decision to join a union is not an easy one. Some nurses consider union activity unprofessional. They see negotiations for wages and working conditions as obstructing, rather than facilitating, quality patient care. Others hesitate to trust their economic and professional welfare to an organization, preferring to deal directly with employers as individuals. Still others find the cost of union dues and the commitment of time and effort more than they are willing to give (*Nurses' Legal Handbook* 1985).

How nurses go about securing economic status and working conditions that meet their personal and professional needs depends on many factors. Joining a union may or may not be the best way to achieve career goals. If you, like Sue, know little about contracts, union organizations, collective bargaining, and how disputes are settled, read on.

Contracts

Many nurses sign employment contracts without reading all the words. Even when they read all the words they may not understand the terms, recognize implied conditions, or notice if crucial elements are missing. Understanding these matters helps nurses avoid problems and function within defined limits. Table 11-1 lists some key terms used in contracts.

♬ *Table 11-1*

Key Terms Used in Contracts

breach of contract   Failing to perform all or part of the contracted duty without justification

contract   Legally binding agreement between two or more people to do, or not do, something

contract violations   Actions that break mutually agreed-on rules

expressed contract   Verbal or written agreement between two or more people to do, or not do, something

implied contract   Verbal or written agreement, inferred rather than expressed, between two or more people to do, or not do, something

invalid contract   Any contract concerning illegal or impossible actions; no legal obligation exists

terminate   To fulfill all contractual obligations or absolve onself of the obligation to fulfill them

Reprinted with permission from Nurse's Reference Library. *Practices*. Springhouse, 1984.

Essential Features of Contracts

Every contract, to be enforceable as law, must have four essential features: (1) promises made between two or more legally competent parties to do or not to do something, (2) mutual understanding of the terms and obligations of the contract by all parties, (3) compensation in the form of something of value in exchange for an action or inaction, and (4) a lawful purpose (Creighton 1986).

As a legally binding agreement between two or more people to do or not do something, a contract can be enforced by court action. Of course, if fraud, coercion, or an illegal act is involved, the contract is *invalid* or *void* and the courts will not enforce it. If either party to a legal contract fails to perform their part of an agreement, the damaged party can seek relief in the courts. They can also seek penalties for noncompliance with the contract. For example, if Sue borrows money from a bank but fails to make agreed-on payments, the bank can take her to court to enforce the contract. If her hospital agrees to pay Sue $15 per hour, but actually pays a different rate, she can take the hospital to court to force it to fulfill the agreement. On the other hand, if someone fails to keep a social or moral contract, they rarely go to court, either because the agreement lacked some essential feature of a legal contract or because the wronged party does not seek redress through the legal system.

Types of Contracts

Individual and Collective

Contracts with employers may be *individual* (those negotiated personally by individuals) or *collective* (those negotiated by a labor union for employees). Most individual contracts are negotiated informally and therefore are less precise. Collective contracts, on the other hand, are negotiated formally, spelling out specifics in detail. While such precision leaves less room for interpretation, it also leaves less room for flexibility in real-life situations involving the delivery of nursing care.

Formal and Simple

A *formal contract* is one required by law to be in writing. In order to prevent fraudulent practices, each state has a statute of frauds that requires that certain contracts be written, such as deeds and mortgages. Some formal contracts also must be *under seal,* that is, they must be written on paper imprinted or stamped with an official seal. All other contracts are called *simple,* whether they are written or oral (Creighton 1986).

Written and Oral

Oral contracts are just as binding as written contracts, but they may create problems. Since the terms and conditions of oral contracts are not written down, they are subject to memory and interpretation. The passage of time and changes in policies or personnel of an institution may blur the original meaning, causing disagreement between the parties about the terms of the contract. As a result, most state courts do not consider oral contracts valid unless the terms can be fulfilled within a year (Nurse's Reference Library 1984).

Expressed and Implied

An *expressed contract* may be written or oral. For example, during a job interview Melanie is offered a position as a staff nurse for a certain shift at a particular salary. If she agrees verbally to the offer, she enters into an *oral expressed contract*. If she signs a contract she enters into a *written expressed contract*. On the way home Melanie stops by a hair salon. Even though she does not sign an agreement or discuss the price, by having her hair cut, Melanie enters into an *implied contract* and must pay for the service she receives.

Most contracts contain implied conditions, elements of agreement that are not explicitly stated but are assumed to be part of the contract. For example, hospitals assume that registered nurses will practice in a safe, competent manner, as defined by the state nurse practice act. Nurses assume that the hospital will staff the units with qualified personnel and will provide necessary supplies and equipment for them do to their job (*Nurses' Legal Handbook* 1985).

If a nurse decides to accept an employment contract, the nurse can sign the contract, verbally agree to it, provide a written acceptance of it, or simply report for work. By reporting for work the nurse gives *implied agreement* to the terms of the contract. However, if a nurse fails to respond in any way to an employment offer, there is no contract. The employer is free to withdraw the offer at any time before it is accepted without penalty (Nurse's Reference Library 1984).

Termination and Breach of Contract

It is important for nurses to know how to end, or *terminate a contract*. One way is for each party to fulfill all the terms of a contract or for both parties to agree to end it. Another way is for one party to release the other from further obligation to the contract. Some contracts provide for termination at the end of a fixed time or on the occurrence of an event, such as completion of a project. Most individual employment contracts do not state termination dates, but employees and employers may end them by following procedures prescribed in the contract.

When people *breach a contract*, they have unjustifiably failed to perform all or part of their contractual duty. A substantial breach of contract is never lawful (Nurse's Reference Library 1984). If John signs a contract agreeing to work the night shift for a minimum of six months but after two months refuses to do so, he is breaching his contract. The hospital can discharge him and seek an injunction against him. An *injunction* is a court order to refrain from taking some particular action, such as working for any other hospital. Since obtaining an injunction is complex and expensive, hospitals rarely seek injunctions against nurses. Even so, breaching a contract may damage John's reputation and make it difficult for him to get a job at other hospitals.

Elements of a Sound Employment Contract

When nurses go to work for an institution with a union contract, they sign an individual contract, agreeing to a work assignment, a beginning classification, and to abide by the terms of the contract in effect at that time. It is important to recognize and understand the features of a sound employment contract. If nurses go to work for a nonunion agency, such knowledge is even more vital. However, they may decide to have an attorney read the contract and explain its implications.

Collective contracts are written by the representatives of organized employees and their employers. Each contract looks different from any other. Even the names vary. One may be called an agreement, another a memorandum of understanding, and still another a contract. Although the items may appear in a different sequence and be called by different words, a sound employment contract includes certain items:

1. *Date and parties to the agreement.* The contract declares who is entering into a contract and when, as "This Memorandum of Understanding was made and entered into July 1, 1989, by and

between the California Nurses Association . . . and the Petaluma Valley Hospital District . . . and covers all Registered Nurses . . . in those classifications specified in Article II" (CNA 1989b).

2. *Preamble or purpose.* The contract states the overall reason for the contract, as "Both parties recognize that it is to their mutual advantage and for the protection of the patients to have efficient and uninterrupted operation of the Hospital. This Agreement is for the purpose of establishing such harmonious and constructive relationships between the parties that such results shall be possible" (CNA 1989b).

3. *Recognition of representatives.* The contract states that the employer formally recognizes the legal authority of union representatives, as "The Hospital recognizes the Association as the exclusive representative of the Nurses covered by this Agreement for the purpose of establishing mutual satisfactory conditions of employment" (CNA 1989b).

4. *Coverage.* The contract stipulates which employees are covered by the contract, as "This Agreement covers all Registered Nurses, excluding Head Nurses and Supervisors, as defined in the National Labor Relations Act" (CNA 1989a). Often first-level nurse managers are covered unless specifically excluded.

5. *Hospital rights.* The contract affirms areas of authority reserved by the institution, as "The Hospital retains all the rights, powers, and authority exercised or had by it except as may be limited by a specific provision of the Agreement" (CNA 1989b).

6. *Association rights.* The contract affirms specific rights of the union regarding membership, dues collection, and access to members. In an *agency shop,* membership in the union is mandatory. New hires must join within a specific period of time to continue working. The employer may also agree to deduct membership dues from employee paychecks, as authorized, to remit the money to the union, and to permit the union to visit the agency, post notices, and to use meeting rooms as available.

7. *Classifications of nurses.* The contract describes the various levels of nurses, such as Staff Nurse I, II, and III, and how to advance from one level to the next. Such a clinical ladder is critical for career advancement.

8. *Scheduling categories.* The contract defines full time, part time, per diem, on call, call back, other categories, how nurses may

change from one category to another, and how fringe benefits are calculated. This section may be long and detailed.

9. *Compensation*. The contract addresses wages and salaries, often with a grid of classifications, scheduling category, and years of service, stating specific dollar amounts. It may have subsections stipulating credit for tenure, academic degrees, special certification, shift, holiday, special services, and relief for higher classifications and on-call differentials.

10. *Hours of work*. The contract describes normal shift schedules, mandatory shift rotation, if any, weekends off, extra shifts, rest periods, lunch periods, overtime, double shifts, late calls, posting the schedule, reporting pay, guaranteed hours of work per pay period, the right to object to a work assignment, and the method to register that objection.

11. *Education and training*. The contract addresses educational leaves, inservice education, and mandatory recertification.

12. *Holidays*. The contract lists recognized holidays and specifies compensation for working on those days.

13. *Vacations*. The contract states accrual rate of vacation hours and addresses the issue of holidays and sickness during vacations and vacation time carry-over.

14. *Sick leave*. The contract states accrual rate of sick leave, when it begins, and when it can be used.

15. *Leaves of absence*. The contract recognizes that bereavement, medical, maternity, military, parental, jury duty, and personal leaves may be needed and stipulates procedures to apply for them.

16. *Insurance*. The contract describes available dental, vision, medical, disability, and life insurance, stating the amount or the percentage of the premiums paid by the agency.

17. *Retirement and pension*. The contract describes retirement and pension plans available through the agency and amounts paid by the agency. Desirable features are pension plans that move if the nurse moves and retirement accounts to which employers contribute that have immediate vesting and portability.

18. *Seniority*. The contract defines seniority, how it is accrued, how it affects temporary and permanent work reductions (lay-offs) and advancement, and how it is lost. An affirmation of the principle of "last hired, first fired" is desirable.

19. *Posting and filling of vacancies.* The contract describes the method of announcing staff vacancies, criteria for filling them, and means for employees to bid for work assignments.

20. *Professional performance committee (PPC).* The contract authorizes the formation of a PPC and defines its composition, meetings, purpose (to improve patient care), and role, if advisory. If the PPC is empowered, the contract defines its limits of power and the enforcement process.

21. *Discipline for cause with due process.* The contract describes the procedure for discipline, suspension, and discharge of nurses who do not meet performance criteria. "For cause" ensures that discipline is not frivolous. "Due process" provides a mechanism for correction of deficiencies and endorses rehabilitation programs for impaired nurses. Managers must follow these procedures precisely when they discipline staff.

22. *Grievance procedure.* The contract defines a grievance as "any dispute, claim, or complaint involving the interpretation or application of any of the provisions of this Agreement, except of those Articles or provisions which state that they are not subject to the grievance procedure" (CNA 1989b). The contract states that individuals or the union may file a grievance. It affirms that individuals may be represented at any meeting or hearing they think may lead to disciplinary action and describes the grievance procedure in detail.

23. *No strike or lockout.* The contract stipulates that there will not be a strike, slowdown, or other work stoppage by the nurses or a lockout by the hospital during the life of the agreement.

24. *Terms of agreement.* The contract states the effective dates of the contract, often "extending it from year to year thereafter without change or amendment unless either party serves notice in writing to the other party" (CNA 1989a).

Union Organizations

Historical Background

While the customs that regulated medieval guilds may be the distant kin of modern labor laws, the Act of 1824 by the British House of Commons is a direct forebear. That act recognized the "desirability of relieving tension . . . by conceding the right of workers to form combinations for 'collective bargaining' with their masters" (Wells 1956).

Nearly 100 years later, during the late nineteenth and early twentieth centuries, trade unions grew in numbers and strength. Violent clashes between employee groups and employers disrupted social order, crying out for legal intervention. In response, the United States Congress passed the National Labor Relations Act (NLRA) of 1935. Known as the Wagner Act, the NLRA gave workers the legal right to organize for better working conditions and required employers to bargain with labor unions. However, the act used the term *labor organization,* which was interpreted to exclude nursing and other professions such as medicine and teaching. The act created a quasijudicial body called the National Labor Relations Board (NLRB) to administer and enforce its provisions. In recent years in their quest for improved wages and working conditions nurses have learned the importance of that body.

In 1946, the American Nurses' Association (ANA) launched its Economic Security Program, setting up national salary guidelines. It passed a resolution encouraging state nurses' associations to act as exclusive bargaining agents for members. However, the concept of *professional collectivism* was not widely accepted. In 1950, out of concern for the image of nursing, the ANA adopted a no-strike policy that was not rescinded until 1968.

In the years between 1946 and 1974, a number of federal and state laws affecting collective bargaining and employee rights were enacted. In 1947, the National Labor Management Relations Act (NLMRA), known as the Taft-Hartley Act, established the Federal Mediation and Conciliation Services (FMCS) and expanded some employee rights, but it excluded nonprofit hospitals from the legal obligation to bargain with employees. In 1959, the Landrum/Griffin Act regulated the internal affairs of unions and established a bill of rights for union members. In 1962, federal employees were given the right to bargain collectively. In 1964, the Civil Rights Act forbade job and wage discrimination based on religion, race, sex, or ethnicity and in 1967, age was added to the list by the Age Discrimination in Employment Act. During the 1960s several states passed laws granting bargaining rights to employees of nonprofit hospitals. Not until 1974, in the Health Care Amendments to the

Taft-Hartley Act, were employees of nonprofit hospitals through-out the United States granted the right to bargain collectively.

Union Representation

After nurses everywhere won the right to bargain with employ-ers, many unions wanted to represent them. To many nurses it seemed only natural that their own professional organization would serve as their bargaining agent. Others viewed the arrangement as a potential conflict of interest, because both staff nurses and super-vising nurses are members of the ANA. Today state nurses' asso-ciations serve as bargaining agents for 139,000 of the 180,000 or-ganized nurses in the United States. Although the door is now open for nurses to organize, only about 18% of all employed registered nurses are members of any labor organization (The American Nurse, 1991). Perhaps this small percentage is due to a lack of understanding of labor union terminology, procedures for organiz-ing a union, or the process of bargaining collectively.

Terminology

Many terms employed by labor organizations seem foreign to nursing. They are. They originated in factories generating prod-ucts, not service. Over the years the words have taken on new meanings to better fit the health-care industry and nurses have learned to understand them (see Table 11-2).

Administration and Enforcement of Labor Laws

The National Labor Relations Board (NLRB) is especially im-portant to nurses because it administers and enforces national la-bor laws. It decides appropriate bargaining units for employee groups, conducts elections for employee representatives, protects the rights of both employees and employers, and resolves disputes between labor and management. In 1989, the NLRB voted to rec-ognize the following bargaining units within health-care agencies: (1) RNs and permittees; (2) MDs, excluding house staff; (3) all other professionals, such as pharmacists; (4) technical workers, such as LPNs; (5) skilled maintenance personnel, such as plumbers; (6) business clerical staff; (7) nonskilled maintenance and service employees such as nurse aides; and (8) security guards. The NLRB action was blocked by a US district court ruling. ANA appealed to the US Supreme Court, and in 1991 the Court decided in favor of the eight units (the American Nurse 1991).

Employer Protection

The NLRB ensures that employers have the freedom to explain election rules to employees, tell them about union drawbacks, and encourage them to vote against unionization. The NLRB protects employers and employees from unfair labor practices of unions. Specifically, unions may not (1) restrain or coerce employees from exercising rights guaranteed by labor laws, (2) refuse to bargain collectively with an employer if the union is the certified representative, (3) attempt to cause an employer to discipline an employee who is out of favor with the union, (4) engage in unlawful strikes, (5) require employees to pay excessive membership fees, and (6) attempt to coerce an employer to pay the union for services not performed (Epp 1976).

Employee Union Protection

The NLRB ensures that employee (labor) unions have the freedom to explain election rules, extol the advantages of union membership, and encourage employees to vote for the union in an election. The NLRB protects unions and employees from unfair labor practices of employers. Specifically, employers may not interfere, dominate, discriminate, or refuse to bargain in good faith.

Interfere means to (1) threaten to close down a facility if a union is elected, (2) make intimidating statements relative to participation in union activities, (3) question employees about union activities, (4) spy on union meetings or suggest that spying may occur, and (5) unilaterally improve benefits or wages during a union campaign to sway employees to vote against a union.

Dominate means to (1) give union leaders special benefits or compensation, (2) organize a competing union, and (3) pay the expenses of a certain union.

Key Terms Used in Collective Bargaining

agency shop   A business where employees may either pay union dues or agency fees to a collective bargaining agent; nonmembers are required to join the union as a condition of employment

arbitration   Procedures for settling labor disputes using the services of a third party. See binding arbitration definition

arbitrator, arbiter   Person chosen by agreement of both parties to decide a dispute between them

authorization cards   Cards employees sign to authorize representation by a specific union. See Figure 11-1

bargaining agent   A group or person accepted by an employer and chosen by members of a bargaining unit to represent them in collective bargaining

bargaining unit   An employee group that the state or NLRB recognizes as an appropriate division for collective bargaining

binding arbitration   When both parties agree to abide by the decision of an arbitrator

certification   Official recognition by a labor organization as the exclusive bargaining agent for employees of a specific bargaining unit

contract violations   Actions that break the terms of a contract

collective bargaining   A legal process by which representatives of organized employees negotiate with an employer about wages and related concerns, resulting in an employment contract

deadlock   A stall in the negotiation process because of an issue about which neither party is willing to compromise

decertification   Withdrawal of official recognition of a union as the exclusive bargaining agent for a group of workers

grievance   Any complaint by an employer or union concerning any aspect of the employment relationship

grievance procedures   Steps both sides agree to follow to settle disputes. See Chapter 11 text

injunction   A court order that requires a person to take or refrain from taking a specific action

mandatory bargaining issues   Subjects such as wages and working conditions, about which employers must bargain in good faith

mediation   A process for settling labor disputes, whereby a mediator assists the parties to reach their own decision

mediator   A person chosen by both parties to help them agree

open shop   A business where employees are not required to become members of a union as a condition of employment

past practice/precedent   Established customs that have existed over time, enforceable because they are in essence a part of the "whole" agreement, though not mentioned in the contract

Table 11-2 (continued)

Key Terms Used in Collective Bargaining

professional collectivism   The concept of members of a profession joining together to bargain for wages and working conditions

supervisor   Any individual having authority, in the interest of the employer, to hire, transfer, suspend, lay off, discharge, recall, promote, assign, reward, or discipline other employees, or responsibility to direct them or adjust their grievances, or effectively to recommend such action, if in connection with the foregoing, the exercise of such authority is not of a merely routine or clerical nature but requires the use of independent judgment (Public Law 93-360, Sec. 2, 1974)

unfair labor practices   Illegal strategies employers or unions may use against each other to harass or punish, see Chapter 11 text

union steward   An employee who assumes a leadership role among his/her peers regarding collective bargaining/union concerns

voluntary bargaining issues   Subjects such as noneconomic fringe benefits, about which employers are not obliged to bargain

From Mary Foley, RN, and the Center for Labor Relations, ANA.

Discriminate means to (1) enforce rules unequally between employees who are involved in union activities and those who are not, (2) refuse to hire anyone who belongs to a union or has been a union organizer, (3) discharge, discipline, or threaten an employee for joining a union or for encouraging others to join, and (4) refuse to reinstate or promote employees who testify at a NLRB hearing.

Refuse to bargain in good faith means to (1) refuse to meet for negotiation at regular times with the intent to resolve disputed issues, (2) demand to negotiate a voluntary issue, (3) refuse to negotiate a mandatory issue, and (4) take unilateral action affecting employment conditions that are covered by an existing contract or included among legally mandated areas of bargaining.

Organizing a Union

Nurses may ask, "How, then, do we go about organizing a union that the NLRB will recognize?" The process is as follows:

1. A group of nurses meets informally and decides to form a bargaining unit in their institution and to ask an established employee union such as a state nurses' association (SNA) to represent

California Nurses Association

AUTHORIZATION TO REPRESENT

I hereby authorize the California Nurses' Association to be my exclusive representative with my employer for the purpose of negotiating all matters related to salaries, hours of work, and other terms and conditions of employment.

Signature _____ Hospital _____

Date _____ Position _____

Name _____ Area _____
(Please print)

Mailing address _____ Shift _____

_____ Soc. Sec # _____
City   Zip

Home Telephone _____

Reproduced with permission of the California Nurses Association.

Figure 11-1 *Typical Authorization Card*

them. The economic and general welfare division of the SNA, not local regions, provide this service. When invited, the union assigns an organizer-representative to the group of nurses.

2. The union representative provides the nurses with *authorization cards* (see Figure 11-1). If not already members of the union, the nurses join, sign authorization cards, and recruit other staff nurses to do so as well. If 50% of eligible nurse members sign the cards, no election is required. However, if the nurses can get only 30% of eligible members to sign cards authorizing a union to represent them, whether a competing union has entered the picture or not, an election to select a representative union must be held.

3. The nurses sign and deliver the authorization cards to the union. When sufficient cards are collected, the union petitions the NLRB for recognition. The NLRB appoints a representative to referee and organize an election, if necessary.

4. If either side challenges the eligibility of certain nurses to be counted as employee members of the union and not supervisors,

the NLRB representative schedules a hearing. (See definition of a supervisor in Table 11-2.) Disputed eligibility is settled by reviewing the job description and actual supervisory functions of the nurses in question. The regional director of the NLRB makes the decision and declares the percent of eligible members who authorized a particular union.

5. If an election is necessary, the NLRB representative announces a date and place. Within seven days of the announcement, the employer must give the NLRB representative a list of the names and addresses of all eligible nurses. The NLRB forwards this list to the union and any competing unions.

6. The employer and other competing unions begin campaigning to gain the vote of eligible nurses. On election day the nurses vote by secret ballot for no representation or one of the competing unions. Two representatives from each competing union and the NLRB representative supervise the election.

7. NLRB representatives count the ballots in the regional office and send the tabulation to the NLRB General Council in Washington, DC. No matter how many nurses were eligible to vote, the one with the most votes is the winner. If "no representation" gets the most votes or ties with a union, the employer ("no") wins. Another election involving a union is prohibited by law for one year.

8. If any one of the competing unions receives the most votes, the NLRB *certifies* the winner as the official representative of employees. That representative is then legally bound to represent all eligible employees, regardless of their loyalty prior to the election. An election to *decertify* a union follows the same process as the one to certify a union.

Collective Bargaining

The Process

Formation of a union is just the beginning. A satisfactory contract is yet to be negotiated through the process of collective bargaining, as follows:

1. Immediately after the election, contract negotiations begin. Both parties select a negotiating team. The employer team of a health-care facility often includes a labor law expert, nursing di-

rector, personnel director, administrator, and department heads where union employees work. The employee union team includes union representatives, attorney, and employees selected to serve on the negotiation team.

2. In consultation with its members, the union creates a "wish list," called "demands," which it gives to the employer prior to the first negotiation session. The list includes mandatory bargaining issues as well as voluntary issues (see Table 11-2).

3. Face-to-face meetings of the two sides begin. Negotiations may be item-by-item or all-or-none. The all-or-none system gives negotiators more room to bargain right up to the final agreement (Werther and Lockhart 1976). The process may move along smoothly or may be long and arduous. Each side keeps its constituents informed. If all goes well, the parties reach agreement on every issue and negotiating team members initial the proposed contract.

4. The proposed contract is printed, distributed to union members, and a vote is scheduled. If a majority of union members accepts it, the contract is *ratified*. The negotiating teams sign the document and the contract becomes effective on a certain day.

When Negotiations Break Down

Mediation

If negotiations break down and neither side will compromise, bargainers have several options. The least coercive way to resolve disputes is through *mediation*. The two sides may invite a mediator to join their talks to assist them to reach agreement. Professional mediator-arbitrators may be requested from several sources. The American Arbitration Association is a nonprofit, nonpartisan agency that for a nominal fee provides a list of qualified persons. Various state mediation and conciliation services and the Federal Mediation and Conciliation Service (FMCS) also provide mediation services.

Strikes and Lockouts

If mediation fails to bring about agreement, employees may decide to strike to convince the employer to make concessions or the employer may decide to lock out or lay off employees to convince them to make concessions. Because of the critical nature of health care, the NLRB requires many more steps by these institutions than nonhealth-care institutions before a strike can be called or a lockout imposed, as follows:

1. If the employees or the employer wish to modify or terminate an existing contract, they must notify the other side of intended changes 90 days before the contract is due to expire. During that time the two sides meet to negotiate a new agreement.

2. If after 30 days the two sides have not reached agreement, or if the parties are negotiating a contract for the first time and have reached an impasse, the parties must notify the FMCS and a state agency.

3. Within 30 days, the FMCS appoints a mediator/arbitrator to gather information from both sides and to submit the findings to the FMCS regional director for evaluation. The FMCS may then appoint a Board of Inquiry (BOI).

4. Within 15 days of appointment the BOI conducts hearings and issues a written report with its findings and recommendations for resolution of the dispute. The report is given to both sides.

5. If after 15 more days the parties don't agree, the employees may plan to strike or the employer to lock out the employees.

6. If a strike vote has not yet been held, it is conducted at this time. If a majority of employees vote to strike, the union must send the employer a notice at least ten days before, stating the exact date, time, and place of the strike.

7. A strike cannot be scheduled before a contract expires. If employees ignore the rules and engage in an illegal strike, they lose NLRB protection and may be fired by the employer. The NLRB can decertify a union that sanctions an illegal strike.

8. After scheduling a strike a union may delay it for up to 72 hours if it feels the extra time will help resolve the impasse.

9. To delay a strike employees must give employers written notice at least 12 hours before a strike is scheduled to begin. If an initial strike date passes during negotiations, the union must issue another ten-day strike notice. If a contract expires during negotiations, the parties remain bound by the old contract.

10. If a strike is called, both sides must abide by strict rules of conduct. They cannot threaten nonstriking employees, attack em-

ployer representatives, or physically block other nurses and personnel from entering or leaving the facility.

11. Negotiations may be broken off for a time, but eventually must be reinstituted and continue until a settlement is reached. Sometimes the negotiators reach such an impasse that they submit the disputed issue to *binding arbitration*, using the services of a private or FMCS arbitrator described earlier. Settlements often include a guarantee that striking employees will be rehired after the strike, called *reinstatement privilege*.

Strikes cause serious disruptions of services to patients, deep divisions between staff members, and lost income for both employers and employees. Strikes and lockouts are measures of last resort, undertaken only when all else fails. For this reason, contracts may include "no-strike, no-lockout" clauses whereby both sides agree to follow grievance and arbitration procedures throughout the life of the contract.

Grievances and Arbitration

When an employer and employee bargaining agent sign a contract, they agree to follow the specific provisions of the contract. Since they cannot anticipate every possible difficulty they agree on grievance procedures to resolve disputes. Often arbitration is the final step in the grievance procedure.

Each contract defines a *grievance*. Most describe a grievance as any dispute, claim, or complaint that involves violations of any part of a contract, of past practice, or precedent. A grievance may also be a complaint of an unfair labor practice, such as interference, domination, discrimination, refusal to bargain in good faith, or encouraging employees to do any of these things.

Contract violations are actions that break mutual agreements stipulated in the contract. For instance, Joan is working under a contract that states that if two or more equally well qualified nurses bid for an open position, the one with most seniority will be chosen. Although she is equally well qualified and the most senior nurse, Joan was not selected for the open position. She filed a grievance on the basis of a contract violation.

Violations of precedent or past practice are unilateral changes in established policies or procedures. For example, although not mentioned in the contract, for at least ten years normal work shifts in a local hospital were 8:00–4:30, 4:00–12:30, and 12:00–8:30. One day the director of nurses announced that, beginning in one week, normal work shifts would be 7:00–3:30, 3:00–11:30, and 11:00–7:30. The nurses filed a grievance based on a past practice violation.

Both employers and employees may file grievances against the other. Employers file grievances against employees in the form of *disciplinary action* for such things as failure to perform assigned tasks, chronic tardiness, excessive sick leave, and negative relationships with co-workers. Employees file grievances against supervisors for unequal or unfair treatment. These complaints often involve issues such as promotion, vacation time, shift assignment, and merit pay raises. Many grievances result from unwitting contract violations such as poorly thought-out work load decisions by nurse managers (Nurse's Reference Library 1984). Nurse managers can avoid some of these disputes by gaining a thorough knowledge of the contract, consulting with resource persons, and using a participatory instead of authoritarian management style.

Grievance Procedure

Because the purpose of grievance procedures is to resolve disputes, they usually provide (1) time limits for filing a grievance and making a decision, (2) opportunities for both sides to investigate complaints, (3) procedures for appealing to higher authority with a plan for ultimate resolution, and (4) assignment of priority to more serious complaints. The one who files the complaint, the *grievant,* has a right to be assisted by legal and union counsel at each step of the grievance procedure.

Grievance procedures typically follow a series of steps:

1. The grievant discusses a claim, complaint, or dispute with the immediate supervisor. The supervisor renders a decision within a specified number of days.

2. If not satisfied with the decision the grievant may submit the issue in writing to the next level of authority, often the director of nursing service. The director meets with the grievant to try to resolve the matter and renders a written decision within a specified number of days.

3. If not satisfied with the decision, the grievant may submit a written appeal to the highest level of authority, often the hospital administrator. The administrator meets with the grievant to try to resolve the issue and renders a written decision within a specified number of days. If the grievant is not satisfied with the decision, the next step is arbitration.

Arbitration Process

Arbitration is a process that settles a labor dispute by presenting evidence to a neutral labor relations expert, usually an employee of a private or government agency (*Nurses' Legal Handbook* 1985). The process may be clearly defined in the contract, but since an arbitration clause is not required, not all labor contracts include it. Without such a clause, all these arrangements must be negotiated at the time of a dispute.

When the process is defined in the contract and a grievant is not satisfied with the outcome of step 3 of the grievance procedure, the grievant, in consultation with the union, may submit a written request for arbitration to the employer. The contract stipulates the source of an arbitrator, such as from a list supplied by the Federal Mediation and Conciliation Service, and the method of selection. A date, time, and place for the arbitration hearing is set.

The arbitration hearing is similar to a court case, although not as formal. The side requesting the arbitration has the burden to prove that a contract has been violated, except in cases of disciplinary action, in which the employer must prove its case. Both sides may call witnesses and cross-examine them. After the hearing, the arbitrator can issue a summary judgment shortly after the proceedings or a written decision to both sides within a month (Marriner-Tomey 1988). Often, both parties share the costs of arbitration.

Both employers and unions prefer arbitration to a court trial because it is faster and less costly. However, when a dispute goes to arbitration, both sides lose control of the outcome. In the United States the arbitrator's decision is binding. The other side can challenge the decision in court, but courts rarely overturn an arbitrator's decision (Nurse's Reference Library 1984).

Amicable labor relations require that both sides honor the contract and demonstrate good will in using grievance procedures.

Both sides must carefully consider when to retreat, press forward, or compromise. Union representatives may be able to defuse complaints early in the process. They must distinguish between a substantive complaint involving a contract violation and a personal problem of an employee. Employers must separate contract violations from personal problems of supervisors. Of course, sometimes unions and employers pursue groundless complaints to harass the other or to pursue political ends. Both sides must remember that it is to their advantage to respect the needs of one another and resolve disputes with minimum conflict.

Other Grievances

Most grievances arise from contract violations and are settled through the grievance process. However, when either employers or unions believe the other one has engaged in "unfair labor practices" as described earlier, they can complain to the NLRB. After investigating, the NLRB may conduct a hearing to review the evidence and issue a decision. Either employer or union may challenge the NLRB ruling in court.

All employees, whether union members or not, can file complaints with the Equal Employment Opportunity Commission (EEOC) and comparable state agencies if they believe they have been descriminated against because of race, religion, national origin, age, or sex. Union members may also file a grievance as stipulated in their employment contract. The EEOC handles violations of a number of antidiscrimination laws, including: (1) the Equal Pay Act of 1963, forbidding wage discrimination based on sex; (2) the Civil Rights Act of 1964, forbidding job and wage discrimination on the basis of religion, race, sex, or ethnic background, and forbidding sexual harassment; and (3) the Age Discrimination in Employment Act of 1967, forbidding discrimination based on age.

Preventing Discontent

If so few nurses in the United States are unionized, and so many have strong feelings against professional collectivism, why do any nurses join labor unions?

Nurses join labor unions because they are dissatisfied with the status quo and feel powerless as individuals to change the system (Marriner-Tomey 1988). They may have tried many approaches but have been frustrated. Finally, like Sue in the vignette, they turn to a union for help.

If employers want to avoid the intervention of unions in their relationships with employees, they need to pay attention to the reasons nurse become discontented. Othman and Chaney suggest that nurses join unions because employers fail to meet their needs for security, benefits, and leadership (1987). They listed actions employers take or fail to take that create discontent. Turning that list around, we suggest that employers can prevent discontent by:

- Treating all employees fairly and equally
- Offering opportunities for advancement
- Recognizing people as valued individuals
- Making the workplace safe and pleasant
- Offering special training/education
- Giving economic security with adequate and competitive wages; fair work hours; vacation, sick, holiday, severance, overtime, and bereavement pay; and retirement, medical, and life insurance
- Providing adequate supervision and leadership
- Instituting grievance procedures
- Opening two-way channels of communication
- Giving opportunities for self-expression
- Maintaining high standards of care
- Encouraging autonomy and innovation

By these actions employers demonstrate respect for their professional nursing staff. When employers, like Sue's, fail to demonstrate such respect, the collective power of the labor organization becomes an important ally.

Summary

Nurses turn to employee unions to help them achieve economic security and satisfactory working conditions. Work contracts, like other legal contracts, include promises, mutual understandings, compensation, and a lawful purpose. State nurses' associations serve as union representatives for 72% of organized nurses. The National Labor Relations Board (NLRB) administers and enforces national labor laws, ensuring that both employers and employees abide by the rules and avoid unfair labor practices. Unions organize in a prescribed sequence, climaxed by certification of the NLRB. Work contracts are negotiated through collective bargaining. When disputes arise, a grievance procedure is followed; if it fails, arbitration may be necessary. Amiable working relations require that both sides honor the contract and demonstrate good will.

Learning Activities

1. Visit the regional office of a state nurses' association; ask to see copies of employment contracts of hospitals in your area and compare them.

2. Go to the personnel office of a local hospital and request a copy of the employment contract that is currently in force.

3. Interview a director of nursing service and ask him/her to state the disadvantages of labor organizations.

4. Interview a state nurses' association labor representative or member of a bargaining team and ask him/her to state the advantages of labor organizations.

5. In a group discussion, make a "wish list" for an ideal employment contract; then, prioritize the items on the list.

Annotated Reading List

Bagwell M, Clements S: The art of negotiating. Chapter 6 in: *A Political Handbook for Health Professionals*. Little, Brown, 1985.

This chapter provides a practical discussion of the questions: "What is negotiation? When do I use it? Where do I use it? How do I use it?" The authors define negotiation as the "effort to resolve disagreements on specific issues." They describe the two forms of negotiation (trade-off and problem-solving), discuss major errors in negotiation, and provide a concrete example of the negotiations that occured relative to a bill for third-party payment for Arizona nurses. Though brief, the chapter is clearly focused and readable.

Flanagan L: *Earn What You're Worth. A Nurse's Guide to Better Compensation.* ANA, 1989.

This brief, meaty pamphlet provides nurses with "key background information, directions, and guidelines for taking concrete steps to improve the compensation packages offered to them by employers." Its six chapters offer specific strategies to (1) learn to articulate nursing's value, (2) enhance marketability by acquiring business savvy, (3) collect data to build a case for greater compensation, (4) assess compensation packages and present proposals, (5) become involved in various tactics to gain better pay and fringe benefits.

McFarland GK, Leonard HS, Morris MM: Job satisfaction and the nurse employee. Chapter 14 in: *Nursing Leadership and Management, Contemporary Strategies.* Wiley, 1984.

Although written in scholarly language, this chapter presents important research on how nurse managers can increase staff motivation and job satisfaction. The authors discuss findings about three aspects of job satisfaction: the job, individual work, and interaction of individuals and their jobs. The 20 items reproduced from the Minnesota Job Description Questionnaire plus "autonomy" provide readers with an excellent "wish list" for nurses planning collective bargaining.

References

California Nurses Assocation: *Agreement Between Doctor's Hospital of Pinole and the California Nurses' Association.* CNA, 1989a.

California Nurses Association: *Memorandum of Understanding Between Petaluma Valley Hospital and the California Nurses Association.* CNA, 1989b.

Creighton H: *Law Every Nurse Should Know,* 5th ed. Saunders, 1986.

Epp D: *Labor Law.* Oceana Publications, 1976.

Facts About Nursing 86-87. ANA, 1987.

Hemelt MD, Mackert ME: *Dynamics of Law in Nursing and Health Care,* 2nd ed. Reston, 1982.

Marriner-Tomey, A: *Guide to Nursing Management,* 3rd ed. Mosby, 1988.

Nurses' Legal Handbook. Springhouse, 1985.

Nurse's Reference Library. *Practices.* Springhouse, 1984.

Othman JE, Chaney HS: Labor relations in union and nonunion environments. In: *Management Concepts for the New Nurse,* Vestal KW, Lippincott, 1987.

Supreme Court okays all-RN unit. *Am Nurs,* June 1991.

Wells, HG: *Outline of History,* Vols I, II. Garden City, 1956.

Werther, WB, Lockhart CA: *Labor Relations in the Health Professions: The Basis of Power, The Means of Change.* Little, Brown, 1976.

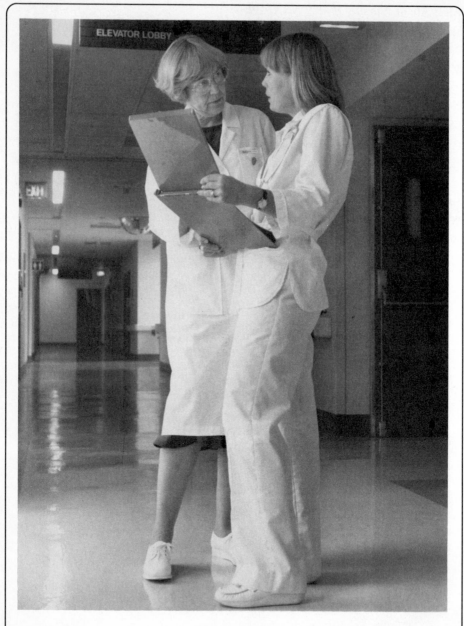

A staff nurse consults with a clinical specialist. Such collegial relationships support professional growth and pave the way for nurses to achieve their career goals. (Photograph by Chuck O'Rear, Westlight)

CHAPTER 12

Career Management

LEARNING OBJECTIVES

1. Compare a job perspective with a career perspective.

2. Describe sources of information nurses can use to make a life-work plan.

3. Discuss the personal characteristics and aspects of the profession to assess when planning a career in nursing.

4. Discuss the implementation phase of career management, describing specific actions.

5. Explain the value of management strategies and the concepts of marketing, relationships, production, and control strategies.

6. Compare resumes and curricula vitae and list rules for writing each.

7. State the purpose of cover letters and state rules for writing them.

8. Discuss the interviewing process and its follow-up from an interviewee's perspective.

9. Describe some strategies for negotiating, networking, and maintaining collegial relationships.

10. Explain why continuing education and occupational health and safety are production strategies.

11. Discuss the value of control strategies in helping nurses manage their careers and survive in the real world of nursing.

Excitement *was high in class that day. Applications for the licensing exam had just arrived and everyone was talking about where they would apply for their first job. Casey listened silently. She felt a sense of urgency and confusion. As class ended Casey picked up her books and hurried from the room. The chatter around her was upsetting. She needed to think alone.*

For years Casey had dreamed and worked toward the day she would be a registered nurse. Now, at last, she was almost there. Why was she feeling so anxious? Maybe the goal had been so large she hadn't seen beyond it. Maybe she was just insecure about her ability to function as a nurse. Casey hurried along in a daze, trying to analyze the situation. "I could go full time at the convalescent hospital where I've worked for the last three years . . . I could take a job in the local community hospital or commute to where the pay is better . . . I really liked psychiatry, but people say new grads should do a year of med-surg before they specialize . . . Maybe I should just go for another degree right away . . . What do I really want to do? . . . How should I go about deciding? . . . There is so much I don't know . . . I'm not even sure how to write a resume or apply for a 'real' nursing job!"

Casey stopped her anxious pace. "My whole life is ahead of me and I don't want to mess it up. I've got to get more information." Casey turned and began walking back to the nursing department, sure that someone there could help her.

Graduation from a nursing program brings the realization of a long-cherished goal. It heralds the completion of one phase of life and the beginning of another. Therefore, graduation is an opportune time to make a personal and professional work-life plan. Making such a plan is quite different from finding a job. A *job perspective* is short-term. It only meets immediate needs. With it "nurses comply with the terms of a contract, perform tasks according to a job description, and depend on the employer for benefits and opportunities" (Henderson and McGettigan 1986).

By contrast, a *career perspective* is long term. It meets lifelong needs in accord with a work-life plan. With such a plan nurses design and promote skills and act on values in a contract with themselves to provide self-fulfillment and to realize personal and professional goals. Henderson and McGettigan suggest that a "career perspective is not limited by a day-to-day focus but is built on a variety of positions, directed toward the future" (1986). Career management addresses problems related to living and working. It uses the management process to solve problems and management strategies to achieve career goals.

Systematic Problem-solving

In the vignette, even though Casey was excited about graduating, she felt anxious and confused. In nursing process terms, her problem was an alteration in work-life processes, related to graduation from a nursing program, manifested by anxiety and confusion. To solve such a problem, Casey and other nurses like her need to collect and assess data, set goals, make plans, implement them, and evaluate their level of satisfaction.

Data Collection

The first step in systematic problem-solving is data collection. Since the problem involves a career, information about career choices is needed. This information is available from audiovisual media, individuals, organizations, personal assessment, and appraisal of the profession.

Audiovisual Media

Each year professional nursing organizations and publishers produce periodicals, books, AV tapes, and computer programs to help with career planning. Nursing periodicals such as the *American Journal of Nursing, RN Magazine,* and *Nursing* publish classified sections listing particular employment offerings. Information about specific topics is indexed in references such as the *International Nursing Index, Cumulative Index to Nursing and Allied Literature, Index Medicus,* and *Hospital Literature Index,* and computerized data bases such as the *National Library of Medicine (NLM Medline)* and *Educational Resources Information Center (ERIC).*

Individuals and Organizations

Individuals and organizations are a rich source of information about careers in nursing. These include: (1) staff nurses, mentors, nursing leaders, and instructors; (2) representatives of professional organizations; (3) the regional office of the American Nurses' Association; (4) placement agencies; (5) recruitment offices of the United States armed services; (6) career fairs, where many health-care providers set up exhibits to recruit nurses; (7) bibliographies of workshop speakers; (8) networking with peers at workshops; (9) recruitment offices: the Peace Corps, Washington, DC 20525; World Health Organization, Avenue Appia, 1211 Geneva 27, Switzerland; Nursing Abroad, c/o The International Council of Nurses, Box 42, 1211 Geneva 20, Switzerland; and Intercristo, Box 33487, Seattle, WA 98109.

Personal Assessment

Socrates admonished his followers to "know thyself" because "an unexamined life is not worth living." Indeed, to make a work-life plan, Casey and others like her must first know themselves.

𝄜 **Exercise 12-1**   *Assessment of the Physical Self*

Stand in front of a full-length mirror dressed as you are at work. Rate yourself on a scale of 1 to 5: 1 = unkempt, unprofessional to 5 = well-groomed, professional.

Appropriateness of dress for practice area	1	2	3	4	5
Cleanliness of clothing, including shoes	1	2	3	4	5
Cosmetics and jewelry	1	2	3	4	5
Energy level	1	2	3	4	5
Facial expression	1	2	3	4	5
General size and shape of body	1	2	3	4	5
Grooming, neatness	1	2	3	4	5
Posture	1	2	3	4	5

Go back and look at the features you marked 1 or 2. Ask yourself if that is the picture you want to portray to others. Though you cannot change genetics, you can change behaviors.

Exercises 12-1 to 12-7 will help you assess and summarize your personal preferences and characteristics.

Appraisal of the Profession

As nurses plan their careers, they need information about their profession and how aspects of nursing practice affect personal work satisfaction. These include patients, settings, payment for services, work hours, health problems, human responses, nursing functions, and nursing roles.

PATIENTS.   As consumers of nursing service, patients present a variety of health problems and human responses. Although nurses cannot allow personal preference to interfere with ethical practice, they experience greater satisfaction when they work with certain types of patients. These preferences are due to personal values, interests, and psychosocial traits. Although these preferences change

𝒞 **Exercise 12-2** *Values and Needs Assessment*

(1) Select the 10 items that are of HIGH value or need for you.
(2) From those 10, select the 5 that are of HIGHEST value or need.

	HIGH	HIGHEST
Achievement, accomplishment, recognition	_____	_____
Adventure, risk, exploration	_____	_____
A meaningful love relationship	_____	_____
Authenticity, genuineness, honesty	_____	_____
Beautiful home in a choice setting	_____	_____
Being a change agent	_____	_____
Education, self-growth, development	_____	_____
Equal opportunity for everyone	_____	_____
Expertness, skillfulness in a task	_____	_____
A happy, contented family	_____	_____
Independence, personal freedom	_____	_____
Intelligence, a bright mind	_____	_____
Leadership, influence, power	_____	_____
Leisurely life without pressure	_____	_____
Long life	_____	_____
Meaningful, purposeful work	_____	_____
Physical appearance that brings pride	_____	_____
Physical health	_____	_____
Security, stability	_____	_____
Self-confidence, emotional strength	_____	_____
Service, contributing to others	_____	_____
Spirituality, religious beliefs	_____	_____
Unlimited wealth	_____	_____
Wisdom, maturity, insight	_____	_____

✐ Exercise 12-3 *Psychosocial Behavior and Attribute Assessment*

Consider how often each of the characteristics listed below describes you. In the space write a (0) if never or not at all, (1) if sometimes or somewhat, and (2) if continually.

_____ Arrive on time for work and other appointments

_____ Believe I am treated fairly

_____ Consider myself a rebel

_____ Cry when I am angry

_____ Display a hot temper

_____ Enjoy speaking out, being in the spotlight

_____ Experience numerous physical symptoms

_____ Fear authority figures

_____ Feel angry and misunderstood

_____ Feel anxious and tense

_____ Feel discouraged and hopeless

_____ Feel inferior to others

_____ Feel left out of things

_____ Feel shy, hesitate to voice an opinion

_____ Get along with everyone

_____ Have an intense need to be perfect

_____ Identify with "underdogs" and unfortunates

_____ Like to manage other people and activities

_____ Prefer to work alone, independent of others

_____ Say "yes" when I really want to say "no"

_____ Seek out and enjoy taking responsibility

_____ Suffer migraine headaches or a nervous stomach

_____ Talk less than anyone else in a group

_____ Talk more than anyone else in a group

_____ Think of myself as unworthy or ugly

_____ Use sarcasm and indirect ways to express anger

_____ Vacillate when I need to make a choice

Now go back and look at the items where you placed a (0) or a (2). You may want to hold on to these traits and choose a career where they are assets. You may conclude that they are a detriment and decide to change them. The decision is yours to make.

✔ Exercise 12-4   *Assessment of Interests*

For each of the activities listed below indicate your interest as: 1 = low, 2 = moderate, 3 = high. Add the scores for each category of activity and write the total in the space provided.

Activities	Score	Activities	Score
Creative-artistic		*Investigative*	
Acting	_____	Assessing	_____
Composing music	_____	Analyzing	_____
Designing	_____	Clarifying	_____
Drawing	_____	Diagnosing	_____
Generating ideas	_____	Evaluating	_____
Photographing	_____	Experimenting	_____
Sculpting	_____	Researching	_____
Writing	_____	Using logic	_____
Creative-artistic score	_____	Investigative score	_____
Management		*Ordering*	
Assigning tasks	_____	Classifying data	_____
Coordinating	_____	Filing	_____
Competing in games	_____	Finance record keeping	_____
Implementing policies	_____	Following directions	_____
Managing conflicts	_____	Inventorying	_____
Planning change	_____	Managing budgets	_____
Leading meetings	_____	Organizing records	_____
Scheduling events	_____	Processing forms	_____
Management score	_____	Ordering score	_____
Physical		*Social*	
Biking	_____	Care giving	_____
Dancing	_____	Counseling	_____
Hiking	_____	Entertaining	_____
Running	_____	Group sports	_____
Sailing	_____	Listening	_____
Singing	_____	Meeting in groups	_____

Exercise 12-4   *(continued)*

Physical		*Social*	
Skiing	_____	Telephoning	_____
Swimming	_____	Writing letters	_____
Physical score	_____	Social score	_____

Scoring Summary

Scoring Key

Interest	*Score*	Score range	Interest level
Creative-artistic	_____	0–8	Low
Investigative	_____	9–16	Moderate
Management	_____	17–24	High
Ordering	_____		
Physical	_____		
Social	_____		

Scoring: 1. Write the score for each category of interest in the blank.
2. Use the key to interpret the extent of your interest. Are your interests grouped in one or two categories or are they distributed in several categories? Are the results consistent with your self-perception? How might this data affect a career decision?

Adapted from Henderson FC, McGettigan BO: *Managing Your Career in Nursing,* pp 86–88. Addison-Wesley, 1986.

with time, they are legitimate and deserve recognition. Exercise 12-8 will help you assess patient preferences.

SETTINGS.   Nurses practice in many different settings. In 1982, three out of four nurses worked in hospitals or nursing homes (Nurses today 1982). That proportion is changing. As a result of social and economic forces, increasing numbers of nurses practice in nontraditional settings. When planning a career it is important to consider aspects of work settings that affect work satisfaction.

Type of industry has to do with whether a setting is or is not part of the health-care industry. Hospitals, nursing homes, clinics, and companies that sell health-care products or services are part

---

🖍 Exercise 12-5   *Assessment of Proficiency*

Assess your level of nursing proficiency (ability, competency, skill) based on the five levels identified by Benner.

Level I, Novice:

No experience in situations where a nurse is expected to perform; relies on rules to guide actions

Level II, Beginner:

Limited recurring experience; relies on concrete guidelines from experience of others; performs basic assessment skills but has limited ability to discern importance

Level III, Competent:

Minimum of two years' experience in stable situations; systematically solves problems and analyzes situations

Level IV, Proficient:

Minimum of three to five years' experience with similar patient population; demonstrates ability to perceive situations as wholes with speed and flexibility due to reflection on previous experience

Level V, Expert:

More than five years' experience with similar patient population and setting; demonstrates immediate and intuitive grasp of situation due to experience and mastery of previous complex situations

My experience level is: _____

From Benner P: *From Novice to Expert*, pp 20–30. Addison-Wesley, 1984.

of the health-care industry. Schools, government agencies, recreational facilities, and most businesses are not part of that industry. Autonomy and opportunity may be greater in agencies not associated with health care.

Kind of care refers to whether health care is provided through an inpatient facility, ambulatory center, or home care agency. The role of nurses is significantly affected by the kind of care. Inpatient institutions provide 24-hour care; patients are sicker and more de-

✿ Exercise 12-6 *Assessment of Education, Credentials, and Experience*

Although retention of knowledge varies, one way to assess and verify it is to compile a list of formal and informal learning experiences. You will use this information to write your resume.

Education

List all schools where you have studied since high school, their locations, attendance dates, major areas of study, and the certificate or degree earned in each.

Special Knowledge and Skills

Describe special knowledge and skills; state how they were learned; indicate locations, dates, and circumstances.

Licenses, Credentials, and Certificates

List licenses, credentials, and certificates you possess; indicate the official number and expiration date.

Organizational Memberships

List the names of professional and personal organizations to which you belong if they might be an asset; indicate the offices you have held or committees on which you have served.

Publications

List articles, books, papers, videos, and computer programs you have created, such as teaching modules, procedures, and policies; indicate the title, date, and publisher.

Special Achievements

List significant professional or personal awards, honors, and unique projects in which you have participated; name, describe, and give date of achievement.

Documentation

Collect and preserve in a safe place the following:

All past or present resumes
Applications for nursing positions and schools
Awards and letters of commendation
Certificates of completion
Course descriptions of higher education courses from college
Catalogs and continuing education brochures
Current continuing education certificates
Performance evaluations
Published materials you have authored
Transcripts from educational institutions

✔ **Exercise 12-7**   *Summary of Personal Characteristics*

Summarize your findings from Exercises 1 through 6:

My physical appearance is: _____

_____

_____

My highest values and needs are: _____

_____

_____

My persistent psychosocial behaviors and attributes are: _____

_____

_____

My primary interests are: _____

_____

_____

My proficiency level is: _____

_____

_____

My areas of greatest knowledge and skill are: _____

_____

_____

---

pendent, but there are more support services. Ambulatory centers serve patients for brief periods; patients may be more independent and not as acutely ill. Home care agencies serve patients for longer periods; patients must be independent or have home attendants, and nursing practice is more holistic, less structured, and requires more innovation.

Labor organizations provide collective bargaining services for their members. In general, nurses enjoy higher salaries, more autonomy, and better working conditions where there are collective bargaining agreements. In return, they pay dues and abide by union rules. (See Chapter 11, Collective Bargaining.)

✂ Exercise 12-8 *Assessment of Patient Characteristic Preferences*

Place an X beside characteristics you prefer in patients.

Age: _____ premature infants   _____ adolescents (13 to 19)

     _____ infants (birth to 1 yr)   _____ young adults (20 to 39)

     _____ young children (1 to 5)   _____ middle-age adults (40 to 64)

     _____ school age (6 to 12)   _____ older adults (65+)

Sex: _____ female   _____ male

Sexual preference: _____ bisexual _____ heterosexual

     _____ homosexual

Culture and racial origin:

     _____ African   _____ Middle Eastern

     _____ Anglo-Saxon   _____ Micronesian-Polynesian

     _____ counter-culture   _____ Native American

     _____ East Indian   _____ Northern European

     _____ Hispanic   _____ Asian

     _____ Mediterranean   _____ other:

Religion:

     _____ agnosticism-atheism   _____ Moslemism

     _____ Buddhism   _____ Protestantism

     _____ Greek Orthodoxy   _____ Roman Catholicism

     _____ Hinduism   _____ other:

     _____ Judaism

Social class:

     _____ famous, privileged, inherited great wealth

     _____ famous, unsophisticated, recently acquired great wealth

     _____ professional, educated, possesses moderate wealth

     _____ professional, educated, possesses modest wealth

     _____ white collar, technically skilled, possesses modest wealth

     _____ blue collar, technically skilled, possesses modest wealth

     _____ laborer, uneducated, possesses little wealth

     _____ unskilled, unemployed, destitute

     _____ other:

Organizational profile has to do with the size, type of service, structure, management style, and ownership of an institution. Size reflects the location and resources of the facility, often affecting atmosphere and structure. Structure influences the operation of an agency and its ability to change. Management style affects the degree of autonomy given to staff members. Ownership of a health-care agency may be vested in governments, investors for profit, religious groups, charitable organizations, or educational institutions. Owners have ultimate control. Consequently, the philosophy and management style of owners affects every aspect of an institution.

Autonomy for nurses increases as the profession more clearly defines its roles and functions. More and more nurses are self-employed, working as nurse practitioners, midwives, and clinical specialists in private practice and as independent contractors with hospitals and clinics. Autonomy for nurses within health-care institutions varies greatly from setting to setting. For this reason, nurses need to assess the degree of autonomy in specific settings and their preference in this regard.

Orientation and socialization programs for new staff members are indicators of the commitment an institution has to quality care. Generally, the longer an orientation, the greater the commitment. Morale is higher when an institution assists its staff to succeed. Chapter 10, Management-leadership, describes orientation and socialization programs in greater detail. Exercise 12-9 will help you assess work setting preferences.

PAYMENT FOR SERVICES.   Payment for nursing services is an indication of the value an employer places on nursing care. Nurses deserve to be paid for their knowledge, skill, and hard work. Their pay should be comparable to other professionals of like preparation, risk, and responsibility within a geographic area. Differential pay can be expected for evenings, nights, and overtime work. In addition to wages, employers offer various benefits such as health care, vacation time, sick leave, disability insurance, continuing education, and opportunities for advancement. Benefits should be assessed carefully in the light of personal needs because they may be more important to a nurse than wages.

✒ Exercise 12-9   *Assessment of Settings*

Place an X beside characteristics of work settings you prefer.

Type: _____ associated with the health-care industry
_____ not associated with the health-care industry

Kind: _____ inpatient (patients more dependent, sicker)
_____ ambulatory (patients less dependent, brief contact)
_____ home (patients sometimes less dependent, nursing functions are
holistic, innovative, less structured)

Labor organizations: _____ state nurses' association
_____ other organization _____ not organized

Organizational profile:
Ownership: _____ for-profit corporation _____ government
_____ nonprofit corporation _____ community

Profit motive: _____ high _____ moderate _____ low

Management style: _____ authoritarian _____ democratic
_____ laissez faire

Size: _____ small (100 or less employees)
_____ medium (101 to 600 employees)
_____ large (601 to 1500 employees)
_____ very large (1501 or more employees)

Resources: _____ extremely limited
_____ somewhat limited
_____ almost unlimited

Structure: _____ informal _____ formal _____ highly codified

Autonomy of nurses: _____ great _____ moderate _____ little

Orientation and socialization programs for new staff members:
_____ less than 2 weeks _____ 3 to 8 weeks _____ more than 8 weeks
_____ preceptorship _____ mentorship _____ buddy system

✔ Exercise 12-10   *Assessment of Pay and Working Conditions*

Fill in the wages, benefits, and hours you consider minimum requirements.

Wages per hour _____

Evening/night differential _____

Weekend/holiday differential _____

Overtime pay _____

Health care _____

Dental care _____

Salary increments _____

Vacation credits _____

Sicktime credit _____

Disability insurance _____

Career ladder options _____

Continuing education _____

Shift: days, evenings, nights _____

Hours per shift _____

Shifts per week _____

Other benefits (eg, child care) _____

WORKING CONDITIONS.   In ambulatory and home care agencies where health care is offered during normal working hours, nurses usually work five eight-hour weekdays. However, in hospitals providing 24-hour, seven-day-a-week care, some nurses must work evenings, nights, and weekends. Some agencies require all nurses to work all shifts. Others give them choices. When not enough people choose to work the less desirable shifts, agencies often use length of employment to decide who works these shifts. Thus, new graduates can expect to work evenings and nights. Some facilities offer such options as four ten-hour shifts and three 12-hour shifts per week. Exercise 12-10 will help you assess payment and working conditions.

HEALTH PROBLEMS.   Health problems are classified as acute, chronic, developmental, and environmental. They also are described by

---

✒ Exercise 12-11   *Assessment of Health Problems*

Place an X by the type of health problems and medical specialties you find most challenging.

Category: _____ acute _____ chronic _____ developmental
         _____ environmental

Medical specialty:

_____ allergy	_____ orthopedic surgery
_____ cardiology	_____ otorhinolaryngology
_____ dermatology	_____ pathology
_____ endocrinology	_____ pediatric diseases
_____ gastroenterology	_____ physical medicine and rehabilitation
_____ geriatrics	_____ plastic and reconstructive surgery
_____ hematology	_____ preventive medicine
_____ infectious diseases	_____ psychiatry
_____ infertility	_____ pulmonary diseases
_____ nephrology	_____ radiation therapy
_____ neurology	_____ rheumatology
_____ neurosurgery	_____ surgery
_____ nutrition	_____ urology
_____ ophthalmology	_____ obstetrics

---

medical specialties. The type of health problem nurses find challenging is a personal matter. Nursing functions differ from one health problem to another. Acute conditions demand immediate action; work is exciting but more stressful. Chronic and developmental disorders call for great patience and deliberate actions. Cultural and environmental problems require holistic approaches and involvement with bureaucracies. Exercise 12-11 will help you identify health problems that interest you most.

HUMAN RESPONSES.   The unique concern of nursing practice is to promote useful, adaptive, and effective human responses to health problems. Nursing diagnoses are the terms used to describe ineffective responses to health problems. Since its beginning in 1973,

---

✎ Exercise 12-12   *Assessment of Human Responses to Health Needs*

Place an X beside the category of human responses that particularly interests you.

_____ activity-exercise   _____ role-relationship

_____ cognitive-perceptual   _____ self-perceptual/self-concept

_____ coping-stress tolerance   _____ sexuality-reproductive

_____ elimination   _____ sleep-rest

_____ health-perception/management   _____ value-belief

_____ nutrition-metabolic

---

the North American Nursing Diagnosis Association (NANDA) has been creating a taxonomy of diagnoses. In 1982, Gordon organized them into eleven categories: activity-exercise, cognitive-perceptual, coping-stress tolerance, elimination, health-perception/management, nutrition-metabolic, role-relationship, self-perceptual/self-concept, sexuality-reproductive, sleep-rest, and value-belief.

Although nurses view humans holistically, they have different experiences and values. For this reason they may have greater interest in one category of human responses than another and may wish to focus their practice in that area. For example, a nurse who is interested in activity-exercise may choose to work in a neuro-rehabilitation unit. One who is interested in sexuality-reproduction may choose to work in women's health clinics. Exercise 12-12 will help you assess which human responses interest you most.

NURSING FUNCTIONS.   Nursing functions are actions taken to comfort and sustain suffering persons, prevent and treat health problems, and teach and encourage healthful living. These functions are carried out by applying the nursing process to patient problems and providing service at various levels of prevention. Since nursing actions can be performed by different individuals, nurses can choose to perform those functions they find most challenging. For example, a nurse who enjoys assessment and diagnosis may choose to work in triage in an emergency department. One who prefers planning, implementing, and evaluating may choose to work in an inpatient care unit.

✔ **Exercise 12-13**   *Assessment of Nursing Functions*

Place an X beside the nursing functions that interest you the most.

Nursing process:	Services:	Prevention:
_____ assessment	_____ direct	_____ primary
_____ diagnosis	_____ semidirect	_____ secondary
_____ planning	_____ indirect	_____ tertiary
_____ implementing		
_____ evaluating		

Services to clients may be direct, semidirect, or indirect (Archer and Fleshman 1979). *Direct services* to clients include all those direct care functions nurses do for and with clients. *Semidirect services* include functions such as supervising or educating others to give direct care to clients. *Indirect services* include functions nurses perform working politically and administratively to influence patient care.

Levels of prevention are termed primary, secondary, and tertiary. In *primary prevention,* nurses promote health and prevent health problems by activities such as prenatal teaching. In *secondary prevention* they seek to minimize complications of acute conditions by activities such as ambulating postoperative patients. In *tertiary prevention* nurses work to prevent complications of chronic conditions by such things as teaching foot care to clients with diabetes. Exercise 12-13 will help you identify nursing functions that give you the most satisfaction.

NURSING ROLES.   A role is defined as a set of behaviors expected of a person holding a position. Usually, nurses function in one or more of four roles: administrator, clinician, educator, and researcher. Administrators manage nursing service, clinicians provide direct patient care, educators teach, and researchers conduct scientific studies. Aptitudes and expected behaviors vary for each of the roles. Since all nurses begin as clinicians, education and experience affecting clinical roles is discussed more fully in Chapter 2, Education for Nursing. As nurses complete their initial education and

---

❝ **Exercise 12-14** *Assessment of Roles*

Place an X by the role that particularly appeals to you.

Role:	Expected Behaviors:
_____ Administrator	Manages nursing service, establishes budgets, collaborates with other units, oversees implementation of standard policies and procedures, evaluates personnel, provides leadership, and represents the institution in the community
_____ Clinician	Provides care of patients, using the nursing process to assess, diagnose, plan, implement, and evaluate care
_____ Educator	Develops curricula, lesson plans, and learning activities; maintains clinical and educational currency; participates in professional activities
_____ Researcher	Develops proposals for funding; plans and carries out research within theoretical frameworks; presents findings for critique

---

go on to plan a career, they may wish to consider additional roles open to them. Exercise 12-14 will help you identify the role you prefer.

SUMMARY OF APPRAISAL OF THE PROFESSION. Before going on to set goals and make a work-life plan, use Exercise 12-15 to summarize your assessment of the nursing profession as the various aspects relate to you.

Goal Setting

Goals are as essential to career plans as destinations are to journeys. They serve as guides for a work-life plan. Without goals nurses are vulnerable to economic pressure and employment expe-

❧ **Exercise 12-15**   *Summary of Aspects of the Nursing Profession*

My preference of patient characteristics: _____

_____

_____

My preference of setting characteristics: _____

_____

_____

My requirements for wages and working conditions: _____

_____

_____

Health problems I find most challenging: _____

_____

_____

Human responses I find most interesting: _____

_____

_____

Nursing functions I prefer: _____

_____

_____

Nursing roles I find most appealing: _____

_____

_____

dience. Setting goals involves making a general statement of intent and checking it against personal characteristics. A general statement of intent is made from information collected during the assessment process. Exercise 12-16 provides a framework for this statement.

Checking Goals Against Personal Traits

The next step is to check general statements of intent against personal characteristics identified earlier to see if they match. Ask

---

ℓ **Exercise 12-16**   *General Statement of Intent*

Based on my assessment of various aspects of the nursing profession,

I see myself focusing on these health problems and human responses:

_____

_____

_____

performing these nursing functions: _____

_____

_____

for these patients: _____

_____

_____

in these settings: _____

_____

_____

practicing in this role: _____

_____

_____

for this compensation: _____

_____

_____

and doing these personal activities to enrich my life: _____

_____

_____

Adapted from Henderson FC, McGettigan BO: *Managing Your Career in Nursing*, p 161. Addison-Wesley, 1986.

yourself, "Do my intended goals match my values, needs, interests, psychosocial behaviors, proficiency level, and physical capacities? Are my tentative goals realistic?"

CASE STUDY 1.   Connie sees herself in an acute care obstetrics unit, concerned with sexuality-reproductive human responses, providing direct service to young women as a nurse-midwife in private practice, with an income equal to other professionals.

Connie has an associate degree in nursing and is a single mother supporting three young children. She believes parenting is her God-given responsibility and places high value on spending maximum time with her children. To fulfill her tentative goal Connie needs several more years of education. To do this she would need to work full time and go to school evenings and weekends, leaving her children in the care of others. As a result Connie would experience conflict between her role as mother and her role as student. Her tentative goal is not realistic at this time. Until her children are older, Connie decides to modify her goal and become an expert clinician in the maternity unit of her local hospital.

CASE STUDY 2.   Harvey sees himself focusing on developmental psychiatry and cognitive-perceptual human responses, providing indirect service to people as an administrator at a mental health facility, with an income equal to other top-level managers.

Although Harvey is bright and motivated, he has difficulty with assertive communication and authority and calls himself a "loner." To fulfill his tentative goal, Harvey will need to deal with and become an authority figure himself. He will need to communicate assertively and work with people. Even if Harvey undergoes psychotherapy to work through his authority issues and enrolls in an assertiveness class, he may feel more successful if he alters his career goal and becomes an independent practitioner.

CASE STUDY 3.   Sondra sees herself focusing on preventive medicine, environmental issues, and health perception/management responses, providing direct services to employees in a large industrial plant as an occupational health nurse practitioner, with an income equal to professionals in similar positions.

Sondra is grossly overweight, has a serious self-esteem problem, and avoids leadership roles. To fulfill her tentative goal Sondra needs to become a role model of health and to learn management-leadership skills. Even if she initiates therapy to deal with her obesity and self-esteem problems, Sondra may find greater satisfaction if she alters her career goal to becoming a clinician in a health-care institution, where she could function as a team member rather than a leader.

Making Changes

It is important to recognize that personal characteristics can and do change. Some can be changed deliberately. For example, after Connie's children were reared she decided to return to school for further education. As a result of Harvey's psychotherapy and course work, he learned to deal with authority and to communicate assertively. Because of Sondra's resolve, she lost 95 pounds. Her self-esteem increased and she decided to pursue her goal of becoming an occupational health nurse.

Some personal characteristics change coincidentally, causing change in career plans. For instance, one of Connie's children developed leukemia. Because of her involvement in his care, Connie became interested in pediatric oncology. When she returned to school she became a pediatric nurse practitioner instead of a midwife. One summer Harvey took a job at a camp for developmentally disabled boys. Until then he had never cared for outdoor activities. He found the experience exhilarating. Over time, Harvey became an avid outdoorsman and decided to start a ranch for developmentally disabled children. When Sondra lost so much weight she needed new clothes. To save money she learned to sew, became involved in fashion design, and developed a fulfilling avocation. Thus, both deliberate and coincidental change in personal traits may affect work-life plans.

Planning

Once goals have been clarified, planning can begin. The first step of planning is to identify necessary education and experience. This information can be obtained from the American Nurses' Association and various specialty organizations (see Chapter 4). For example, Sondra contacted the Council on Primary Health Care Practitioners of the American Nurses' Association and the American Association of Occupational Health Nurses. She discovered that the preferred educational requirement for top-level occupational health positions is a master's degree in community health nursing with a specialty in occupational health (AAOHN 1986). Recommended minimum work requirements are one year each of acute medical-surgical nursing, emergency care, and community health nursing.

When nurses know the requirements of a goal, they compare their education and experience with those requirements and identify what more they need. These needs then become specific objectives in the career plan. For example, Sondra had an associate degree but needed a bachelor's and master's degree in nursing. She had worked a year in acute medical-surgical nursing but needed a year of emergency and a year of community health nursing experience.

Besides education and work experience, nurses should consider other interests that contribute to a well-rounded life and fit these into their work-life plans. For example, Sondra wanted to do some traveling and to develop a love relationship.

The final step in the planning process is to make a timeline to accomplish specific objectives, including education, work, and social activities. Thus, Sondra decided to combine school, work, and recreation rather than do only one thing at a time. She calculates that she can achieve all of her objectives and reach her goal in seven years. Exercise 12-17 will help you summarize your career plan.

It is never too late to make a work-life plan. Whether you are 18 or 80 years of age, the process is the same. Begin where you are, assess yourself and your work, identify goals, use past education and experience, and make a career plan.

Implementing a Career Plan

The beginning date of a career plan is important. It signals the end of dreaming and the start of doing, the time when action replaces planning. However, after a while the excitement of implementing a career plan wears off and reality sets in. Returning to school or acquiring new experience requires sacrifice. Discouragement is common. To reduce melancholy and maintain enthusiasm: (1) post the goal somewhere; (2) take time to sleep, exercise, and eat; (3) develop a support system; and (4) periodically reward yourself.

⟅ Exercise 12-17   *A Career Plan*

My professional goal is: _____

Educational requirements: _____

_____

Experiencial requirements: _____

_____

Educational needs (objectives): _____

_____

Experiencial needs (objectives): _____

_____

My personal goal is: _____

Personal needs (objectives): _____

_____

Cost of living: _____

_____

Sources of funding: _____

_____

Timeline to achieve specific objectives: _____

_____

Date I will begin implementing my plan: _____

_____

Accomplished by the end of one year: _____

_____

Accomplished by the end of two years: _____

_____

Accomplished by the end of three years: _____

_____

Evaluating a Career Plan

As nurses go about implementing a career plan it is important to evaluate not only the goal, but progress toward the goal. For example, Sondra found that returning to school and working part-time was more difficult than she anticipated. After a month of working 20 hours a week and taking 12 units at the university, she decided to drop 3 units and revise her timeline accordingly. The adjustment made her life more manageable.

Things went well and Sondra completed her bachelor's degree on the revised schedule. When she applied for graduate school she found that federal money had become available for graduate students in the mental health major. Sondra thought long and hard about changing her major, because such a change would greatly affect her career plan. After checking the job market and counseling with people working in mental health, Sondra decided to become a clinical specialist in mental health nursing. The revised goal eased Sondra's financial burden, gave her an opportunity to explore her interest in eating disorders, and allowed her to use her experience to help others.

Management Strategies

The same tactics used by institutions to achieve agency goals can be used by nurses to achieve career goals. These tactics are marketing, relationship, production, and control strategies.

Marketing

Marketing is the process of selling goods or services to prospective buyers. Nurses may feel uncomfortable with the idea of marketing themselves, yet that is exactly what they do when they go about seeking employment. They present their knowledge and skill to a prospective employer for the purpose of selling their services. While nurses may think of patient caregivers in altruistic terms, the health-care industry thinks in terms of market value, asking, "What is your expertise worth to me?" Some professionals, such as actors and athletes, hire agents to market their services. Most nurses, however, serve as their own agents. For this reason they need to learn the essential written communication and interviewing skills of marketing.

Written Communication

RESUMES AND CURRICULA VITAE. Resumes and curricula vitae are valuable tools in the marketing process. Both instruments provide a summary of qualifications. However, they have different uses and formats.

A *resume* is a summary of education and experience most relevant to a specific career objective. It is written to attract attention and obtain an interview. Formats of resumes vary, depending on the position for which they are written. Some resumes use a chronological format, listing positions held, education, experience, special accomplishments, and skills, beginning with the most recent. Some resumes use a functional format, state a career objective, and follow it with a summary of education and experience. Some resumes combine the features of chronological and functional formats to fit a special situation.

A *curriculum vitae* (CV) is a precise formal account of scholarly achievements and activities. It is most often used by educators when they apply for an academic appointment, promotion, tenure, or honor. Curricula vitae (the plural form) are written to engender respect and admiration. The format is relatively fixed.

Some general rules for writing resumes and CVs are as follows:

1. Decide on a format that presents you to your best advantage and is appropriate for the position you are seeking.

2. Use precise phrases with action verbs, such as directed, solved, led, built, and taught; avoid wordy descriptions.

3. Do not be afraid to use the vocabulary of nursing, such as primary nursing, or triage.

4. Use numbers to show quantitative results, such as nosocomial infection rates dropped 52%.

5. Omit personal information such as birthdate, marital status, religion, health status, and politics; never use "I," "me," or "my" in a resume or curriculum vitae.

6. Never use gimmicks or try to be cute with such things as smiling faces; these devices trivialize your marketing efforts.

7. Never mention the salary of prior positions or the salary expected in a new position; that comes during negotiation.

8. Be prepared to give names as references; ask colleagues and supervisors for their permission in advance.

9. Be aware that employers may ask questions about long gaps of unemployment or numerous, brief periods of employment.

✐ **Exercise 12-18**   *Framework for a Chronological Resume*

Name (First, middle initial, and last):   (Do not state birthdate)

Address: Home Phone:

Education (degrees or certificates earned; school, beginning with the most recent; do not include high school):

Licenses and Certificates (eg, RN #07253, California):

Other Skills (eg, speak Spanish language):

Professional Experience (beginning with the most recent, state the dates, employer, position, and a brief job description, using action verbs in phrases; do not use "I," "me," or "my"):

Special Accomplishments and Honors (go ahead, brag, list recent or outstanding achievements, eg, 1991 recipient Nurse of the Year Award, Sutter Hospital, Albany, CA):

Continuing Education (recent or relevant):

Other Activities (that show your specialness, eg, coordinator, Health Faire 1990 and 1991; volunteer, Meals-on-Wheels, 1989):

References Available on Request (never include names in resume).

---

10. Use white, gray, or cream-colored, letter-size, high-quality paper; center data and use only one side of the paper; use clear, clean type. Word processors produce flawless copies at little cost and facilitate updating.

11. Proofread to eliminate misspelled words, typographical errors, or grammatical mistakes; never underline for emphasis or make corrections in ink after the resume has been reproduced (Schuman and Lewis 1987).

12. Never attach transcripts, letters of recommendation, or photographs to a resume or CV; do attach a resume or CV to a cover letter.

13. Make resumes brief, preferably one page long, so that employers can scan them in 30 to 45 seconds.

Exercises 12-18, 12-19, and 12-20 provide frameworks for resumes and curricula vitae.

𝒞 Exercise 12-19   *Framework for a Functional Resume*

Name (First, middle initial, and last):   (Do not state birthdate)
Address: Home Phone:

Professional Objective (optional, should stress employer-valued benefits rather than applicant-valued benefits, eg, "to demonstrate creative leadership as a nurse manager"):

Summary of Qualifications (eg, *author* of numerous articles on role of nurse managers, *appointee* to state council on health-care costs):

Significant Qualifications (eg, *Administration:* Top administrative officer in a health-care institution; *Clinical practice:* Expert clinician in pediatric oncology):

Professional Development (work experience: beginning with the most recent, state title, dates, name and address of each institution):

Education (beginning with the most recent, state the school and degree or certificate earned):

Professional Affiliations (eg, American Nurses' Association):

References Available on Request (never include names in resume).

COVER LETTERS.   The purpose of a cover letter, or *letter of inquiry,* is to introduce the writer, to express interest in a position, and to point to the enclosed resume. It is written for a certain job, and when possible, addressed to a specific person where the job is located. The cover letter accompanies a resume, personalizes it, and allows the nurse to emphasize a particular area of expertise or interest. Employers use cover letters as screening tools, to get a "feel" for applicants (Schuman and Lewis 1987). Here are some general rules for a well-written cover letter:

1. Whenever possible, address the letter to a specific person.

2. State the reason for the letter and where or how the writer heard of the opening; "I," "me," and "my" may be used.

3. Explain your interest in the position in terms of what employers value rather than what you value (e.g., challenge and growth rather than location and money).

✔ Exercise 12-20   *Framework for a Curriculum Vitae*

Name (First, middle, last):   (Do not state birthdate)

Address (may use academic address):   Phone (that matches address):

Education (begin after high school, state degree, major, and school, but no dates, eg, BS, Nursing, Stanford University; MS, Community Health Nursing, University of California, San Francisco; EdD, University of San Francisco):

Experience (begin with first nursing position, state time span, title, institution, eg, 8/80 – 9/81, staff nurse I, oncology, Peralta Hospital, Oakland, CA; 11/81 – 6/83, staff nurse II, oncology, Peralta Hospital, Oakland, CA; instructor, VN program, Laney College, Oakland, CA):

Professional Memberships (eg, American Nurses' Association, California Nurses' Association, National League for Nursing):

Publications (list alphabetically as in a bibliography):

References Available on Request (never include names in CV).

4. Highlight major career accomplishments and refer the prospective employer to your resume for further details.

5. Indicate a desire for an interview and suggest a plan for arranging it.

6. Close with appreciation for consideration of your application and a final statement of enthusiasm and interest.

7. Use high-quality, letter-size stationary, and clean, clear type; center letter on page; proofread for errors of spelling, grammar, or punctuation (see Exercise 12-21).

APPLICATION FORMS.   Even though nurses send cover letters and resumes to prospective employers, they should be prepared to fill out an application form of the institution. These forms vary in length, detail, and format. They often ask for information not included on resumes, such as names and addresses of references. Although it may seem redundant to copy data from a resume onto an application, it has a valid purpose. A form provides employers with a

---

✿ Exercise 12-21   *Framework for Cover Letter*

Name and Degrees (eg, Nancy Preven, RN, BS)
Address
Phone Number
Date
Name of Person Responsible for Employing Nurses (if unknown, tele-
phone the institution and obtain correct spelling and title, eg, Suzanne
Santos, RN, MS, Director)
Name of Institution
Address
Dear (Mr., Ms, or Dr.) last name:

I (say how you heard or read of a position in the institution, eg, read
your advertisement for a camp nurse at the Clara Barton Camp for Girls
with Diabetes in the February, 1990, issue of *RN Magazine*) with great
interest. My career includes (tell of special experiences that relate to the
prospective position, eg, five years in pediatric nursing, the past two
working with diabetic children and their parents in an outpatient clinic).

I am (tell of special knowledge and education as it relates to the position, eg, knowledgeable of current treatment protocols for childhood
diabetes and teaching techniques for children. I hold a BS in Nursing
and an ANA certificate as a pediatric nurse).

I am (suggest a plan to follow up on this letter, eg, looking forward to
an opportunity to discuss the camp nurse position). I will be calling you
a week from today to set up a time to meet with you.

Thank you for your consideration of my application. I am eager to
put my talents to work for (clients and staff of the institution, eg, Clara
Barton campers and staff).
Sincerely,

(Full signature) _____
Name and Degrees (typed below name, eg, Nancy Preven, RN, BS)

---

standardized means to compare candidates, thus facilitating the selection process. It is acceptable to attach a resume to an application form, but it is not acceptable to line through the form and
write "see attached," at least, not if you are serious about the
position.

RECORD KEEPING.   It is helpful to keep a copy of every resume or CV, cover letter, application form, and letter of resignation you write. When it is time to revise a resume, or write another cover letter, old ones are useful. They include names and addresses of former employers and dates of education and experience.

Interviewing

If a resume or CV accomplishes its purpose, the applicant is invited to a job interview. The resume or CV has persuaded the institution that the nurse it describes has the knowledge and skill it is seeking. The interview confirms and reinforces that description. An interview is a purposeful, goal-directed interaction between people. Job interviews aim to determine if the applicant's services and personal needs match the institution's wages and needs. The goals of both interviewees and interviewers are to learn more about the other, to present themselves in the best light, and to determine if there is a match. Success for both parties requires careful preparation, skillful participation, and energetic follow-up.

PREPARATION.   To prepare for a job interview, wise applicants gather information about the institution, take stock of themselves, and reduce as many stressors as possible.

Information about a prospective employer can be gleaned from informal conversations with staff members and published materials available from the personnel department, such as newsletters, official histories, and policy manuals.

A good way to take stock of oneself is to use the personal assessment exercises found at the beginning of this chapter. Gerberg (1986) suggests that applicants take time to develop a vocabulary of key words and short phrases that describe their accomplishments and personal strengths, such as conscientious, objective, tolerant, resourceful, energetic, reliable, logical, productive, discreet, forward-thinking, and perceptive.

Careful planning can reduce the fear associated with a job interview. Here are some suggestions:

1. Role-play answering often-asked questions, such as: What are some of your accomplishments at your present job? What is

your greatest strength, weakness? What are your short-range and long-range career objectives? Why are you leaving your present job?

2. Bring a list of questions to ask interviewers, such as: What is the management philosophy of this institution? Is professional growth encouraged and rewarded? What opportunities are there for advancement? What happened to the last person in the position? How would you describe ideal behavior in the position? What is the best thing, worst thing, about this institution?

3. Avoid last minute crises: make a practice run to the institution; note the route, driving time, and parking; try on the clothes you plan to wear; gather together and take: a job description, your resume, cover letter, correspondence from the institution, and a notepad listing your questions.

4. Go to bed early the night before; start the day by eating easily-digested food; just before the interview, go to the restroom and take a few moments to gain composure and control. You know who you are, what you can do, and what you want.

PARTICIPATION.   Applicants may be interviewed by one person, by a series of individuals, or by a group of people. The opening of an interview includes introduction of participants to one another, clarification of the purpose of the interview, and agreement on guidelines, such as the allotted time and screening process. Here are some suggestions for skillful interview participation:

1. Arrive no more than 10 minutes early. If you are unavoidably delayed, phone and ask for another appointment time. If you are kept waiting more than 20 minutes, ask for another appointment and excuse yourself.

2. Dress well, but conservatively. A suit is a good choice for both men and women, although in some areas more casual attire is acceptable. Avoid faddish clothes, excessive jewelry or make-up, and strong perfume. Torn or soiled clothing, dirty hair, body odor, or bad breath are unacceptable. Avoid fumbling with a heavy coat or packages. Ask to place them in an

out-of-the-way place before the interview begins. Remember, your appearance speaks louder than words. When you feel good about your appearance, you will be more confident.

3. Remain calm and cordial. Speak clearly and slowly. Be brief, positive, and enthusiastic. Think before speaking. Avoid "and-ahs," "you-knows," and other nervous noises.

4. Take brief notes to help you remember names or information.

5. Be truthful. If your background includes substance abuse or a felony offense, volunteer only what you must reveal legally. If asked, tell the truth without defensiveness. You are now a healthy, competent professional. Title VII of the 1964 Civil Rights Act as amended by the 1972 Equal Employment Opportunity Act requires that employer inquiries be position-related. This means you can respectfully decline to answer questions unrelated to job performance, such as age, religion, race, handicaps, and marital status. Chapter 10, Management-leadership, identifies questions interviewers cannot ask.

6. Use a soft sell; underplay your need for the job; emphasize your assets and accomplishments.

7. Maintain professional dignity and emotional control. Do not criticize, condemn, complain, or divulge confidences of your present employer.

8. Be a good listener. Avoid acting bored or impatient. When a period of silence occurs, ask questions that demonstrate your knowledge and experience.

9. The interview is as much for you to "get a feel" for the institution as for the institution to "get a feel for you." Ask your prepared questions and any others that occur to you.

10. The initial interview is rarely the time to negotiate wages; however, salary is always part of the discussion. Do not initiate the subject too early, as you may appear over-eager. Before the interview ends, ask about the salary range, benefits, employee-employer contract, and if membership in a labor union is required. If the institution offers you a position at the interview, give yourself time to consider it. For middle and higher level

positions, salary is never discussed with a search committee. It is negotiated later with other officials.

11. At the close of the interview, thank the people, by name; confirm when you can expect to hear their decision; make sure the interviewer knows when, where, and how to contact you.

EVALUATION.   Evaluation of interviews helps nurses learn from experience and become more skillful. Soon after the interview ask yourself:

1. Did I gather sufficient information about the institution and myself ahead of time? What did I lack?

2. Did I reduce stressors sufficiently? What else could I have done to bolster my composure and sense of control?

3. Was I dressed appropriately? Did I talk too much, too little? Did I present my knowledge and skill accurately? Did I watch for nonverbal or verbal clues and adjust my behavior accordingly? What will I do differently in the future?

Evaluation of the position and institution involves comparing it to an ideal one and to others you have visited. Exercise 12-9, Assessment of Settings, may help with this task. So, too, might Exercise 12-16, General Statement of Intent.

FOLLOW-UP.   Follow-up of an interview is vital. It is done to demonstrate social skills, to confirm interest in the position, and to remind interviewers of applicant qualifications. A follow-up letter should be written after every interview, and if applicants are interested in a position, they should telephone interviewers as well as write. Make both follow-up messages brief and focused. Express appreciation for the interview, indicate continued enthusiasm and interest in the position, and remind interviewers of your qualifications (see Exercise 12-22).

Relationships

Relationship strategies pave the way for nurses to achieve career goals. They include negotiating, networking, maintaining collegial relationships, and discriminating.

*✒ **Exercise 12-22**   *Framework for an Interview Follow-up Letter*

Name and Degrees (eg. etc)
Address
Phone Number
Name of Person Who Conducted the Interview, Degrees, and Title
Name of Institution
Address
Dear (Mr., Ms, or Dr.) last name:

   It was a pleasure to meet with you and members of the screening committee on (state the day and date). I found the interview informative and (state any other positive experience or idea with which you agreed, eg, enjoyed the tour of the new wing).

   I am enthusiastic about (state anything you wish to emphasize about the institution and how you would fill its needs, eg, the challenge available at General Hospital in interdisciplinary care of developmentally disabled children). I would welcome the opportunity to (whatever it is you want to do, eg, be involved in setting up a program in the new unit).

   I look forward to hearing from you in the near future.
Sincerely,

(Full signature)_____
Name and Degrees (typed below etc.)

Negotiating

   Negotiating is mutual discussion aimed at reaching an agreement. It is open communication between individuals for the purpose of reaching an agreement (Henderson and McGettigan 1986). Negotiations between nurses and employers usually involve salary, benefits, and working conditions.

   Until recently, nurses never discussed salaries openly. It was deemed unprofessional to place importance on financial rewards. The nurse's primary reward was supposed to come from providing expert nursing care to clients (Norwak and Grindel 1984). Today, it is appropriate to discuss a beginning salary. Here are some strategies for negotiating:

1. Before negotiations begin, learn what this employer needs and find out what other institutions are offering for the same work.

2. Set realistic goals; when you change positions, a salary increase of more than 25% is unrealistic.

3. Start with a salary range, not a specific figure; the employer will negotiate *down* from your figure.

4. Avoid negotiating from your present salary. Instead, emphasize unique credentials (experience, education, past achievements) you will bring to the position.

5. Be positive about everything except salary, expressing both enthusiasm and sincerity about salary needs.

6. If the salary is fixed and seems low, try for other things, such as an automatic increase in six months, continuing education time and tuition, reimbursement for moving expenses, and medical insurance (Norwak and Grindel 1984).

Networking

Networking is the cultivation of relationships with others for the purpose of sharing information and resources. The overriding function of networking is to help people build their careers. Networking serves as a resource to balance demands and reduce the stresses of a busy life (see Chapter 9). A network provides a sense of belonging and acceptance, social companionship, concrete assistance, information, and advice. A network is made up of a variety of people in and out of nursing. In practice, networking means sharing a tidbit of information, listening to a painful story, contributing to a special need, and giving advice to a neophyte. Whenever people need mutual assistance to build their careers, networking can help.

Maintaining Collegial Relationships

Collegial relationships are based on a professional connection but are closer than those found in networks. Colleagues are co-workers, allies, collaborators, teammates, peers, and mentors (as discussed in Chapter 10, Management-leadership). They share knowledge, provide support, and challenge one another to new ways of thinking. Colleagues may have varying experiences, educational backgrounds, and even belong to different professions. They can be expected to give advice and assistance when asked, such as writing letters of reference (Kelly 1987).

Discriminating

To *discriminate* means to make a distinction on a categorical basis rather than according to actual merit (*The Random House College Dictionary* 1975). Discrimination can be helpful or harmful. It is helpful when a choice must be made between equally valuable things. For example, the career goal of Ulla is to become an educator. She is offered two positions, one in education and one in administration. Ulla chooses the education position, not because of intrinsic merit, but because of its category relative to her career goal.

When discrimination denies people equal opportunity to pursue career goals, it is harmful. In the United States, discrimination on the basis of age, sex, religion, politics, physical disability, and marital status is unlawful in the workplace. However, subtle discrimination continues, discouraging women from becoming administrators and men from becoming nurses. In many arenas, outright discrimination on the basis of sexual preference is still lawful.

Production

Production strategies are tactics that increase the skill, knowledge, and effectiveness of nurses as providers of nursing service. Two such strategies are continuing education and occupational health and safety.

Continuing Education

In many states continuing education (CE) is mandatory for relicensure (see Chapter 2). Yet even when it is not required, nurses must continually update their knowledge and skill to stay current. When they wish to make either lateral or vertical career moves, nurses need further education. For example, Pat wants to transfer to a rehabilitation unit. To support her request she is taking a series of CE courses in rehabilitative nursing. Sam wants to make a vertical move into management. To advance his career Sam is pursuing a master's degree in administration. In the broadest sense, CE includes degree programs, certificate programs, and single subject courses, all of which increase productivity.

Occupational Health and Safety

The maintenance of personal health and safety is an essential production strategy for nurses. Without health, career planning is futile. As nurses go about caring for the sick and injured they may forget to safeguard their own health and safety. Yet they are exposed to dangerous pathogens, physical strain, assaultive patients, hazardous radiation, potent chemicals, and emotional stressors. It is not enough for health-care employers to comply with national and state codes. Nurses must safeguard their own health. They need to get adequate exercise, nutrition, stress-reducing activity, physical checkups, and immunizations.

Control

Control strategies are mechanisms nurses and persons in authority use to achieve goals. These strategies include setting standards, evaluating performance as compared to the standards, and correcting behavior if it deviates (McFarland et al 1984).

Setting Standards

To manage their careers effectively, nurses need to set standards by which they can measure progress toward their goals. Here are some suggested standards:

1. Data collection is systematic and continuous.

2. The career plan includes clearly stated long-term goals and short-term objectives.

3. Actions needed to achieve a career plan are clearly defined and prioritized.

4. Progress or lack of progress toward career goals and objectives is determined by the nurse alone.

5. Periodically the nurse evaluates progress toward career goals, reorders priorities, sets new goals, and revises the plan of action.

Evaluating Performance

When nurses accept employment they can expect employers to evaluate their performance. Often new employees are hired with probationary status for two to six months. At the end of the period their performance is evaluated. Thereafter, agencies evaluate performance at designated intervals unless special problems arise. To evaluate performance, some institutions use peer reviews made by co-workers. Others use administrative reviews made by supervisors.

Because performance evaluations affect salary, professional advancement, and self-esteem, they produce great anxiety. Here are some guidelines to improve performance and reduce fear:

1. During orientation to the agency, obtain a list of evaluation criteria. Nurses need advanced knowledge of the standard by which they will be measured. Ideally, evaluation criteria are stated as behaviors, such as "communicates pertinent patient information at shift change."

2. During the probationary period, review evaluation criteria to remind yourself of valued behaviors.

3. When it is time for a regular evaluation interview, or if a problem arises and a "counseling session" is scheduled, take a moment to relax and become centered. Expect negative comments.

4. No matter what is said or written do *not* exhibit hostility. Do *not* appear defensive. *Do* listen to the supervisor's comments carefully. If you feel the feedback is exaggerated or not true, say so in a matter-of-fact way. Without admitting fault, assure the supervisor that the errant behavior will not happen in the future. You share the same goal as the institution: to deliver high-quality nursing care. If you are deficient in some way, enlist the supervisor's assistance to change.

Only nurses themselves can evaluate progress toward career goals. However, performance evaluations may open new career options. For example, in several reviews, Ulla's supervisor commended her for her teaching ability. Until then, Ulla had never seriously considered a teaching career. These evaluations encouraged her to enroll in a master's degree program in nurse education.

Termination and Resignation

Control strategies involve terminating old positions and moving on to new ones. Like the feedback loop of the nursing process, where evaluation serves as reassessment, terminating one position serves as the beginning of a new employment cycle. Terminations may be initiated by an employer as a firing or layoff or by the nurse as a resignation.

When performance evaluations identify behaviors that do not meet standards, employers follow the process spelled out in the employer-employee contract. Often the steps include: counseling, written warnings, and opportunities for change. If these measures fail, the nurse is terminated (fired). Common reasons for nurse terminations are: poor job performance, tardiness, absenteeism, substance abuse, inappropriate behavior, and staff reductions. Reasons for immediate terminations are: patient or visitor abuse, drug possession, intoxication, theft, disorderly conduct, record falsification, willful property destruction, and sleeping on duty (Marriner-Tomey 1988).

Termination is especially difficult when nurses are laid off through no fault of their own. Nurses who are hired into highly visible and vulnerable positions sometimes anticipate layoffs and make "termination agreements" in advance, stipulating continuation of benefits or salary for a certain time (Norwak and Grindel 1984). Many hospitals follow industry's lead, offering "outplacement counseling" for terminated staff members. The purpose of this counseling is to help nurses deal with their loss and grief and find other employment. Rituals such as going-away parties facilitate the termination process (Marriner-Tomey 1988).

No job lasts forever. Eventually all nurses resign from their work positions. Even so, resignation should not be impulsive or precipitous. Neither should it be delayed endlessly because of guilt or misplaced loyalty. Moving on toward goals means saying good-bye to the old and familiar. Before you talk or write to anyone about leaving consider these suggestions:

1. Check your employee-employer contract regarding benefits, accrued sick leave, and vacation time. It is important to comply with legal agreements and ethical commitments. Advance notice should be given for at least the number of days of the pay period; more notice is given for more responsible positions.

2. Check with personnel to determine current accrued time.

3. Be considerate of co-workers; try to complete projects you have begun and prepare helpful guides to assist your successor.

4. Write a letter of resignation using these guidelines:
   (a) State your intention to leave, the effective date of resignation and last working day, a reason for leaving, some sincere positive experience in the position, and an offer to assist in the transition.
   (b) Use precise wording; avoid being maudlin or malicious; mention people by name who have been especially helpful.
   (c) Address letter to the top nursing administrator, such as the nursing director, with a copy to the immediate supervisor.
   (d) Proofread for correct spelling, punctuation, and grammar.
   (e) Use high-quality, letter-size paper; center text on page; use one side only with clean, clear type.
   (f) Remember, resignation letters are like epitaphs on tombstones. They leave a final impression of the writer; better you say nothing than make bitter or inappropriate statements.

5. Before you deliver a resignation letter to the administrator, courtesy dictates that you meet with your immediate supervisor; give the essential facts stated in the letter of resignation and express your personal appreciation. (See Exercise 12-23.)

✐ **Exercise 12-23**   *Framework for a Letter of Resignation*

Name and Degrees (eg, Donna Parks, RN, BS)
Address
Date

Name of Top Nursing Service Administrator, Degrees, Title, (eg, Sandra Haber, RN, MS, Vice-president of Nursing Service)
Name of Institution (eg, General Hospital)
Address

Dear (Mr., Ms, or Dr.) last name:

  I have decided to (state plan of action, eg, return to school for a MS degree in nursing at the University of Texas). Therefore, I wish to resign effective (state the date that will include all accrued leave days): Since I have ____ accrued vacation days, my last working day will be (state the date).

  Working with the patients and staff at (name of institution) has been a satisfying personal and professional experience. I have (say something positive, eg, learned so much about pediatric nursing care). I particularly appreciate (name someone, if true) because (state act or attitude). I am proud to have been a part of (name of institution) because (state why). (Omit the last sentence if it is not true.)

  If there is something I can do to help in the transition, I will be happy to do so.

Sincerely,

(Full signature) _____

Name and Degrees (typed below name, etc), eg, Donna Parks, RN BS)
Name of Immediate Supervisor

Summary

  Career management means making a work-life plan to provide self-fulfillment and realize personal and professional goals. To make such a plan nurses collect and assess data about themselves and their profession. With this information they set goals, make plans, implement them, and evaluate progress. To sell themselves to prospective employers nurses use the marketing strategies of written communication and interviewing. They use relationship, production, and control strategies to succeed in a demanding profession. With a work-life plan, nurses experience successful, fulfilling careers.

----------------------------------- ✆ -----------------------------------

Learning Activities

1. Make a personal and professional assessment using Exercises 12-1 to 12-15.

2. Write your career goals and tentative plan using Exercises 12-16 and 12-17.

3. Write a resume or curriculum vitae using Exercises 12-18, 12-19, or 12-20 as a guide.

4. Write a cover letter to accompany your resume or curriculum vitae using Exercise 12-21 as a guide.

5. Visit a career center at a college or university. Find out what services they offer students and graduates.

6. Visit a career fair or recruiting office of a military service. Collect information about nursing opportunities.

7. Make a list of questions to ask at a job interview.

8. Interview the nurse recruiter or personnel manager at a local hospital. Ask what that person looks for in nurse applicants.

Annotated Reading List

Norwak JB, Grindel CG: Contracts and salary negotiations. Chapter 6 in: *Career Planning in Nursing*. Lippincott, 1984.

This useful chapter describes the process of salary negotiation from the viewpoint of an individual nurse negotiating with an employer without the benefit of a union contract. It includes strategies for negotiating a salary increase, what to do when the employer counters your salary range, and how to handle more than one offer.

Nurse's Reference Library: Your choices about your job. Chapter 9, *Practices*. Springhouse, 1984.

This chapter is written from a job perspective. It gives a condensed view of how nurses can make employment changes. Its graphic displays help readers identify important points. For example, there are "key term" charts and devices such as colored notes superimposed on sample forms to emphasize content.

Winstead-Fry P: *Career Planning: A Nurses's Guide to Career Advancement*. National League for Nursing, 1989.

This useful text offers first-hand views of career choices open to nurses with baccalaureate and advanced degrees as well as strategies for achieving success in such fields as nurse-midwifery, independent practice, community health, administration, research, and education. Drawing on both interviews and questionnaires, the author offers detailed guidance on career planning, especially for careers outside the traditional hospital setting.

References

American Association of Occupational Health Nurses: *Guidelines for Developing Job Descriptions in Occupational Health Nursing*. AAOHN, 1986.

Archer S, Fleshman R: *Community Health Nursing*, p. 461. Duxbury Press, 1979.

Benner P: *From Novice to Expert*, pp. 20–30. Addison-Wesley, 1984.

Gerberg RJ: *Robert Gerberg's Job Changing System, World's Fastest Way to Get a Better Job*. Andrews, McMeel, & Parker, 1986.

Gordon M: *Nursing Diagnosis*, pp. 327–328. McGraw-Hill, 1982.

Henderson FC, McGettigan BO: *Managing Your Career in Nursing.* Addison-Wesley, 1986.

Kelly LY: *The Nursing Experience: Trends, Challenges, and Transitions.* Macmillan, 1987.

Marriner-Tomey A: *Guide to Nursing Management,* 3rd ed. Mosby, 1988.

McFarland GK, Leonard HS, Morris MM: *Nursing Leadership and Management, Contemporary Strategies,* p. 122. Wiley, 1984.

Norwak JB, Grindel CG: *Career Planning in Nursing.* Lippincott, 1984.

Nurses today: A statistical portrait. *Am J Nurs* 1982, 448–451.

The Random House College Dictionary. Random House, 1975.

Schuman N, Lewis W: *Revising Your Resume.* Wiley, 1987.

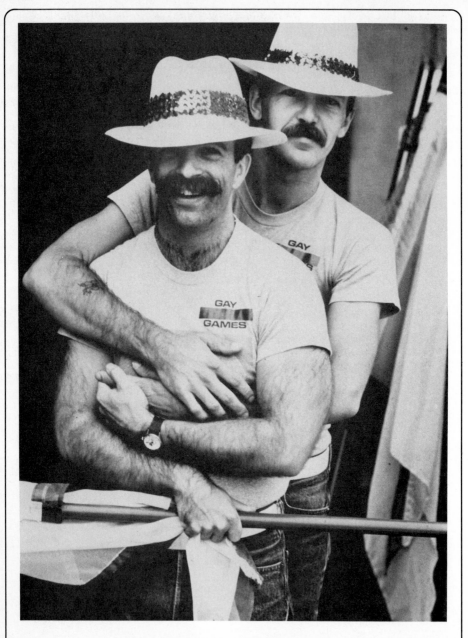

Homosexual men and women share the joys and sorrows of life just as heterosexual people. Yet, nurses may find it difficult to care for individuals whose life style differs from their own.

AFTERWORD

Afterword: Current Realities

Billy Jo *peeled off her gloves and left the room. She felt dirty, nauseated, ill. "Those disgusting homosexual creeps," she thought. "They come here and expect sympathy! Dying of AIDS is horrible, but they deserve it. Why didn't they think of that when they had sex with other men!" Billy Jo shuddered. She went to the sink and turned on the water, as if to wash away her disgust. A co-worker saw the look on her face and asked, "What's the matter? Are you afraid you'll get AIDS, or do you just hate gays?" Billy Jo pretended to ignore the taunt, but she knew the answer to both questions was "Yes." She also knew she felt guilty. Nurses weren't supposed to have disease or patient phobias. Just the same, Billy Jo believed homosexuality was wrong, that homosexual acts were repulsive. She decided to take her break.*

In the cafeteria Billy Jo sat by two nurses from another unit. One was joking about a drunk with cirrhosis and the other was bemoaning homeless riff-raff who are too lazy or crazy to work. Billy Jo had no sympathy for substance abusers or people who didn't work. Her father was an alcoholic and she'd been self-supporting since she was sixteen. Eagerly, Billy Jo joined the discussion, adding her condemnation of homosexuality as a social blight. It felt good to vent her emotions and to be accepted by nurses with other prejudices. Somehow it helped reduce her guilt.

Even so, as Billy Jo walked back to her unit she realized that her conscience bothered her. Nurses weren't supposed to feel so hostile toward patients. How could she reconcile her personal beliefs with her professional ideals?

The first chapter of this text described how war, politics, religion, culture, technology, and medicine influenced the practice of nursing throughout history. This afterword describes three realities that impact nursing today: homelessness, substance abuse, and sexually transmitted diseases, particularly AIDS. It addresses the prejudice these realities expose in nurses and offers a remedy for such judgmental attitudes.

Homelessness

An estimated two to three million people are homeless in the United States today. Although homelessness has existed in every era, in recent times the number of homeless people in industrialized societies has risen dramatically. This increase is attributed to economic depression, unaffordable housing, substance abuse, family breakdown, and fewer institutions to house the mentally ill. About 60% of the homeless are single adults, a third of whom are mentally ill. The other 40% of the homeless are emancipated minors and families, most of whom are single mothers with children (Barrick 1990). Many homeless people work but cannot afford housing. Their children are educationally deprived and exist in "degrading conditions that take a profound and lasting toll" (Berne 1989). Emancipated minors are an especially tragic group of the homeless. Most come from violent, impoverished, and chaotic families whose parents are either unable or unwilling to care for them. To survive, they live in abandoned buildings, sleep in 24-hour theaters, sell drugs, panhandle, and work as prostitutes (Rafferty 1989).

The health of homeless people is in constant jeopardy. Many diseases afflict homeless adults, especially tuberculosis. Youths and children suffer upper respiratory infections, nutritional deficiencies, sexually transmitted diseases, and a pregnancy rate twice the national average (Coalition for the Homeless 1987). The human immunodeficiency virus (HIV), which causes AIDS, infects thousands. Rodgers and Aron estimated that in New York City alone 10,000 homeless people were infected with HIV (1989). Assault, substance abuse, and injury add to the misery and peril of these hapless people.

Substance Abuse

Substance abuse has reached crisis proportions in the United States today. It affects all ages, socioeconomic classes, and cultural groups. It destroys individuals and families and invades every area of life. The causes of substance abuse are illusive, but the impact is catastrophic, personally affecting one of every two United States families. One in ten workers in the general population and one in five nurses abuse substances. Four million people use cocaine. One in five high school students "does drugs" on a weekly basis. Substance abuse, chiefly alcohol, increases the rate of work-related injuries, auto crashes, absenteeism, suicides, and teenage pregnancies. Alcohol kills more people under 25 years of age than anything else because it causes more than 8000 deaths and 40,000 serious injuries from vehicle crashes (Hutchinson 1988).

Sexually Transmitted Diseases

The incidence of sexually transmitted diseases (STDs) in the United States has reached epidemic levels. This rate is due in part to ignorance of the dangers of sexual activity, changing social standards, and a notion that there is an easy cure for every disease. A variety of bacteria, fungi, parasites, and viruses cause STDs. However, the most serious STD is acquired immune deficiency syndrome (AIDS), caused by HIV. Because HIV destroys the body's defense system, victims become vulnerable to rare opportunistic diseases, such as *Pneumocystis carinii* pneumonia; toxoplasmosis, a parasitic encephalitis; Kaposi's sarcoma, a malignant skin cancer; and *cryptosporidiosis,* a severe gastroenteritis (Bateson and Goldsby 1988). Surprisingly, HIV is *not* highly infectious. It must enter the blood stream to produce infection. The virus does this by vaginal or rectal sexual contact with an infected person, by inoculation with infected blood or blood products, or by transmission from a mother to an infant during gestation or birth.

In 1981, the US Center for Disease Control reported the first deaths from AIDS. By 1991, 171,876 cases had been reported and 1.3 million people were believed to be infected (US Center for Disease Control 1991). At first, the disease spread among homosexual men in urban areas at an alarming rate. In San Francisco, for example, the virus spread at the rate of 20% per year. By 1990, this rate had fallen to 1% per year, but many people still consider AIDS a homosexual problem. About 60% of infections in men come from sexual contact. Most infections in women come from contaminated IV paraphernalia and 80% of pediatric cases come from infected mothers (Winkelstein et al 1987).

Although antibiotics help fight opportunistic infections and some new drugs slow the advancing disease, there is no known cure for AIDS. Major efforts are underway to develop a vaccine and drugs to prevent and cure the disease. However, until an effective treatment is developed, the only defenses against this terrible scourge are prevention and education.

Many nurses react to clients' struggling with AIDS, homelessness, and substance abuse as did Billy Jo and the nurses of the vignette. They dread the effects of these realities and they blame the victims. Like Billy Jo, many nurses feel guilty about their phobias. They do not understand what prejudice is, nor do they know how to overcome the alienation it creates.

Prejudice

Prejudice is a belief, attitude, or opinion formed beforehand, without knowledge, thought, or reason (*Random House Dictionary* 1975). Unless an event or influential person comes along to change a prejudice, it may remain throughout life.

Prejudice is not a modern phenomenon. In 1790, Charles Lamb said, "each person seems to be a bundle of prejudice" (McGuire 1969). People *learn* prejudgments from single and repeated experiences. They also learn them from their parents and society, by words and by deeds. In the musical *South Pacific*, Rodgers and Hammerstein immortalized this truth in the song, "You've Got to be Carefully Taught":

> "You've got to be taught before it's too late,
> before you are six, or seven, or eight,
> to hate all the people your relatives hate,
> You've got to be carefully taught!" (1949).

Prejudice involves believing, feeling, and acting for or against someone or something. Usually the belief comes first. People hold fixed beliefs about other people or things. They experience a range of emotions associated with those beliefs. Then, because of their beliefs and feelings, they behave in typical ways. Billy Jo *believes* that homosexuality is wrong. As a result she *feels* uncomfortable in the presence of people she thinks are homosexuals. Then she *acts* out her feelings in hostile ways.

Prejudice is expressed openly or covertly. Some groups act out their prejudice without shame. For example, the Ku Klux Klan makes no secret of their hostility toward people of color, homosexuals, Jews, and Roman Catholics. Other people harbor just as much hatred, but they express it in more subtle ways.

Prejudice serves several functions. It is a means to an end, a way of thinking, and a mode of emotional release. As a *means to an end,* prejudice may be used to make people feel superior to others, to gain favor, or to get rid of a threat. As a *way of thinking,* prejudice generalizes and simplifies life. It strips people of their personhood, blurs their faces, and makes them into objects. As a *mode of emotional release,* prejudices provide a focus for a wide range of emotions, from intense anticipation to paralyzing fear. Regardless of its functions, prejudice replaces objective evidence with subjective belief and subverts rational thought.

Caring: The Essential Function of Nursing

When Billy Jo became aware of her prejudice she wondered how she could reconcile her personal beliefs with her professional ethics. Happily, Billy Jo does not need to choose between the two. However, to overcome her prejudice she must affirm her commitment to the essential function of nursing, *to care* (Leininger 1981).

Caring means responding to others as unique individuals, sensing their emotions, and accepting them as they are, unconditionally. It means extending to other persons accurate empathy, genuineness, and nonpossessive warmth, regardless of their homelessness, substance abuse, or diagnosis. Caring makes a connection with another human being and breaks down the alienation that prejudice creates.

We nurses do not have to choose between professional ideals and personal beliefs. When we truly care we affirm the ethical principles of beneficence (doing good), justice (treating people equally), and autonomy (respecting individual rights). We care for and love people, not their deeds. Thus, we do not need to give up personal beliefs, although our beliefs may change with time.

As nurses connect with others, we find ourselves mirrored in their eyes, each of us longing for acceptance, understanding, and recognition. As we respond to the needs of others and extend our love toward them, we find our own needs being met. The love we give to others returns to us a thousand fold and our mutual reward is joy.

References

Barrick, B: Light at the End of the Decade. *Am J Nursing*, 1990; 90: 37–40.

Bateson MC, Goldsby R: *Thinking AIDS*. Addison-Wesley, 1988.

Berne A et al: *The Health and Mental Health of Homeless Families*. Paper presented at the International Quadrennial Congress of Nursing, Seoul, Korea, June 1989.

Coalition for the Homeless. *Safety Network* Feb. 1987; 5:2.

Hutchinson SA: Applying the nursing process for clients with psychoactive substance use disorders. In: Wilson HS, Kneisl CR: *Psychiatric Nursing*, 3rd ed. Addison Wesley, 1988.

Leininger M (ed): *Caring: An Essential Human Need.* Slack, 1981.

McGuire WJ: The nature of attitudes and attitude change. In: Lindzey G, Aronson E (editors): *Handbook of Social Psychology,* 2nd ed, vol 3, 1969.

Rafferty M: Standing up for America's homeless. *AJN* 1989; 89:12, 1614–1617.

Random House Dictionary. Random House, 1975.

Rodgers D, Aron R: AIDS in the United States: Patient care and politics. *Daedalus: J Amer Acad Arts and Sci* Spring 1989; 116:48.

Rodgers, R and Hammerstein, O: "You've Got to be Carefully Taught." Copyright © 1949 by Richard Rodgers and Oscar Hammerstein II. Copyright renewed. International copyright secured. Williamson Music owner of publication and allied rights throughout the world. Used by permission. All rights reserved.

US Center for Disease Control, Center for Infectious Diseases. *HIV/AIDS Surveillance Report.* USCDC, 1991.

Winkelstein W Jr, et al: Reduction in human immunodeficiency virus transmission among homosexual/bisexual men: 1982–1986. *Am J Publ Health* June 1987; 76:685–689.

Appendix A

Members of the National Council
of State Boards of Nursing

Alabama Board of Nursing
500 Eastern Blvd., Suite 203
Montgomery, AL 36117

Alaska Board of Nursing
Department of Commerce and Economic Development
Division of Occupational Licensing
3601 C Street, Suite 722
Anchorage, AK 99503

American Samoa Health Service Regulatory Board
LBJ Tropical Medical Center
Pago Pago, American Samoa 96799

Arizona State Board of Nursing
2001 W. Camelback Road, Suite 350
Phoenix, AZ 85015

Arkansas State Board of Nursing
1123 South University Drive
Little Rock, AR 72204

California Board of Registered Nursing
P.O. Box 944210/1030 13th Street
Sacramento, CA 94244

California Board of Vocational Nurse and Psychiatric Technician
    Examiners
1414 K Street, Room 103
Sacramento, CA 94244

Colorado Board of Nursing
1560 Broadway Street, Suite 670
Denver, CO 80202

Connecticut Board of Examiners for Nursing
150 Washington Street
Hartford, CN 06106

Delaware Board of Nursing
Margaret O'Neill Building
P.O. Box 1401
Dover, DE 19901

District of Columbia Board of Nursing
614 H Street, NW
Washington, DC 20001

Florida Board of Nursing
111 Coastline Drive, East
Jacksonville, FL 32202

Georgia Board of Nursing
166 Pryor Street, SW
Atlanta, GA 30303

Georgia State Board of Licensed Practical Nurses
166 Pryor Street, SW
Atlanta, GA 30303

Guam Board of Nurse Examiners
P.O. Box 2816
Agana, Guam 96910

Hawaii Board of Nursing
P.O. Box 3469
Honolulu, HI 96801

Idaho Board of Nursing
280 North 8th Street, Suite 210
Boise, ID 83720

Illinois Department of Professional Regulation
320 West Washington Street
Springfield, IL 62786

Indiana State Board of Nursing
Health Professions Bureau
One American Square, Suite 1020
Box 82067
Indianapolis, IN 46282

Iowa Board of Nursing
State Capitol Complex
1223 East Court Avenue
Des Moines, IA 50319

Kansas Board of Nursing
Landon State Office Building
900 SW Jackson Street, Suite 551-S
Topeka, KS 66612

Kentucky Board of Nursing
4010 Dupont Circle, Suite 430
Louisville, KY 40207

Louisiana State Board of Nursing
  907 Pere Marquette Building
  150 Baronne Street
  New Orleans, LA 70112

Louisiana State Board of Practical Nurse Examiners
  Tidewater Place
  1440 Canal Street, Suite 2010
  New Orleans, LA 70112

Maine State Board of Nursing
  35 Anthony Avenue
  State House Station #158
  Augusta, ME 04333

Maryland Board of Examiners of Nurses
  4201 Patterson Avenue
  Baltimore, MD 21215

Massachusetts Board of Registration in Nursing
  Leverett Saltonstall Building
  100 Cambridge Street, Room 1519
  Boston, MA 02202

Michigan Board of Nursing
  Department of Licensing and Regulation
  Ottawa Towers North
  611 West Ottawa/P.O. Box 30018
  Lansing, MI 48909

Minnesota Board of Nursing
  2700 University Avenue, West #108
  St. Paul, MN 55114

Mississippi Board of Nursing
  239 N. Lamar Street, Suite 401
  Jackson, MS 39206

Missouri State Board of Nursing
  P.O. Box 656/3524-A North Ten Mile Drive
  Jefferson City, MO 65102

Montana State Board of Nursing
  Department of Commerce
  Arcade Building, Lower Level
  111 North Jackson
  Helena, MT 59620

Nebraska Bureau of Examining Boards, Department of Health
  P.O. Box 95007/301 Centennial Mall South
  Lincoln, NE 68509

Nevada State Board of Nursing
1281 Terminal Way, Suite 116
Reno, NV 89502

New Hampshire Board of Nursing
Health & Welfare Building
6 Hazen Drive
Concord, NH 03301

New Jersey Board of Nursing
1100 Raymond Blvd., Room 508
Newark, NJ 07102

New Mexico Board of Nursing
4253 Montgomery Blvd., Suite 130
Albuquerque, NM 87109

New York State Board of Nursing
State Education Department
Cultural Education Center, Rm. 3013
Albany, NY 12230

North Carolina Board of Nursing
P.O. Box 2129/3724 National Drive
Raleigh, NC 27602

North Dakota Board of Nursing
919 South 7th Street, Suite 504
Bismark, ND 58504

Northern Mariana Islands Commonwealth Board of Nurse Examiners
Public Health Center
P.O. Box 1458
Saipan, MP 96950

Ohio Board of Nursing Education and Nurse Registration
77 South High Street, 17th Floor
Columbus, OH 43266

Oklahoma Board of Nurse Registration and Nursing Education
2915 North Classen Blvd., Suite 524
Oklahoma City, OK 73106

Oregon State Board of Nursing
10445 S.W. Canyon Road, Suite 200
Beaverton, OR 97005

Pennsylvania Board of Nursing
P.O. Box 2649
Harrisburg, PA 17105

Rhode Island Board of Nurse Registration and Nursing Education
  Cannon Health Building, Rm. 104
  Providence, RI 02908

South Carolina State Board of Nursing
  220 Executive Center Drive, Suite 220
  Columbia, SC 29210

South Dakota Board of Nursing
  304 South Phillips Avenue, Suite 205
  Sioux Falls, SD 57102

Tennessee State Board of Nursing
  283 Plus Park Blvd.
  Nashville, TN 37217

Texas Board of Nurse Examiners
  9101 Burnet Road, Suite 104
  Austin, TX 78758

Texas Board of Vocational Nurse Examiners
  9101 Burnet Road, Suite 105
  Austin, TX 78758

Utah State Board of Nursing
  Division of Occupational and Professional Licensing
  P.O. Box 45802/Herber M. Wells Building, 4th Floor
  160 East 300 South
  Salt Lake City, UT 84145

Vermont State Board of Nursing
  Redstone Building
  26 Terrace Street
  Montpelier, VT 05602

Virgin Islands Board of Nursing
  Knud Hansen Complex
  Charlotte Amalie
  St. Thomas, Virgin Islands 00801

Virginia State Board of Nursing
  1601 Rolling Hills Drive
  Richmond, VA 23229

Washington State Board of Nursing
  Department of Health
  P.O. Box 1099
  Olympia, WA 98507

Washington State Board of Practical Nursing
  1300 S.E. Quince Street, EY-27
  Olympia, WA 98507

West Virginia Board of Examiners for Registered Nurses
Embleton Building, Suite 309
922 Quarrier Street
Charleston, WV 25301

West Virginia State Board of Examiners for Practical Nurses
Embleton Building, Suite 506
922 Quarrier Street
Charleston, WV 25301

Wisconsin Bureau of Health Professions
P.O. Box 8935/1400 East Washington Avenue
Madison, WI 53708

Wyoming State Board of Nursing
Barrett Building, 2nd Floor
2301 Central Avenue
Cheyenne, WY 82002

List courtesy of the National Council of State Boards of Nursing, 625 N. Michigan Ave., Suite 1544, Chicago, IL 60611

Appendix B

Directory of Selected Nursing and Health-related Organizations

International

International Committee of Catholic Nurses and Social Assistants
43, Sq. Vergote, 1040 Brussels, Belgium

International Council of Nurses and the Florence Nightingale
International Foundation
3, Place Jean Marteau, 1201 Geneva, Switzerland

Pan American Health Organization, Pan American Sanitary Bureau,
WHO Regional Office for the Americas
525 23rd Street NW, Washington, DC 20037

People to People Health Foundation (Project HOPE)
Millwood, VA 22646

Sigma Theta Tau, International Honor Society of Nursing
550 W. North Street, Indianapolis, IN 46202

World Health Organization
Avenue Appia, 1211 Geneva 27, Switzerland

National

Alpha Tau Delta National Fraternity for Professional Nurses
5207 Meseda Street, Alta Loma, CA 91701

American Academy of Nurse Practitioners
45 Foster Street, Suite A, Lowell, MA 01851

American Academy of Nursing
2420 Pershing Road, Kansas City, MO 64108

American Assembly of Men in Nursing
P.O. Box 31753, Independence, OH 44131

American Association of Colleges of Nursing
Suite 530, One Dupont Circle, Washington, DC 20036

American Association of Critical-Care Nurses
101 Columbia, Aliso Viejo, CA 92656

American Association of Neuroscience Nurses
218 N. Jefferson, Suite 204, Chicago, IL 60606

American Association of Nurse Anesthetists
216 Higgins Road, Park Ridge, IL 60068

American Association of Nurse Attorneys
720 Light Street, Baltimore, MD 21230

American Association of Occupational Health Nurses, Inc.
50 Lenox Pointe, Atlanta, GA 30324

American Cancer Society
1599 Clifton Road NE, Atlanta, GA 30329

American College of Nurse-Midwives
1522 K Street NW, Suite 1000, Washington, DC 20005

American Heart Association
7320 Greenville Avenue, Dallas, TX 75231

American Hospital Association
840 N. Lake Shore Drive, Chicago, IL 60611

American Journal of Nursing Company
555 W. 57th Street, New York, NY 10019

American Nurses' Association
2420 Pershing Road, Kansas City, MO 64108

American Nurses' Foundation
1101 14th Street NW, Suite 200, Washington, DC 20005

American Organization of Nurse Executives
840 N. Lakeshore Drive, 10-E, Chicago, IL 60611

American Psychiatric Nurses' Association
6900 Grove Road, Thorofare, NJ 08086

American Public Health Association
1015 15th Street NW, Washington, DC 20005

American Red Cross, National Headquarters
17th and D Streets NW, Washington, DC 20006

American Society of Plastic and Reconstructive Surgical Nurses, Inc.
N. Woodbury Road, Box 56, Pitman, NJ 08071

American Society of Post Anesthesia Nurses
11512 Allecingie Parkway, Richmond, VA 23235

Association for Practitioners in Infection Control
505 E. Hawley Street, Mundelein, IL 60060

Association of Operating Room Nurses
10170 E. Mississippi Avenue, Denver, CO 80231

Association of Rehabilitation Nurses
5700 Old Orchard Road, First Floor, Skokie, IL 60077

Catholic Health Association of the US
4455 Woodson Road, St. Louis, MO 63134

Commission on Graduates of Foreign Nursing Schools
   3600 Market Street, Philadelphia, PA 19104

Dermatology Nurses Association
   N. Woodbury Road, Box 56, Pitman, NJ 08071

Drug and Alcohol Nursing Association, Inc.
   113 W. Franklin Street, Baltimore, MD 21201

Emergency Nurses Association
   230 E. Ohio Street, 6th Floor, Chicago, IL 60611

Frontier Nursing Service
   Wendover, KY 41775

Joint Commission on Accreditation of Healthcare Organizations
   One Renaissance Boulevard, Oakbrook Terrace, IL 60181

NAACOG: The Organization for Obstetric, Gynocologic, and
   Neonatal Nurses
   409 12th Street SW, Washington, DC 20024

National Alliance of Nurse Practitioners
   P.O. Box 44707, L'Enfant Plaza SW, Washington, DC 20026

National Association for Health Care Recruitment
   P.O. Box 5769, Akron, OH 44372

National Association for Practical Nurse Education and Service
   1400 Spring Street, Suite 310, Silver Springs, MD 20910

National Association of Hispanic Nurses
   6905 Alamo Downs Parkway, San Antonio, TX 78238

National Association of Neonatal Nurses
   191 Lynch Creek Way, Suite 101, Petaluma, CA 94952

National Association of Orthopaedic Nurses, Inc.
   N. Woodbury Road, Box 56, Pitman, NJ 08071

National Association of Pediatric Nurse Associates and Practitioners
   1101 Kings Highway Route, Suite 206, Cherry Hill, NJ 08034

National Association of School Nurses, Inc.
   P.O. Box 1300, Lamplighter Lane, Scarborough, ME 04074

National Black Nurses Association, Inc.
   1012 Tenth Street NW, Washington, DC 20001

National Council of State Boards of Nursing
   676 N. St. Clair, Suite 550, Chicago, IL 60611

National Federation of Licensed Practical Nurses, Inc.
   P.O. Box 18088, Durham, NC 27619

National Federation of Specialty Nursing Organizations
   875 Kings Highway, West Deptford, NJ 08096

National Flight Nurses Association
P.O. Box 8222, Rapid City, SD 57709

National League for Nursing
350 Hudson Street, New York, NY 10014

National Organization for the Advancement of Associate
Degree Nursing
2033 Sixth Avenue, Suite 804, Seattle, WA 98121

National Student Nurses' Association
555 W. 57th Street, New York, NY 10019

North American Nursing Diagnosis Association
3525 Caroline Street, St. Louis, MO 63104

Nurses Christian Fellowship
6400 Schroeder Road, P.O. Box 7895, Madison, WI 53707

Nurses House, Inc.
350 Hudson Street, New York, NY 10014

Oncology Nursing Society
1016 Greentree Road, Pittsburgh, PA 15220

Society for Nursing History
Nursing Education Department, Box 150, Teachers' College,
Columbia University, New York, NY 10027

Society for Peripheral Vascular Nursing
309 Winter Street, Norwood, MA 02062

Society of Gastroenterology Nurses and Associates
1070 Sibley Tower, Rochester, NY 14604

Society of Respiratory Nursing
5700 Orchard Road, First Floor, Skokie, IL 60077

Transcultural Nursing Society, Department of Nursing,
Madonna College
36600 Schoolcroft Road, Lwonia, MI 48150

Visiting Nurse Association of America
3801 E. Florida Avenue, Suite 806, Denver, CO 80210

Government

Air Force Nurse Corps, HQ USAF/SGN
Bolling Air Force Base, Washington, DC 20332

Alcohol, Drug Abuse, and Mental Health Administration
5600 Fishers Lane, Rockville, MD 20857

Army Nurse Corps, Office of the Surgeon General
5111 Leesburg Pike, Room 623, Falls Church, VA 22041

Center for Disease Control
1600 Clifton Road NE, Atlanta, GA 30333

Department of Health and Human Services, Regional Offices
   I: John F. Kennedy Federal Bldg., Boston, MA 02203
   II: 26 Federal Plaza, New York, NY 10278
   III: P.O. Box 13716, Philadelphia, PA 19101
   IV: 101 Mariette Tower, Atlanta, GA 30323
   V: 300 S. Wacker Drive, Chicago, IL 60606
   VI: 1200 Main Tower Bldg., Dallas, TX 75202
   VII: 601 E. 12th Street, Kansas City, MO 64106
   VIII: 1961 Stout Street, Denver, CO 80294
   IX: Federal Office Bldg., 50 United Nations Plaza, San Francisco, CA 94102
   X: 2901 3rd Avenue, Seattle, WA 98121

Department of Veterans Affairs Nursing Service
810 Vermont Avenue NW, Washington, DC 20420

Federal Bureau of Prisons, Director of Nursing Service
320 First Street NW, Rm 1018, Washington, DC 20032

Food and Drug Administration, Center for Devices and
Radiological Health
1390 Piccard Drive, Rockville, MD 20850

Health Resources and Services Administration, Bureau of Health
Professions, Division of Nursing
5600 Fishers Lane, Rm. 14-05, Rockville, MD 20857

Indian Health Service, Division of Nursing
12300 Twinbrook Metro Parkway, Suite 100,
Rockville, MD 20852

National Center for Nursing Research
9000 Rockville Pike, Bldg. 31, Rm 5B-03, Bethesda, MD 20892

National Institute for Occupational Safety and Health, Robert A.
Taft Laboratories
4676 Columbia Parkway, Cincinnati, OH 45226

National Institutes of Health
9000 Rockville Pike, Bethesda, MD 20892

Navy Nurse Corps, Bureau of Medicine and Surgery, Code 00NC,
23rd and E Streets, NW, Washington, DC 20372

Office of Human Development Services, Office of Policy, Planning,
and Legislation
200 Independence Avenue, SW, Washington, DC 20201

Peace Corps, Office of Recruitment
1990 K Street, NW, 9th Floor, Washington, DC 20526

US Office of Personnel Management
1900 E Street, NW, Washington, DC 20415

US Public Health Service, DHHS, Office of the Assistant Secretary of
Health: OFFICE OF THE SURGEON GENERAL
5600 Fishers Lane, Rm. 18-67, Rockville, MD 20857

Index